SYSTEMIC SCLEROSIS

Edited by **Mislav Radic**

Systemic Sclerosis
http://dx.doi.org/10.5772/63286
Edited by Mislav Radic

Contributors

Manuel Rubio-Rivas, Simone Parisi, Aniko Rentka, Krisztina Koroskenyi, Gabriella Szucs, Adam Kemeny-Beke, José Delgado Alves, Maja Spiritovic, Michal Tomcik, Hana Storkanova, Sabina Oreska, Madelon Vonk, Fleur Poelkens, Annelies Van Ede

Published by InTech
Janeza Trdine 9, 51000 Rijeka, Croatia

Publishing Process Manager Edi Lipovic
Technical Editor SPi Global
Cover InTech Design team

First published September, 2017
Printed in Croatia
Legal deposit, Croatia: National and University Library in Zagreb

Additional hard copies can be obtained from orders@intechopen.com

Systemic Sclerosis, Edited by Mislav Radic
p. cm.
Print ISBN 978-953-51-3547-0
Online ISBN 978-953-51-3548-7

For EU product safety concerns:
IN TECH d.o.o., Prolaz Marije Krucifikse Kozulić 3, 51000 Rijeka, Croatia,
info@intechopen.com or visit our website at intechopen.com.

Meet the editor

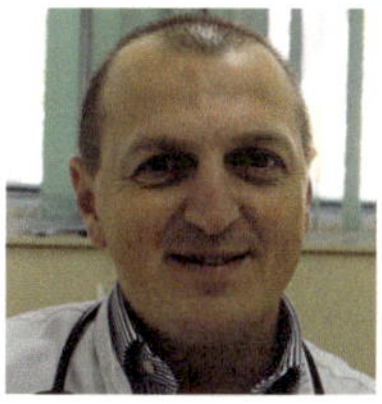

Assistant professor Mislav Radić, MD, PhD, is a young rheumatologist working at the Division of Rheumatology and Clinical Immunology, University Hospital Split, Croatia. His PhD degree thesis was on the correlation of *Helicobacter pylori* infection and systemic sclerosis. He is a member of the Croatian Society for Rheumatology, Croatian Society for Allergology and Clinical Immunology, and EUSTAR and a former EMEUNET Working Group member. In February 2017, he was a chairperson of the local organizing committee for EUSTAR educational scleroderma course, Split, Croatia, supported by both the EUSTAR and World Scleroderma Foundation. He is an author of more than 50 publications. His scientific and clinical interests are systemic sclerosis, osteoarthritis, vasculitis, epidemiology, and imaging tools in rheumatology.

Contents

Preface

Systemic sclerosis, or scleroderma, is a chronic connective tissue disease generally classified as one of the autoimmune rheumatic diseases. Systemic sclerosis is a chronic connective tissue disease of unknown etiology that causes widespread microvascular damage and excessive deposition of collagen in the skin and internal organs. Raynaud phenomenon and scleroderma (hardening of the skin) are hallmarks of the disease. Since systemic sclerosis presents with symptoms similar to other autoimmune diseases, diagnosis is difficult. The typical patient is a young or middle-aged woman with a history of Raynaud phenomenon who presents with skin induration and internal organ dysfunction. Clinical evaluation and laboratory testing, along with pulmonary function testing, Doppler echocardiography, video-capillaroscopy, and high-resolution computed tomography of the chest, establish the diagnosis and detect visceral involvement. Patients with systemic sclerosis can be classified into two distinct clinical subsets with different patterns of skin and internal organ involvement, autoantibody production, and survival. Prognosis is determined by the degree of internal organ involvement. Although no disease-modifying therapy has been proven effective, complications of systemic sclerosis are treatable, and interventions for organ-specific manifestations have improved substantially.

This book covers new insights into genetics of systemic sclerosis; animal models of systemic sclerosis; survival, causes of death, and factors of poor outcome; pulmonary hypertension in systemic sclerosis; cardiovascular risk in systemic sclerosis; possible treatments in systemic sclerosis; video-capillaroscopy in systemic sclerosis; and many more. Contributors include systemic sclerosis experts from all over the world reflecting the collaborative international effort for improved understanding and management of this disease. I am indebted to my colleagues for their dedication, expertise, and timely submissions. Each author must be certain that his or her efforts will benefit to all patients suffering from this serious disease such as systemic sclerosis. It is an honor to be the editor of this book.

I am grateful to Ana Pantar for this kind invitation to be an editor of this book. Furthermore, this book could not have been edited without the dedicated technical assistance of the publishing process manager Edi Lipovic; I would like to thank him for his patience and willingness.

Systemic Sclerosis book is meant to provide the interested clinician and researcher with the most current understanding of this complex and fascinating disease.

Mislav Radić, MD, PhD
Deputy Head of the Center of Excellence for Systemic Sclerosis,
Ministry of Health of the Republic of Croatia,
Division of Rheumatology and Clinical Immunology,
Internal Clinic of Medical School University of Split,
Split, Croatia

Chapter 1

Pulmonary Hypertension in Systemic Sclerosis

Fleur Poelkens, Madelon C. Vonk and
Annelies E. van Ede

Additional information is available at the end of the chapter

http://dx.doi.org/10.5772/intechopen.68535

Abstract

The main cause of death in systemic sclerosis is interstitial lung disease, followed by pulmonary hypertension (PH). Pulmonary hypertension is the result of microvasculopathy which is caused by a disrupted healing process of endothelin damage and is featured by vasoconstriction, proliferation of arterial wall, inflammation, and fibrosis. Reclassification of pulmonary hypertension has led to five distinctive groups. In systemic sclerosis, patients may suffer from pulmonary artery hypertension (PAH, group 1), pulmonary hypertension due to interstitial lung disease (group 3), cardiac disease (group 2), and/or thromboembolic pulmonary hypertension (group 4). Patients endure declining performance during exercise, but symptoms may be variable and nonspecific. Diagnosis is made by right heart catheterization. To select patients for this invasive procedure, several screening tools are discussed, including N-terminal pro-brain natriuretic peptide levels, uric acid levels, spirometry and diffusing capacity for carbon monoxide (DCLO), echocardiography (ECG), and the DETECT algorithm. Depending on features such as disease duration, presence of anti-centromere antibodies, and DCLO, three different flow charts for screening are presented. Based on pathophysiology, several medical treatments have been developed like prostanoids, endothelin receptor antagonists, phosphodiesterase-5 inhibitors, and stimulation of the nitric oxide pathway. Combination therapy as well as lung transplantation and supportive therapy is discussed.

Keywords: systemic sclerosis, pulmonary hypertension, DETECT algorithm, pharmaceutical treatment (prostanoids, endothelin receptor antagonists, phosphodiesterase-5 inhibitors, nitric oxide pathway)

1. Pulmonary hypertension

Pulmonary hypertension (PH) is a progressive disease characterized by an elevated pulmonary arterial pressure and pulmonary vascular resistance. As a consequence of the elevated pulmonary arterial pressure, patients are at risk of right ventricular failure and death. PH is classified in five distinctive groups with similar pathophysiology, patient characteristics, and treatment options. It can occur as a complication in patients with systemic sclerosis, and as such, it is the second main cause of death after pulmonary fibrosis in patients with systemic sclerosis. The estimated 3-year survival among patients with PH associated with systemic sclerosis is approximately 55% compared with 95% in those patients without PH [1]. The diagnosis of pulmonary arterial hypertension is defined at right heart catheterization (RHC) by a mean pulmonary arterial pressure (mPAP) of ≥ 25 mmHg. RHC should be performed in all patients in whom PH is suspected. Early diagnosis and, subsequently, treatment of PH are of utmost importance since they improves survival rates.

1.1. Epidemiology

In patients with systemic sclerosis, approximately 10% develop pulmonary arterial hypertension as a complication of the disease [2, 3]. Prior to the availability of disease-specific PH therapies, the median survival for PH in patients with systemic sclerosis was 1 year following diagnosis [4]. A meta-analysis accomplished in 2013 with the inclusion of 22 studies representing 2244 patients with systemic sclerosis-associated PH showed that the current pooled survival rates after 1,2, and 3 years are respectively 81% (95% confidence interval [95% CI] 79–84%), 64% (95% CI 59–69%), and 52% (95% CI 47–58%) [5]. To note, the prognosis of PH associated with systemic sclerosis is substantially worse than patients with idiopathic pulmonary artery hypertension (PAH) [6]. PH is generally considered a late complication of the disease, but in fact, it can occur at any time following the diagnosis. In a study from Hachulla et al. [7], PH was diagnosed 6.3 ± 6.6 years after the first non-Raynaud symptom of systemic sclerosis. It was also shown that patients with early-onset PH were older at systemic sclerosis diagnosis than patients with late-onset PH (mean age, 58.0 ± 12.5 vs 46.6 ± 12.9 years), and that, early-onset PH was more severe than late-onset PH, with a lower cardiac index and greater total pulmonary resistance. Despite these differences, the mortality however was comparable between the early-onset and late-onset PH groups. In general, patients with limited cutaneous systemic sclerosis are considered to be at greater risk of PH than patients with diffuse cutaneous systemic sclerosis [8, 9]. In these studies, however, the diagnosis of PH was not always based on right heart catheterization but by Doppler echocardiography. In a retrospective cohort analysis from Nihtyanova et al. [10], it was found that the prevalence of RHC confirmed PH was similar in diffuse cutaneous systemic sclerosis (7%) and limited cutaneous systemic sclerosis (8%).

1.2. Classification of pulmonary hypertension

The classification of PH went through a series of changes since the first classification was proposed in 1973 by the World Health Organization (WHO) [11]. This first meeting was organized due to the epidemic of the aminorex-induced PAH. Before this date, there was little knowledge of PH, and there were no effective drugs available resulting in a survival prognosis of several years. Despite the fact that PH was an orphan disease, significant interest from scientists with collaborative effort from the pharmaceutical industry resulted in studies focusing on pathophysiology, molecular biology, epidemiology, and clinical trials.

Prompted by the attained scientific insights, the second world symposium on PH was held in Evian, France. Here, in 1998, the 'Evian' classification was proposed which consisted of five categories which shared pathophysiology, clinical patient characteristics, and pharmacological treatment options [12]. Five years after the Evian conference, the third world symposium on PH was held in Venice where several changes were made to the Evian classification. At this time, there were already three classes of drugs effective in the treatment of PH (prostanoids, endothelin receptor antagonists, and phosphodiesterase type 5 inhibitors), and a specific treatment algorithm was proposed [13]. At the fourth world symposium on PH held in Dana Point, California, the Evian-Venice classification composition was refined, and a few modifications, reflecting new scientific knowledge, were added. The last world symposium on PH was held in Nice, France, in 2013. At that moment, several worldwide experts were divided into 12 task forces, each with a specific topic related to PH [14]. The task force responsible for the clinical classification proposed to include the individual categorization of the persistent PH of neonates, the addition of congenital diseases in groups 2, 3, and 5, and the shifting of PH associated with chronic hemolytic anemia from group 1 to group 5 [15]. **Table 1** shows the last updated clinical classification of pulmonary hypertension proposed in 2015 [16].

In systemic sclerosis, patients may suffer from both pulmonary artery hypertension (PAH, group 1) and from pulmonary hypertension due to interstitial lung disease (group 3), cardiac disease (group 2), and/or chronic thromboembolic pulmonary hypertension (group 4). The diagnosis and evaluation of PH is through a series of testing including pulmonary function testing, such as the measurement of DCLO, chest X-ray, high resolution computed tomography (HRCT) scan, ECG, echocardiography, cardio-pulmonary exercise test, and laboratory testing, including antinuclear antibodies, and is always confirmed by the gold standard, a right heart catheterization.

1.3. Pathophysiology

PH is a hemodynamic abnormality of the pulmonary vasculature most often found in patients with heart and lung diseases. PH is also present in approximately 10% of the patients with systemic sclerosis [2, 3]. The consensus definition of PH, an mean pulmonary arterial pressure (mPAP) of ≥25 mm Hg, originates from the fifth world symposium on PH [17]. The normal physiological upper limit for mPAP is considered 20 mm Hg. The significance and prognosis is unknown so far in patients with a mildly elevated mPAP, that is a resting mPAP between 21 and 24 mmHg. In patients with systemic sclerosis for 3 years and 5 years after diagnosis of systemic sclerosis, respectively, 18.5% (95% CI 8.3–28.7) and 27.1% (95% CI 13.9–40.3) developed PH [18]. This implies that these patients should be carefully monitored.

PH may be due to abnormalities confined to the pulmonary arterial blood vessels (pre-capillary PH), to elevation of pulmonary venous pressure (post-capillary PH), to elevated resistance in the pulmonary capillary bed, to elevated cardiac output, or to a combination of these factors. Pre-capillary pulmonary hypertension is also called pulmonary arterial hypertension (PAH) and is considered one of the major clinical PH subtypes. In PAH, the hemodynamic hallmark states a normal pulmonary venous pressure measured as a pulmonary capillary wedge pressure (PCWP) of 15 mmHg or less and a high mPAP. As a consequence, the transpulmonary

1. Pulmonary arterial hypertension

1.1. Idiopathic PAH

1.2 Heritable PAH

1.2.1. BMPR2

1.2.2. ALK1, ENG, SMAD9, CAV1, KCNK3

1.2.3. Unknown

1.3. Drug- and toxin-induced

1.4. Associated with

1.4.1. Connective tissue disease

1.4.2. HIV infection

1.4.3. Portal hypertension

1.4.4. Congenital heart disease

1.4.5. Schistosomiasis

1.4.6. Chronic hemolytic anemia

1.5. Pulmonary veno-occlusive disease (PVOD) and/or pulmonary capillary hemangiomatosis (PCH)

1.5.1. Idiopathic

1.5.2. Heritable

1.5.2.1. EIF2AK mutation

1.5.2.2. Other mutations

1.5.3. Drugs, toxins, and radiation induced

1.5.4. Associated with:

1.5.4.1. Connective tissue disease

1.5.4.2. HIV infection

1.6. Persistent pulmonary hypertension of the newborn (PPHN)

2. Pulmonary hypertension due to left heart disease

2.1. Left ventricular systolic dysfunction

2.2. Left ventricular diastolic dysfunction

2.3. Valvular disease

2.4. Congenital/acquired left heart inflow/outflow tract obstruction and congenital cardiomyopathies

2.5. Congenital/acquired pulmonary veins stenosis

3. Pulmonary hypertension owing to lung disease and/or hypoxia

3.1. Chronic obstructive pulmonary disease

3.2. Interstitial lung disease

3.3. Other pulmonary diseases with mixed restrictive and obstructive pattern

3.4. Sleep-disordered breathing

3.5. Alveolar hypoventilation disorders

3.6. Chronic exposure to high altitude

3.7. Developmental abnormalities

4. Chronic thromboembolic pulmonary hypertension (CTEPH)

4.1. Chronic thromboembolic pulmonary hypertension

4.2. Other pulmonary artery obstructions

4.2.1. Angiosarcoma

4.2.2. Other intravascular tumors

4.2.3. Arteritis

4.2.4. Congenital pulmonary arteries stenosis

4.2.5. Parasites (hydatidosis)

5. Pulmonary hypertension with unclear multifactorial mechanisms

5.1. Hematological disorders: chronic hemolytic anemia, myeloproliferative disorders, splenectomy

5.2. Systemic disorders: sarcoidosis, pulmonary histiocytosis, lymphangioleiomyomatosis, neurofibromatosis

5.3. Metabolic disorders: glycogen storage disease, Gaucher disease, thyroid disorders

5.4. Others: tumoral obstruction, fibrosing mediastinitis, chronic renal failure, segmental PH

Table 1. Updated clinical classification of pulmonary hypertension in 2015.

gradient is elevated as is the pulmonary vascular resistance. In post-capillary PH, also called pulmonary venous hypertension, the elevated PH is a consequence of an increased resistance to blood flow anywhere downstream from the pulmonary capillaries such as the pulmonary veins, left heart of even the systemic vasculature. This results in an elevated PCWP and most often normal transpulmonary gradient. The presence of solely a high cardiac output rarely results in marked PH since a healthy pulmonary vasculature is highly compliant. So the presence of PH in a situation with high cardiac output always suggests a pulmonary vascular defect.

In patients with systemic sclerosis, each of the PH subtypes may be present to different degrees. **Figure 1** provides a schematic view of the pulmonary vasculature and shows the anatomical location of the clinical subtypes of PH in patients with systemic sclerosis.

It is important to quantify each subtype in a patient, since it provides a prognosis for possible treatment effects. For example, PH associated with interstitial lung disease (ILD) has a worse prognosis compared to PAH in patients with systemic sclerosis [19–21]. A high mPAP in patients with systemic sclerosis can be due to proliferative pulmonary vasculopathy (PAH) featured by pulmonary artery vasoconstriction, proliferation of adventitia and intima wall, inflammation, and, ultimately, fibrosis. The PH may also be a consequence of the associated lung fibrosis due to prominent parenchymal destruction. The differentiation between PAH and pulmonary fibrosis-associated PH is sometimes difficult. In general, lung volumes

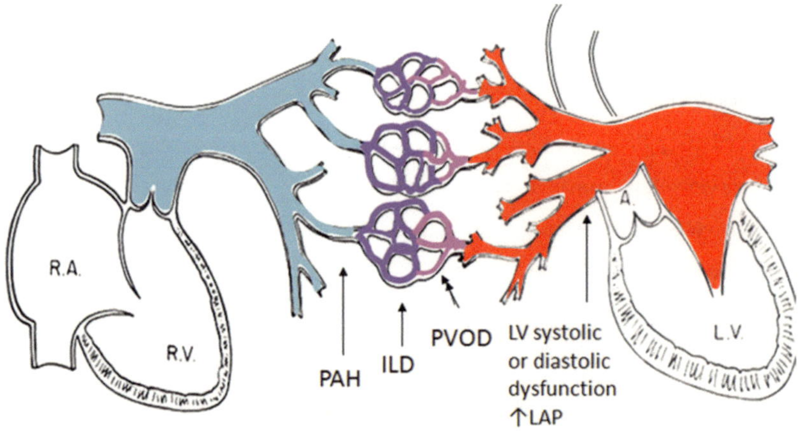

Figure 1. A schematic view of the pulmonary vasculature. RA: right atrium, RV: right ventricle, PAH: pulmonary arterial hypertension, ILD: interstitial lung disease, PVOD: pulmonary veno-occlusive disease, LV: left ventricle, LAP: left atrial pressure, and A: aorta.

(forced vital capacity (FVC) and/or total lung capacity (TLC)) below 60% of the predicted value indicate that PH is more likely to be associated with pulmonary fibrosis. When lung volumes (FVC and/or TLC) are above 70% of the predicted value, the PH is considered more likely to be due to PAH. For lung volumes between 60–70% of the predicted value, the cause is uncertain. Another cause of a high mPAP in patients with systemic sclerosis is pulmonary veno-occlusive disease (PVOD) [22]. This is thought to be the result of a more diffuse nature of the vascular lesions associated with systemic sclerosis and is located in the small venules of the vascular bed. Patients with PVOD often have more severe hypoxemia and a severe decrease in pulmonary diffusion capacity for carbon monoxide (DCLO). Indications for PVOD are typical radiological signs (lymph node enlargement, centrolobular ground glass opacities, and septal lines [23], hemoptysis, and severe hypoxemia). The diagnosis of PVOD is important since it may be harmful to prescribe pulmonary vasodilators since these vasodilators increase the risk for developing pulmonary edema. Also, post-capillary PH is seen in patients with systemic sclerosis, merely as a result of left ventricle diastolic dysfunction due to cardiomyopathy as indicated by an elevated PCWP > 15 mmHg [24, 25].

2. Diagnosis of pulmonary hypertension

2.1. Physical signs and symptoms

The first signs and symptoms of pulmonary hypertension are generally vague and nonspecific. Patients experience tiredness, fatigue, and shortness of breath when performing physical exercise or activities of daily living such as climbing stairs. These symptoms are often ascribed to having a low physical fitness. More severe symptoms such as feeling light headed during exercise, angina, syncope, and/or ankle edema only occur after extensive pulmonary vasculopathy have been developed. Also with physical examination, there are no specific abnormalities detected in patients with mild PH. Only when there is extensive pulmonary vasculopathy resulting in right heart failure, there may be physical signs including a loud P2 cardiac sound, a right ventricle third sound, a murmur of tricuspid regurgitation, raised central venous pressure, and other signs of right heart failure such as an enlarged liver and ankle edema. The lack of symptoms until the PH is already advanced often results in a striking patient and doctor's delay for diagnosis and consecutively effective treatment. As a consequence, the majority of patients at diagnosis are in functional New York Heart Association/World Health Organization (NYHA/WHO) class III or IV (**Table 2**) [2, 26]. This is extraordinarily unfortunate since the prognosis is much worse in NYHA/WHO functional class III–IV compared to class I–II [27].

2.2. Screening for pulmonary hypertension

Patients with systemic sclerosis are at risk of developing pulmonary hypertension. Since the first signs and symptoms of PH are nonspecific and the prognosis of patients diagnosed and treated in less advanced stages is better than those diagnosed late, in recent years, several screening programs have been developed to detect PH as early as possible. Depending on features such as disease duration, results from pulmonary function tests, and echocardiography, three different flow charts will be discussed.

In all newly diagnosed patients with systemic sclerosis, it is advised to perform a yearly screening for PH. After performing a thorough history and physical examination, patients should undergo a series of tests including pulmonary function test (including FVC, TLC, and diffusion capacity for carbon monoxide (DCLO)), chest X-ray, HRCT scan, ECG, echocardiography, and laboratory testing including antinuclear antibodies and N-terminal pro-Brain Natriuretic Peptide (N-terminal pro-BNP). Since the gold standard for diagnosing PH is right heart catheterization (RHC) an algorithm is used to indicate which patients should subsequently undergo the invasive procedure of an RHC [2, 28]. An RHC is recommended for those patients with an FVC/DCLO higher than 1.6 and/or DCLO below 60% of predicted values for those who experience shortness of breath or have a N-terminal pro-BNP more than twice the upper limit of normal (**Figure 2A**). For the patients where the echocardiography shows right atrial or right ventricle enlargement, a tricuspid regurgitant jet velocity (TRJ) higher than 2.8 m/s or a TRJ between 2.5 and 2.8 m/s with shortness of breath, it is also strongly advised to perform an RHC (**Figure 2B**).

For those patients with systemic sclerosis and a disease duration of more than 3 years and a pulmonary DCLO below 60% of the predicted value, the DETECT algorithm as described in

Class I: PH but no symptoms and no limitations in ordinary physical activity, for example, no shortness of breath when walking, climbing the stairs, and so on.
Class II: Mild symptoms (mild shortness of breath and/or angina) and slight limitations during ordinary activity.
Class III: Marked limitations in activity due to symptoms even during a less-than-ordinary activity, for example, walking short distances (20–100 m). Comfortable only at rest.
Class IV: Severe limitations. Experiences symptoms even while *at rest*. Mostly bedbound patients.

Table 2. New York Heart Association/WHO functional class.

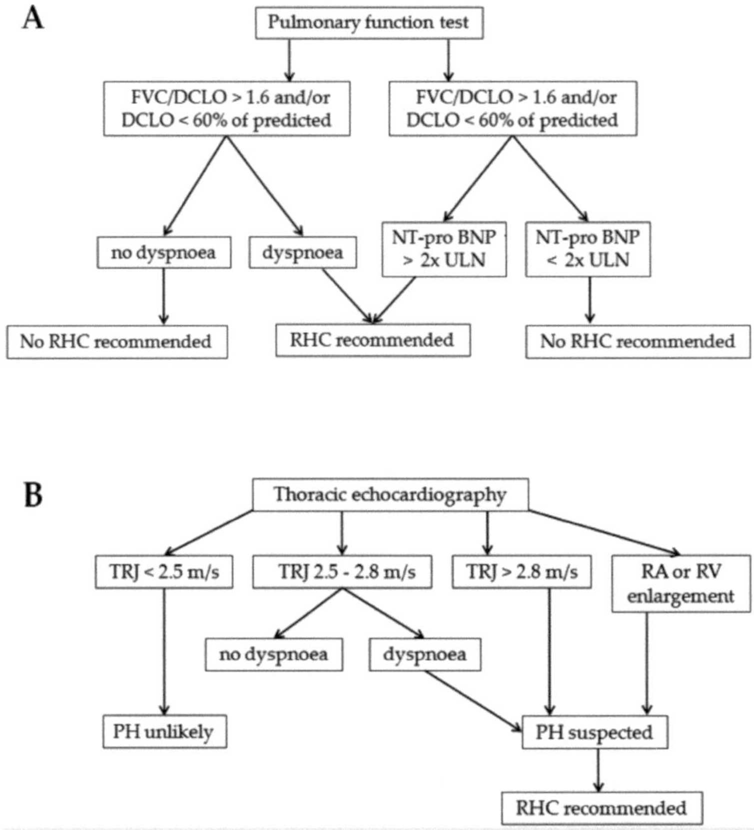

Figure 2. Recommendations when to perform a right-heart catheterization are shown. FVC: forced vital capacity, DCLO: diffusion capacity for carbon monoxide, NT-pro-BNP N-terminal pro brain natriuretic peptide, TRJ: tricuspid regurgitation jet, RA: right atrium, RV: right ventricle, PH: pulmonary hypertension, and RHC: right heart catheterization.

Figure 3 is advised to be conducted yearly [29]. The objective of the DETECT study was to develop the first evidence-based detection algorithm for systemic sclerosis–associated PH. This algorithm would minimize the number of missed PH diagnoses while optimizing the use of diagnostic RHC by determining those patients with systemic sclerosis that will not benefit from catheterization. In the first step of the DETECT algorithm, six relatively simple assessments are used to determine which patients should be referred for an echocardiography. These assessments are a percentage of predicted FVC divided by the percentage of predicted DCLO, the presence of telangiectasia, the presence of anti-centromere antibodies, the serum level of N-terminal pro-BNP, the serum level of urate, and whether there are signs of right-axis deviation on ECG. The total risk score can be calculated at: http://detect-pah.com. In step 2, the step 1 prediction score and two echocardiographic variables, right atrium enlargement and TRJ velocity, determine which patients should subsequently be referred for an RHC. The results from the DETECT study showed that the algorithm recommended RHC in 62% of patients (referral rate) and missed 4% of PAH patients (false negatives). By comparison, when the European Society of Cardiology/European Respiratory Society guidelines were applied to these patients, 29% of diagnoses were missed while requiring an RHC referral rate of 40% [29].

Step 1

- FVC%predicted / DLCO% predicted
- Telangiectasias present yes/no
- Anti-centromere antibody (ACA) present yes/no
- NTproBNP
- Serum urate
- Right axis deviation on ECG present yes/no

→ Calculate on www.detect-pah.com
Total risk score 220-300: no echo recommended
Total risk score 300-400: echo recommended

Step 2 Echocardiography

- Step 1 total risk score
- Right atrium area in cm^2
- TRJ velocity in m/s

→ Calculate on www.detect-pah.com
Total risk score 10-35: no right heart catheterization recommended
Total risk score 35-90: right heart catheterization recommended

Figure 3. DETECT algorithm in patients with systemic sclerosis with more than 3 years of disease duration and DCLO<60%.

For those patients with systemic sclerosis with a disease duration of more than 3 years and a pulmonary diffusion capacity for carbon monoxide (DCLO) above 60% of the predicted value, a yearly screening for PH is recommended by means of a pulmonary function test, including DCLO and, serum level of N-terminal pro-BNP [28–31]. **Figure 4** displays the flow chart and recommends an echocardiography when there is a decline of more than 20% in DCLO within 1 year, a FVC/DCLO ratio below 1.6, or a N-terminal pro-BNP serum level more than twice above the upper limit of normal. Depending on the results of the echocardiography, an RHC is

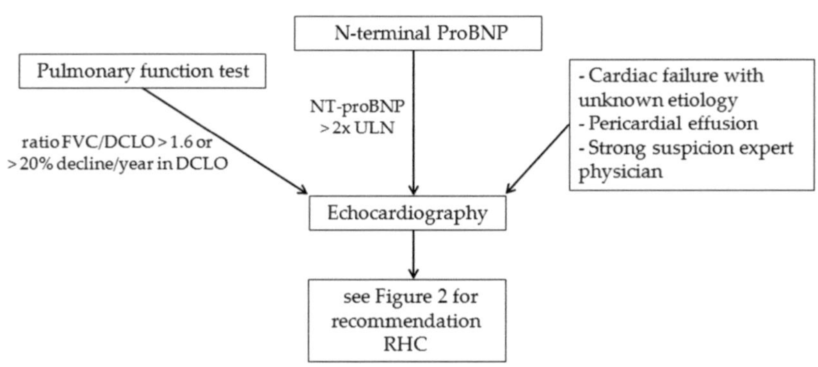

Figure 4. A flow chart for screening PH in patients with systemic sclerosis with more than 3 years of disease duration and DCLO > 60%.

recommended (**Figure 2B**). When there are signs of cardiac failure without a known etiology, signs of pericardial effusion, or a strong suspicion of PH (despite a normal or slightly elevated N-terminal pro-BNP and DCLO above 60% of predicted value), an echocardiography is recommended.

3. Treatment of pulmonary hypertension

The treatment of PH in patients with systemic sclerosis is a complex strategy which consists of a thorough evaluation of the severity of PH and the subsequent response to treatment. The treatment should be done by a team of experts in the field of rheumatology, cardiology, and pulmonary medicine and, in most countries, is restricted to highly specialized hospitals. Before treatment can be initiated, the NYHA/WHO group of PH should be defined in each patient. Vasoactive treatment is only indicated and reimbursed for NYHA/WHO group 1, PAH and NYHA/WHO group 4, and chronic thromboembolic pulmonary hypertension. The treatment strategy for PH can be divided into three main steps [16]. The first consists of general measures, supportive therapy, and referral to a specialized center. The second step includes the initiation of drugs approved for the treatment of PH. The final third step is related to the response to the initial treatment strategy and, in case of an inadequate response, the role of drug-combination therapy and lung transplantation. To note, the initial drug therapy, whether drug mono-therapy or drug-combination therapy for PH, depends on the NYHA/WHO functional class (**Table 2**). In patients with a severe disease (WHO functional class ≥ III), there is a high-estimated 1-year mortality and consequently the urge for a more aggressive treatment strategy [27].

In the first treatment step, general measures should be discussed with patients with systemic sclerosis–associated PH. This includes the encouragement to be physically active within symptom limits and to avoid excessive physical activity that leads to distressing symptoms [32, 33]. The exercise training programs should be conducted in centers which have experience in the care for PH patients. Since PH patients are at risk to develop pneumonia [34], vaccination against influenza and pneumococcal pneumonia is recommended. Patients should also be instructed that when (elective) surgery is necessary, the anesthesiologist is familiar with their PH and when possible local anesthesia or an epidural is preferable [35]. Furthermore, pregnancy should be avoided. As PH has a severe impact on daily living and may be life threatening, psychological, social, and emotional support is advocated [36]. One of the recommendations for supportive therapy for PH in patients with systemic sclerosis is the use of diuretics in those patients who show signs of right heart failure and fluid retention [37]. Although there are no RCTs on the use of diuretics in PH, clinical experience of experts show clear benefits. Continuous long-term oxygen (O_2) therapy is only recommended in PH patients when arterial blood O_2 pressure is consistently below 8 kPa [38], as in patients with chronic obstructive pulmonary disease (COPD). There are no scientific data which suggest that long-term oxygen therapy is beneficial. The evidence for the use of oral anticoagulants in patients with PH is not proven [39] despite the high prevalence of vascular thrombotic events [40] and risk factors such as heart failure, immobility, and coagulation abnormalities [41]. The final recommendation for supportive therapy is iron substitution in those patients with systemic sclerosis–associated PH with known iron deficiencies [42].

The second step in the treatment of PH consists of treatment of the underlying cause or initiating vasoactive therapy if appropriate. In patients with NYHA/WHO group 2 PH, it is due to left heart disease, optimization of cardiac function, and/or valvular disease. In patients with PH associated with lung disease, NYHA/WHO group 3, specific treatment of the cause of this disease is mandatory. PH treatment includes the initiation of drug therapy according to the evidence-based treatment algorithm [16]. In 2012, Nickel et al. [43] showed that goal-orientated therapy, a treatment strategy that uses known prognostic indicators (NYHA/WHO functional class, N-terminal pro-BNP, cardiac index) as treatment targets resulted in better prognosis in the patients achieving these goals. Changes in these established prognostic indicators during the course of the disease provide important prognostic information. In contrast to other causes of PH, such as idiopathic PAH, there is no long-term favorable response to calcium-channel blockers in patients with systemic sclerosis associated-PH [44]. The three pathogenetic pathways targeted by drug therapy in patients with systemic sclerosis–associated PH are the endothelin pathway, the nitric oxide pathway, and the prostacyclin pathway as depicted in **Figure 5** [45].

Endothelin (ET-1) is a peptide produced by endothelial cells which have vasoconstrictive and proliferative effects and is a mediator of vascular hypertrophy and fibrosis. In patients with PH, ET-1 concentrations are elevated and correlated with indices of disease severity [46]. There are two distinct receptor isoforms in the pulmonary vascular smooth muscle cells, the so-called endothelin receptor type A and B. Blocking of these ET-1 receptors by endothelin receptor antagonists (ERAs) has shown to exert beneficial effects on WHO functional class, improved hemodynamics, and an increased time to clinical worsening [47–50]. There are no head-to-head studies comparing the three available ERAs (ambrisentan, bosentan, and

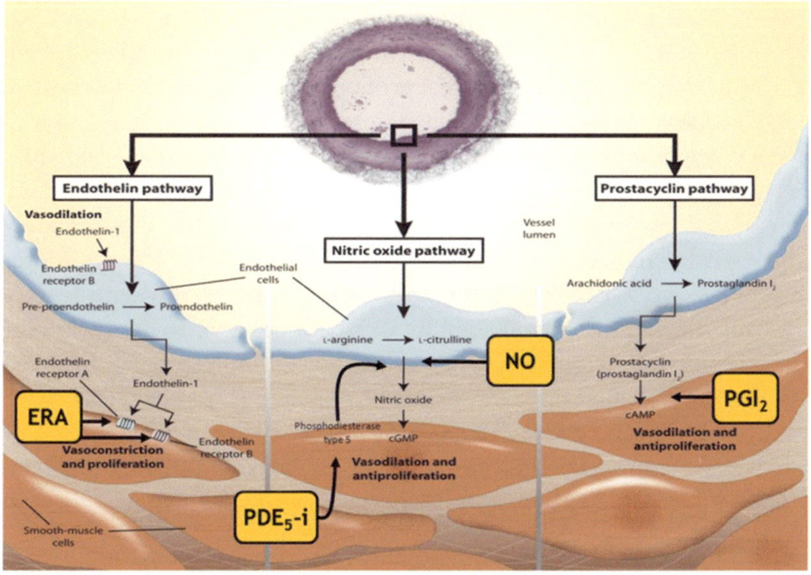

Figure 5. Targeted medical therapy for pulmonary arterial hypertension based on the endothelin pathway, nitric oxide pathway, and prostacyclin pathway. Adapted from Humbert et al. [45]. ERA: endothelin receptor antagonist, PDE_5-I: phosphodiesterase type 5 inhibitor, NO: nitric oxide, and PGI_2: prostacyclin derivates.

macitentan), and they are considered to have similar efficacy. The most serious side effect of ambricentan and bosentan, but not Macitentan, is liver toxicity which was found to be dose dependent and reversible. Monthly liver function assessment is therefore recommended.

The second pathway targeted by drug therapy in patients with systemic sclerosis associated-PH is the nitric oxide (NO) pathway. NO stimulates guanylate cyclase in vascular smooth muscle cells to convert guanosine triphosphate (GTP) to cyclic guanosine monophosphate (cGMP), which ultimately decreases intracellular calcium levels and thereby promotes vascular smooth muscle relaxation [51, 52]. As such, NO is considered a powerful vasodilator. In the pulmonary vasculature, phosphodiesterase type 5 (PDE_5) degrades cGMP. As a consequence, inhibition of PDE_5 by PDE_5 inhibitors (PDE_5-i) results in vasodilation through the NO/cGMP pathway. At the moment, there are two registered PDE_5-i for PH called sildenafil and tadalafil. Both sildenafil [53, 54] and tadalafil [55] have shown beneficial effects such as an improved exercise capacity and prolonged time to clinical worsening in RCTs after 12 weeks of treatment. The soluble guanylate cyclase stimulator, called riociguat, enhances cGMP production and has also shown favorable results on exercise capacity, hemodynamics, NYHA/WHO functional class, and, time to clinical worsening in patients with PH [56].

The final possible targeted pathway in the treatment of PH is the prostacyclin pathway. Prostacyclin is mainly produced by vascular endothelial cells and induces vasodilation of the vascular bed [57] and is a powerful inhibitor of platelet aggregation [58]. Prostacyclin exerts its effects by ultimately increasing the production of intracellular cyclic adenosine monophosphate (cAMP). Unfortunately, it has a very short half-life time of about 3 min. The introduction of stable analogues of prostacyclin with different pharmacokinetic properties but similar pharmacodynamic properties extended the clinical use of prostacyclins. Epoprostenol, a synthetic prostacyclin, has a short half-life time and requires cooling and continuous administration by means of an infusion pump and tunneled venous catheter. In an unblinded Randomized Controlled Trial (RCT), the effects of epoprostenol on 111 patients with PH secondary to the scleroderma spectrum of disease showed an improvement in exercise capacity, cardiopulmonary hemodynamics, and a decrease in mPAP [59]. Serious side effects such as venous catheter infections, sepsis, and pump malfunction have been described and may lead to death. Iloprost is a chemically more stable prostacyclin analogue and can be administered intravenously or via inhalation. Both inhaled iloprost [60] and intravenous iloprost [61] have shown to improve exercise capacity and clinical symptoms. Treprostenil is an analogue of epoprostenol with sufficient chemical stability to be administered without cooling. Both the subcutaneous administration and inhalation of treprostenil have shown beneficial effects in patients with PH [62, 63]. Recently, the first oral selective IP-prostacyclin receptor agonist selexipag was approved. In an event-driven study in 1156 patients, a 40% reduction of mortality and PH-associated complications were found in the selexipag-treated patients [64].

Figure 6 shows the current treatment algorithm for systemic sclerosis associated-PH [16]. Initial drug therapy, whether drug monotherapy or drug-combination therapy for PH, depends on the NYHA/WHO functional class combined with determinants of a worse prognosis such as clinical signs of heart failure, syncope, N-terminal pro-BNP plasma levels above

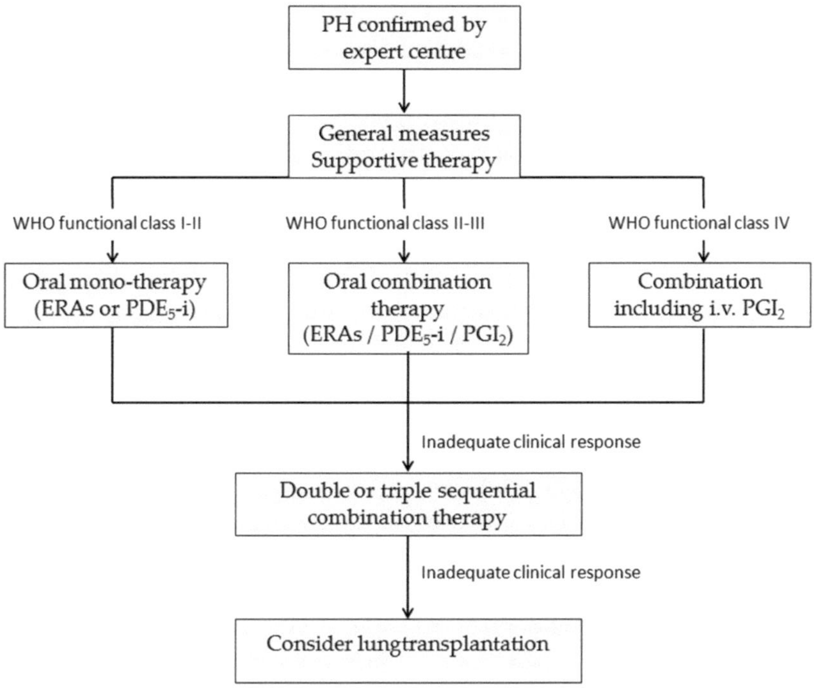

Figure 6. A treatment algorithm for systemic sclerosis associated-PH. ERA: endothelin receptor antagonist, PDE_5-I: phosphodiesterase type 5 inhibitor, and PGI_2: prostacyclin derivates.

300ng/l, echocardiographic signs of right atrial enlargement, 6-min walking distance, and/or low physical fitness levels (VO_2, peak oxygen consumption < 15 ml/min/kg).

3.1. Combination therapy

When initial drug monotherapy in PH patients with WHO functional class I–II fails or when patients with systemic sclerosis associated-PH at first diagnoses are already in WHO functional class II–IV, combination therapy can be applied. Because of the three possible targeted pathways (ET-1-, NO-, and prostacyclin pathway), this was thought to be an attractive option [65]. Combination therapy can be applied sequentially or upfront. Sequential therapy was the most widely used strategy; in case of an inadequate response to monotherapy, a second and subsequently a third drug can be added. Several trials have been conducted which evaluated the efficacy of drug combination therapy compared to monotherapy. A recent meta-analysis on 15 RCTs, with combination of PAH-specific therapies (upfront and sequential add-ons) compared with PAH-specific monotherapy, showed a risk reduction for clinical worsening of 17 versus 28%, respectively [66]. A similar outcome was observed by a meta-analyses from Fox et al. [67] on 18 RCTs. Combination therapy was associated with a reduction in non-fatal end points, an improved 6-min walking distance, improved functional class, and pulmonary hemodynamics. So far, the strongest scientific evidence has been found for the combination therapy of ambrisentan and tadalafil in PH patients with NYHA/WHO functional class II and III [68]. Only recently, the effects of initial triple upfront combination therapy in patients diagnosed with PH has been evaluated [69]. Nineteen newly diagnosed NYHA/WHO functional class III/IV PAH patients initiated on upfront triple combination therapy (intravenous epoprostenol, bosentan, and sildenafil) were collected retrospectively. After 4 months' triple combination therapy, 18 patients significantly improved their 6-min walking distance and hemodynamics. Seventeen patients had improved to NYHA/WHO functional class I or II but most striking was the overall estimated survival of 100% after 1, 2, and 3 years [69].

3.2. Lung transplantation

When patients decline despite aggressive drug therapy and other interventions, lung transplantation can be considered. The first lung transplantation for pulmonary vascular disease was performed in 1982 at Stanford University by Dr. Reitz and colleagues [70]. The timing of transplantation is crucial and depends on several factors, including the cause of PH, stage of the disease, co-morbidities and suitability for operation, possible alternative treatments, and of course, availability of donors. Patients with systemic sclerosis were initially often denied transplantation because of concerns about the short- and long-term outcomes related to the extra-pulmonary manifestations of systemic sclerosis [71]. A systematic review performed by Khan et al. [72] addressed this issue and evaluated the survival of systemic sclerosis patients after lung transplantation. He identified seven observational studies reporting the results of approximately 185 patients with systemic sclerosis who underwent single-lung, double-lung, or heart-lung transplantation. The indication for lung transplantation was both ILD and/or PAH related. The results showed that post-transplantation survival ranged 69–91% at 30 days, 69–85% at 6 months, 59–93% at 1 year, 49–80% at 2 years, and 46–79% at 3 years. He concluded that the short-term and intermediate-term survival after lung transplantation were similar to patients with idiopathic forms of PAH and other causes of ILD requiring lung transplantation. So nowadays, systemic sclerosis is a widely accepted diagnosis for the potential necessary lung transplantation. Remarkable was the considerable variability in survival estimates. This is probably due to different selection criteria of patients and may also be related to survival differences across systemic sclerosis patients with PAH, ILD, or a combination of PAH and ILD. Future work should aim to prospectively study adults with systemic sclerosis as they are evaluated for lung transplantation in order to identify potentially modifiable risk factors that can improve transplant outcomes in this population [73].

Author details

Fleur Poelkens, Madelon C. Vonk and Annelies E. van Ede*

*Address all correspondence to: annelies.vanede@radboudumc.nl

Radboud University Medical Center, Nijmegen, the Netherlands

References

[1] Hachulla E, Carpentier P, Gressin V, Diot E, Allanore Y, Sibilia J, et al. Risk factors for death and the 3-year survival of patients with systemic sclerosis: The French ItinerAIR-Sclerodermie study. Rheumatology. 2009;**48**(3):304-308

[2] Hachulla E, de Groote P, Gressin V, Sibilia J, Diot E, Carpentier P, et al. The three-year incidence of pulmonary arterial hypertension associated with systemic sclerosis in a multicenter nationwide longitudinal study in France. Arthritis and Rheumatism. 2009;**60**(6):1831-1839

[3] Avouac J, Airo P, Meune C, Beretta L, Dieude P, Caramaschi P, et al. Prevalence of pulmonary hypertension in systemic sclerosis in European Caucasians and metaanalysis of 5 studies. The Journal of Rheumatology. 2010;**37**(11):2290-2298

[4] Koh ET, Lee P, Gladman DD, Abu-Shakra M. Pulmonary hypertension in systemic sclerosis: An analysis of 17 patients. British Journal of Rheumatology. 1996;**35**(10):989-993

[5] Lefevre G, Dauchet L, Hachulla E, Montani D, Sobanski V, Lambert M, et al. Survival and prognostic factors in systemic sclerosis-associated pulmonary hypertension: A systematic review and meta-analysis. Arthritis and Rheumatism. 2013;**65**(9):2412-2423

[6] Kawut SM, Taichman DB, Archer-Chicko CL, Palevsky HI, Kimmel SE. Hemodynamics and survival in patients with pulmonary arterial hypertension related to systemic sclerosis. Chest. 2003;**123**(2):344-350

[7] Hachulla E, Launay D, Mouthon L, Sitbon O, Berezne A, Guillevin L, et al. Is pulmonary arterial hypertension really a late complication of systemic sclerosis? Chest. 2009;**136**(5):1211-1219

[8] MacGregor AJ, Canavan R, Knight C, Denton CP, Davar J, Coghlan J, et al. Pulmonary hypertension in systemic sclerosis: Risk factors for progression and consequences for survival. Rheumatology. 2001;**40**(4):453-459

[9] Mukerjee D, St George D, Coleiro B, Knight C, Denton CP, Davar J, et al. Prevalence and outcome in systemic sclerosis associated pulmonary arterial hypertension: Application of a registry approach. Annals of the Rheumatic Diseases. 2003;**62**(11):1088-1093

[10] Nihtyanova SI, Tang EC, Coghlan JG, Wells AU, Black CM, Denton CP. Improved survival in systemic sclerosis is associated with better ascertainment of internal organ disease: A retrospective cohort study. QJM: Monthly Journal of the Association of Physicians. 2010;**103**(2):109-115

[11] Hatano S, Strasser T. Primary Pulmonary Hypertension. Report on a WHO Meeting. Geneva: World Health Organization; 1973

[12] Fishman AP. Clinical classification of pulmonary hypertension. Clinics in Chest Medicine. 2001;**22**(3):385-391

[13] Galie N, Seeger W, Naeije R, Simonneau G, Rubin LJ. Comparative analysis of clinical trials and evidence-based treatment algorithm in pulmonary arterial hypertension. Journal of the American College of Cardiology. 2004;**43**(12 Suppl S):81S–88S

[14] Galie N, Simonneau G. The Fifth World Symposium on Pulmonary Hypertension. Journal of the American College of Cardiology. 2013;**62**(25 Suppl):D1–D3

[15] Simonneau G, Gatzoulis MA, Adatia I, Celermajer D, Denton C, Ghofrani A, et al. Updated clinical classification of pulmonary hypertension. Journal of the American College of Cardiology. 2013;**62**(25 Suppl):D34–D41

[16] Galie N, Humbert M, Vachiery JL, Gibbs S, Lang I, Torbicki A, et al. 2015 ESC/ERS Guidelines for the diagnosis and treatment of pulmonary hypertension: The Joint Task Force for the Diagnosis and Treatment of Pulmonary Hypertension of the European Society of Cardiology (ESC) and the European Respiratory Society (ERS): Endorsed by: Association for European Paediatric and Congenital Cardiology (AEPC), International Society for Heart and Lung Transplantation (ISHLT). European Heart Journal. 2016; **37**(1):67-119

[17] Badesch DB, Champion HC, Sanchez MA, Hoeper MM, Loyd JE, Manes A, et al. Diagnosis and assessment of pulmonary arterial hypertension. Journal of the American College of Cardiology. 2009;**54**(1 Suppl):S55–S66

[18] Valerio CJ, Schreiber BE, Handler CE, Denton CP, Coghlan JG. Borderline mean pulmonary artery pressure in patients with systemic sclerosis: Transpulmonary gradient predicts risk of developing pulmonary hypertension. Arthritis and Rheumatism. 2013;**65**(4):1074-1084

[19] Launay D, Sitbon O, Hachulla E, Mouthon L, Gressin V, Rottat L, et al. Survival in systemic sclerosis-associated pulmonary arterial hypertension in the modern management era. Annals of the Rheumatic Diseases. 2013;**72**(12):1940-1946

[20] Mathai SC, Hummers LK, Champion HC, Wigley FM, Zaiman A, Hassoun PM, et al. Survival in pulmonary hypertension associated with the scleroderma spectrum of diseases: Impact of interstitial lung disease. Arthritis and Rheumatism. 2009;**60**(2):569-577

[21] Condliffe R, Kiely DG, Peacock AJ, Corris PA, Gibbs JS, Vrapi F, et al. Connective tissue disease-associated pulmonary arterial hypertension in the modern treatment era. American Journal of Respiratory and Critical Care Medicine. 2009;**179**(2):151-157

[22] Dorfmuller P, Humbert M, Perros F, Sanchez O, Simonneau G, Muller KM, et al. Fibrous remodeling of the pulmonary venous system in pulmonary arterial hypertension associated with connective tissue diseases. Human Pathology. 2007;**38**(6):893-902

[23] Gunther S, Jais X, Maitre S, Berezne A, Dorfmuller P, Seferian A, et al. Computed tomography findings of pulmonary venoocclusive disease in scleroderma patients presenting with precapillary pulmonary hypertension. Arthritis and Rheumatism. 2012;**64**(9): 2995-3005

[24] Kahan A, Allanore Y. Primary myocardial involvement in systemic sclerosis. Rheumatology. 2006;**45**(Suppl 4):iv14–iv17

[25] Fernandez-Codina A, Simeon-Aznar CP, Pinal-Fernandez I, Rodriguez-Palomares J, Pizzi MN, Hidalgo CE, et al. Cardiac involvement in systemic sclerosis: Differences between clinical subsets and influence on survival. Rheumatology International. 2017;**37**(1):75-84

[26] Humbert M, Sitbon O, Yaici A, Montani D, O'Callaghan DS, Jais X, et al. Survival in incident and prevalent cohorts of patients with pulmonary arterial hypertension. The European Respiratory Journal. 2010;**36**(3):549-555

[27] Chung L, Domsic RT, Lingala B, Alkassab F, Bolster M, Csuka ME, et al. Survival and predictors of mortality in systemic sclerosis-associated pulmonary arterial hypertension: Outcomes from the pulmonary hypertension assessment and recognition of outcomes in scleroderma registry. Arthritis Care & Research. 2014;**66**(3):489-495

[28] Khanna D, Gladue H, Channick R, Chung L, Distler O, Furst DE, et al. Recommendations for screening and detection of connective tissue disease-associated pulmonary arterial hypertension. Arthritis and Rheumatism. 2013;**65**(12):3194-3201

[29] Coghlan JG, Denton CP, Grunig E, Bonderman D, Distler O, Khanna D, et al. Evidence-based detection of pulmonary arterial hypertension in systemic sclerosis: The DETECT study. Annals of the Rheumatic Diseases. 2014;**73**(7):1340-1349

[30] Schwaiger JP, Khanna D, Gerry Coghlan J. Screening patients with scleroderma for pulmonary arterial hypertension and implications for other at-risk populations. European Respiratory Review: An Official Journal of the European Respiratory Society. 2013;**22**(130):515-525

[31] Thakkar V, Stevens W, Prior D, Youssef P, Liew D, Gabbay E, et al. The inclusion of N-terminal pro-brain natriuretic peptide in a sensitive screening strategy for systemic sclerosis-related pulmonary arterial hypertension: A cohort study. Arthritis Research & Therapy. 2013;**15**(6):R193

[32] Galie N, Hoeper MM, Humbert M, Torbicki A, Vachiery JL, Barbera JA, et al. Guidelines for the diagnosis and treatment of pulmonary hypertension: The Task Force for the Diagnosis and Treatment of Pulmonary Hypertension of the European Society of Cardiology (ESC) and the European Respiratory Society (ERS), endorsed by the International Society of Heart and Lung Transplantation (ISHLT). European Heart Journal. 2009;**30**(20):2493-2537

[33] Grunig E, Maier F, Ehlken N, Fischer C, Lichtblau M, Blank N, et al. Exercise training in pulmonary arterial hypertension associated with connective tissue diseases. Arthritis Research & Therapy. 2012;**14**(3):R148

[34] Rich S, Dantzker DR, Ayres SM, Bergofsky EH, Brundage BH, Detre KM, et al. Primary pulmonary hypertension. A national prospective study. Annals of Internal Medicine. 1987;**107**(2):216-223

[35] Meyer S, McLaughlin VV, Seyfarth HJ, Bull TM, Vizza CD, Gomberg-Maitland M, et al. Outcomes of noncardiac, nonobstetric surgery in patients with PAH: An international prospective survey. The European Respiratory Journal. 2013;**41**(6):1302-1307

[36] Guillevin L, Armstrong I, Aldrighetti R, Howard LS, Ryftenius H, Fischer A, et al. Understanding the impact of pulmonary arterial hypertension on patients' and carers' lives. European Respiratory Review: An Official Journal of the European Respiratory Society. 2013;**22**(130):535-542

[37] Cohn JN. Optimal diuretic therapy for heart failure. The American Journal of Medicine. 2001;**111**(7):577

[38] Sandoval J, Aguirre JS, Pulido T, Martinez-Guerra ML, Santos E, Alvarado P, et al. Nocturnal oxygen therapy in patients with the Eisenmenger syndrome. American Journal of Respiratory and Critical Care Medicine. 2001;**164**(9):1682-1687

[39] Olsson KM, Delcroix M, Ghofrani HA, Tiede H, Huscher D, Speich R, et al. Anticoagulation and survival in pulmonary arterial hypertension: Results from the Comparative, Prospective Registry of Newly Initiated Therapies for Pulmonary Hypertension (COMPERA). Circulation. 2014;**129**(1):57-65

[40] Schoenfeld SR, Choi HK, Sayre EC, Avina-Zubieta JA. Risk of pulmonary embolism and deep venous thrombosis in systemic sclerosis: A general population-based study. Arthritis Care & Research. 2016;**68**(2):246-253

[41] Herve P, Humbert M, Sitbon O, Parent F, Nunes H, Legal C, et al. Pathobiology of pulmonary hypertension. The role of platelets and thrombosis. Clinics in Chest Medicine. 2001;**22**(3):451-458

[42] Ruiter G, Lanser IJ, de Man FS, van der Laarse WJ, Wharton J, Wilkins MR, et al. Iron deficiency in systemic sclerosis patients with and without pulmonary hypertension. Rheumatology. 2014;**53**(2):285-292

[43] Nickel N, Golpon H, Greer M, Knudsen L, Olsson K, Westerkamp V, et al. The prognostic impact of follow-up assessments in patients with idiopathic pulmonary arterial hypertension. The European Respiratory Journal. 2012;**39**(3):589-596

[44] Montani D, Savale L, Natali D, Jais X, Herve P, Garcia G, et al. Long-term response to calcium-channel blockers in non-idiopathic pulmonary arterial hypertension. European Heart Journal. 2010;**31**(15):1898-1907

[45] Humbert M, Sitbon O, Simonneau G. Treatment of pulmonary arterial hypertension. The New England Journal of Medicine. 2004;**351**(14):1425-1436

[46] Montani D, Souza R, Binkert C, Fischli W, Simonneau G, Clozel M, et al. Endothelin-1/endothelin-3 ratio: A potential prognostic factor of pulmonary arterial hypertension. Chest. 2007;**131**(1):101-108

[47] Galie N, Olschewski H, Oudiz RJ, Torres F, Frost A, Ghofrani HA, et al. Ambrisentan for the treatment of pulmonary arterial hypertension: Results of the ambrisentan in pulmonary

arterial hypertension, randomized, double-blind, placebo-controlled, multicenter, efficacy (ARIES) study 1 and 2. Circulation. 2008;**117**(23):3010-3019

[48] Galie N, Rubin L, Hoeper M, Jansa P, Al-Hiti H, Meyer G, et al. Treatment of patients with mildly symptomatic pulmonary arterial hypertension with bosentan (EARLY study): A double-blind, randomised controlled trial. Lancet. 2008;**371**(9630):2093-2100

[49] Channick RN, Simonneau G, Sitbon O, Robbins IM, Frost A, Tapson VF, et al. Effects of the dual endothelin-receptor antagonist bosentan in patients with pulmonary hypertension: A randomised placebo-controlled study. Lancet. 2001;**358**(9288):1119-1123

[50] Pulido T, Adzerikho I, Channick RN, Delcroix M, Galie N, Ghofrani HA, et al. Macitentan and morbidity and mortality in pulmonary arterial hypertension. The New England Journal of Medicine. 2013;**369**(9):809-818

[51] Lucas KA, Pitari GM, Kazerounian S, Ruiz-Stewart I, Park J, Schulz S, et al. Guanylyl cyclases and signaling by cyclic GMP. Pharmacological Reviews. 2000;**52**(3):375-414

[52] Pfeifer A, Ruth P, Dostmann W, Sausbier M, Klatt P, Hofmann F. Structure and function of cGMP-dependent protein kinases. Reviews of Physiology, Biochemistry and Pharmacology. 1999;**135**:105-149

[53] Sastry BK, Narasimhan C, Reddy NK, Raju BS. Clinical efficacy of sildenafil in primary pulmonary hypertension: A randomized, placebo-controlled, double-blind, crossover study. Journal of the American College of Cardiology. 2004;**43**(7):1149-1153

[54] Singh TP, Rohit M, Grover A, Malhotra S, Vijayvergiya R. A randomized, placebo-controlled, double-blind, crossover study to evaluate the efficacy of oral sildenafil therapy in severe pulmonary artery hypertension. American Heart Journal. 2006;**151**(4):851 e1-851 e5

[55] Galie N, Brundage BH, Ghofrani HA, Oudiz RJ, Simonneau G, Safdar Z, et al. Tadalafil therapy for pulmonary arterial hypertension. Circulation. 2009;**119**(22):2894-2903

[56] Ghofrani HA, Galie N, Grimminger F, Grunig E, Humbert M, Jing ZC, et al. Riociguat for the treatment of pulmonary arterial hypertension. The New England Journal of Medicine. 2013;**369**(4):330-340

[57] Rubin LJ, Groves BM, Reeves JT, Frosolono M, Handel F, Cato AE. Prostacyclin-induced acute pulmonary vasodilation in primary pulmonary hypertension. Circulation. 1982;**66**(2):334-338

[58] Moncada S, Vane JR. Arachidonic acid metabolites and the interactions between platelets and blood-vessel walls. The New England Journal of Medicine. 1979;**300**(20):1142–1147

[59] Badesch DB, Tapson VF, McGoon MD, Brundage BH, Rubin LJ, Wigley FM, et al. Continuous intravenous epoprostenol for pulmonary hypertension due to the scleroderma spectrum of disease. A randomized, controlled trial. Annals of Internal Medicine. 2000;**132**(6):425-434

[60] Olschewski H, Simonneau G, Galie N, Higenbottam T, Naeije R, Rubin LJ, et al. Inhaled iloprost for severe pulmonary hypertension. The New England Journal of Medicine. 2002;**347**(5):322-329

[61] Higenbottam T, Butt AY, McMahon A, Westerbeck R, Sharples L. Long-term intravenous prostaglandin (epoprostenol or iloprost) for treatment of severe pulmonary hypertension. Heart. 1998;**80**(2):151-155

[62] Simonneau G, Barst RJ, Galie N, Naeije R, Rich S, Bourge RC, et al. Continuous subcutaneous infusion of treprostinil, a prostacyclin analogue, in patients with pulmonary arterial hypertension: A double-blind, randomized, placebo-controlled trial. American Journal of Respiratory and Critical Care Medicine. 2002;**165**(6):800-804

[63] McLaughlin VV, Benza RL, Rubin LJ, Channick RN, Voswinckel R, Tapson VF, et al. Addition of inhaled treprostinil to oral therapy for pulmonary arterial hypertension: A randomized controlled clinical trial. Journal of the American College of Cardiology. 2010;**55**(18):1915-1922

[64] Sitbon O, Channick R, Chin KM, Frey A, Gaine S, Galie N, et al. Selexipag for the treatment of pulmonary arterial hypertension. The New England Journal of Medicine. 2015; **373**(26):2522-2533

[65] Benza RL, Park MH, Keogh A, Girgis RE. Management of pulmonary arterial hypertension with a focus on combination therapies. The Journal of Heart and Lung Transplantation: The Official Publication of the International Society for Heart Transplantation. 2007;**26**(5):437-446

[66] Lajoie AC, Lauziere G, Lega JC, Lacasse Y, Martin S, Simard S, et al. Combination therapy versus monotherapy for pulmonary arterial hypertension: A meta-analysis. The Lancet Respiratory Medicine. 2016;**4**(4):291-305

[67] Fox BD, Shtraichman O, Langleben D, Shimony A, Kramer MR. Combination therapy for pulmonary arterial hypertension: A systematic review and meta-analysis. The Canadian Journal of Cardiology. 2016

[68] Galie N, Barbera JA, Frost AE, Ghofrani HA, Hoeper MM, McLaughlin VV, et al. Initial use of ambrisentan plus tadalafil in pulmonary arterial hypertension. The New England Journal of Medicine. 2015;**373**(9):834-844

[69] Sitbon O, Jais X, Savale L, Cottin V, Bergot E, Macari EA, et al. Upfront triple combination therapy in pulmonary arterial hypertension: A pilot study. The European Respiratory Journal. 2014;**43**(6):1691-1697

[70] Reitz BA, Wallwork JL, Hunt SA, Pennock JL, Billingham ME, Oyer PE, et al. Heart-lung transplantation: Successful therapy for patients with pulmonary vascular disease. The New England Journal of Medicine. 1982;**306**(10):557-564

[71] Massad MG, Powell CR, Kpodonu J, Tshibaka C, Hanhan Z, Snow NJ, et al. Outcomes of lung transplantation in patients with scleroderma. World Journal of Surgery. 2005;**29**(11):1510-1515

[72] Khan IY, Singer LG, de Perrot M, Granton JT, Keshavjee S, Chau C, et al. Survival after lung transplantation in systemic sclerosis. A systematic review. Respiratory Medicine. 2013;**107**(12):2081-2087

[73] Bernstein EJ, Peterson ER, Sell JL, D'Ovidio F, Arcasoy SM, Bathon JM, et al. Survival of adults with systemic sclerosis following lung transplantation: A nationwide cohort study. Arthritis & Rheumatology. 2015;**67**(5):1314-1322

Chapter 2

Atherosclerosis and Cardiovascular Risk in Systemic Sclerosis

Sabina Oreska and Michal Tomcik

Additional information is available at the end of the chapter

http://dx.doi.org/10.5772/67495

Abstract

Atherosclerosis (ATS) has been considered to be a degenerative disease affecting large and medium-sized arteries, resulting in a passive build-up of cholesterol in the artery wall. In the last decade, immune system was proved to play the key role in the pathogenesis of ATS, suggesting ATS to be more progressive and accelerated in chronic inflammatory conditions. Studies in patients with autoimmune diseases, particularly in the most prevalent ones such as rheumatoid arthritis and systemic lupus erythematosus, confirmed the significantly more serious atherosclerotic disease and increased cardiovascular (CV) risk compared to the general population, suggesting these diseases as an independent risk factor for CV diseases. There are only few studies evaluating ATS and CV risk in systemic sclerosis (SSc). Moreover, these studies present contradictory results. Furthermore, it is complicated to differentiate primary vascular affection related to the pathogenesis of SSc from the secondary vascular infliction due to ATS. Nevertheless, most of the studies to date suggest ATS and its clinical manifestations to be more prevalent in SSc. Future studies evaluating larger cohorts of patients are required to determine the relevance of ATS and CV disease and management of these comorbidities in SSc.

Keywords: atherosclerosis, cardiovascular risk, systemic sclerosis

1. Introduction

Accelerated atherosclerosis (ATS) with increased cardiovascular (CV) morbidity and mortality is a well-known complication of many systemic inflammatory diseases such as systemic lupus erythematosus (SLE) and rheumatoid arthritis (RA) [1], resulting in higher rates of CV morbidity and mortality compared to general population [2, 3]. Therefore, ischemic heart disease secondary to coronary ATS is the leading cause of CV mortality in

RA patients and in late stages of SLE (while intercurrent infections are the leading cause in early disease) [4].

There is emerging data that the same process of early accelerated ATS occurs in systemic sclerosis (SSc). Epidemiological studies suggest that a cardiac cause contributes to approximately one-third of the non-SSc-related deaths. Moreover, deaths from CV causes occur in SSc more than a decade earlier than in the general population [5, 6].

In the 1960s and 1970s, the main cause of death in SSc was scleroderma renal crisis (SRC), whereas clinically manifested ATS was rare in SSc patients, and CV involvement was most likely the result of vasospasm of coronary arteries. Thanks to recent advances in the treatment of SRC and pulmonary arterial hypertension (PAH), causes of mortality in SSc have changed. The prevalence of ATS has increased according to recent studies in SSc patients [7–9].

Novel laboratory markers of ATS and non-invasive tools to evaluate subclinical coronary ATS and peripheral artery disease (PAD) have been described. Most of these are used mainly in experimental settings, because of their cost and only partially clear significance of some biomarkers [10].

2. Atherosclerosis

Atherosclerosis (ATS) is a chronic multifactorial process evolving in the medium and large arteries. It figures as a leading cause of cardiac and non-cardiac-related morbidity and mortality worldwide [1]. According to the World Health Organization (WHO) definition, it is a variable combination of changes of the innermost layer of the artery—the intima and is associated with deposits of lipids (mainly cholesterol particles), polysaccharide molecules, and blood elements. The traditional view suggests that ATS results from a passive build-up of cholesterol in the artery wall [11]. In fact, it is a multifactorial disease that can be considered an immune/inflammatory response of intima to tissue damage [4].

Inflammation is a key component of ATS [12]. Even a relatively minor elevation of inflammatory markers (such as C-reactive protein, CRP) is predictive of CV events in the general population [13]. In ATS, endothelial cell dysfunction is the common pathway by which factors (such as elevated low-density lipoprotein (LDL), hypertension, diabetes mellitus, elevated plasma homocysteine, various infectious agents, and exposure to free radicals from smoking) are proposed to contribute to pathogenesis [12]. Endothelial dysfunction leads to upregulation of adhesion molecules on the endothelium and increased vessel wall permeability, which enables the accumulation of the foam cells, that is, lipid-laden monocytes and macrophages. Migration and proliferation of vascular smooth-muscle cells lead to remodeling of the vessel wall and atherosclerotic plaque formation [12].

Cardiovascular diseases (CVDs) have become the most frequent cause of death globally [14]. Myocardial infarction (MI) and ischemic stroke caused by ATS dominate the mortality and disability statistics in all regions of the world [15].

3. Atherosclerosis in rheumatic diseases

Early ATS associated with autoimmune diseases is not fully explained by traditional risk factors such as obesity, smoking, or hyperlipidaemia [16–19]. The acceleration of ATS may be attributed (beside the traditional CV risk factors) also to systemic inflammation and use of pro-atherogenic drugs (**Table 1**) [2]. In addition, various cellular and cytokine pathways have been implicated in the pathogenesis of ATS, as an immuno-inflammatory disease [2, 12, 20–25]. The hyperactivation of the immune system leads to premature ATS, contributes to the formation of atherosclerotic plaque [3], and earlier occurrence of ATS clinical manifestations [4].

There is heterogeneity with respect to autoimmune-inflammatory risk factors. Cytokines, such as tumor necrosis factor alpha (TNF-α), and immune complexes are primarily involved in arthritis, such as RA, ankylosing spondylitis (AS) and psoriatic arthritis (PsA), as well as in SLE. On the other hand, autoantibodies including anti-oxidized low-density lipoproteins (anti-oxLDL), anti-cardiolipin (anti-CL), and anti-beta-2-glycoprotein I (anti-β2GPI) are rather involved in SLE and antiphospholipid syndrome (APS)-associated vascular conditions [26].

Autoimmune rheumatic diseases characterized by systemic inflammation and accelerated ATS are associated with various types of vasculopathies [12, 20, 27]. The characteristics of vasculopathies may significantly differ depending on the underlying disease. While classical accelerated ATS has

Traditional risk factors	**Disease (inflammation) related risk factors**
Age	Disease duration
Smoking	Smoking (RA, SLE)
Hyperlipidaemia	Acute phase reactants (CRP, fibrinogen)
Diabetes mellitus	Autoantibodies (APL, anti-oxLDL, anti-Hsp, etc.)
Obesity	Pro-atherogenic cytokines (e.g. TNF-α, IL-1, IL-6)
Sedentary life style	Chemokines
	Endothelial adhesion molecules (ICAM-1, VCAM-1, E-selectin)
Therapy-related risk factors	Proteases
Methotrexate (bimodal)	Hyperhomocysteinemia, low vitamin B12, and folate
Corticosteroids (bimodal)	Hyperprolactinemia
	Adipokines (resistin, adiponectin, leptin)

Acronyms: RA, rheumatoid arthritis; SLE, systemic lupus erythematosus; CRP, C-reactive protein; APL, antiphospholipid antibodies; anti-oxLDL, anti- oxidized low-density lipoprotein antibodies; anti-Hsp, anti-heat shock protein antibodies; TNF-α, tumour necrosis factor α; IL-1, interleukin-1; IL-6, interleukin-6; ICAM-1, intercellular adhesion molecule-1; VCAM-1, vascular cell adhesion molecule-1.

Adapted from: Soltész et al. [26].

Table 1. Risk factors for atherosclerosis and cardiovascular diseases.

been associated with RA and SLE, obliterative vasculopathy may be characteristic for SSc. All of these diseases greatly differ in vascular pathomorphology and function (**Table 2**) [24, 28–56].

Leading mechanisms	**Disease**
Accelerated atherosclerosis	RA, SpA, SLE, APS (SSc)
Autoantibody-mediated mechanisms	SLE, APS, RA
Proliferative obliteration	SSc, MCTD

Acronyms: RA, rheumatoid arthritis; SpA, spondyloarthritis; SLE, systemic lupus erythematosus; APS, anti-phospholipid syndrome; SSc, systemic sclerosis; MCTD, mixed connective tissue disease
Adapted from: Soltész et al. [26].

Table 2. Different vascular pathogenesis in autoimmune rheumatic diseases.

4. Atherosclersis in SSc

Systemic sclerosis (SSc) is a multi-system autoimmune disease characterized by immune dysregulation, vasculopathy, and fibrosis. In the pathogenesis, three hallmarks have been proposed to play the key role: (1) vasculopathy with the pathognomonic microvascular involvement; (2) fibrosis of skin and visceral organs; (3) systemic inflammation characterized by the presence of circulating autoantibodies and pro-inflammatory cytokines [57, 58].

The etiology of ATS in SSc is unknown. It may be secondary to concomitant multiple factors, including traditional CV risk factors, increased endothelial damage, and disease-specific immunologic and autoimmune factors, which may contribute to both induction and progression of ATS [2, 8, 53, 59–61].

Numerous inflammatory mediators implicated in the pathogenesis of ATS, including TNF-α, interleukin-6 (IL-6), and high-sensitivity C-reactive protein (hsCRP), have been demonstrated to be increased in patients with SSc compared with controls [62]. The relationship between these mediators and CVD in SSc is unclear. However, chronic systemic inflammation probably promotes accelerated ATS. Nevertheless, the level of inflammation in SSc is lower than in RA and SLE, thus the atherosclerotic process may not be so aggressive and easily detectable in small-number studies [63].

Involvement of the microvasculature is one of the earliest features of SSc, preceding and potentially contributing via tissue ischemia to the widespread fibrosis characteristic of this condition. Pathological changes include disruption of the endothelium, mononuclear cell infiltration of the vessel wall, frank obliterative lesions, and progressive loss of capillaries.

Endothelial dysfunction in the capillaries and arterioles, common in SSc, results in disturbed vasomotor regulation [64].

Although macrovascular disease was not originally considered as a feature of SSc, multiple studies have revealed an increased prevalence of large-vessel disease of the upper and lower limbs in patients with SSc [65, 66]. The prevalence of coronary artery and cerebrovascular disease in SSc, however, remains to be elucidated.

4.1. Prevalence of atherosclerosis in SSc

Mortality in SSc was described to be approximately three times increased as compared to the general population, in particular due to cardiopulmonary complications, including pulmonary arterial hypertension (PAH) and interstitial lung disease (ILD) [67]. The 10-year survival of SSc has improved significantly from 54% (1972–1981) to 66–82% (1982–1991), largely due to the early diagnosis and treatments available for PAH and scleroderma renal crisis (SRC) [68]. Emphasis has thus shifted to comorbidities in SSc, such as ATS, that may affect the long-term outcomes of SSc [68] with the substantially increased death rates due to atherosclerotic CVD or cerebrovascular disease [63]. Currently, CV-related deaths are responsible for a 20–30% mortality rate in SSc patients [63].

In particular, the 2010 survey from the European League Against Rheumatism Scleroderma Trials and Research (EUSTAR) database estimated that 26% of SSc-related causes of death were due to cardiac causes (mainly heart failure and arrhythmias) and 29% of non-SSc-related causes of death were due to ATS and CV causes [69].

There are contradictory reports regarding the prevalence of ATS in SSc [70]. According to some authors, the prevalence of ATS of the large epicardial coronary arteries is similar to that of general population [71].

The prevalence of primary cardiac involvement in SSc is variable and difficult to determine because of diversity of cardiac manifestations, presence of subclinical periods, type of applied diagnostic tools, and differences in patient populations [10].

Raynaud's phenomenon, PAH, and SRC represent the main clinical manifestations of microvascular damage (involvement) in SSc, characterized by both vasospasm and structural alterations, pathognomonic features of SSc. All these components are thought to predict macrovascular ATS over time [70, 72].

4.2. Risk factors for atherosclerosis in SSc

There is limited data regarding the prevalence of traditional CV risk factors in SSc. Their prevalence has been found to be either similar [73, 74] or reduced [75–77] when compared with general population. The majority of these studies showed a similar distribution of CV risk factors between SSc patients and controls, thereby suggesting that other factors may contribute to the increased prevalence of CV disease in SSc [77].

In addition to age [75, 77], hypercholesterolaemia [75–77], male gender [77], hypertension [78], and diabetes [78], SSc appears to be an independent risk factor for coronary artery disease (CAD) after adjustment for traditional risk factors [73, 78], including the SSc-related factors: PAH [75, 77], renal involvement [76], and disease duration [75]. Moreover, particularly the disease duration, in addition to age and LDL levels, can act as an independent determinant for more severe coronary calcification [75]. Renal involvement in SSc relates to ischemic heart disease (after exclusion of the impact of age) [76].

Studies mostly failed to show an increased frequency of obesity, hyperlipidaemia, hypertension (there was no difference in blood pressure on 24-hour ambulatory blood pressure monitoring [79]), and diabetes in SSc [7, 73, 75, 79]. These findings were confirmed also in the Australian Scleroderma Cohort Study [77]. Moreover, significantly lower cholesterol levels and diastolic blood pressure were described in SSc compared to controls [75]. On the other hand, one study revealed a slight increase in blood pressure and fasting glucose and a lower BMI in SSc population [80].

Factors contributing to ATS in SSc, beside the traditional risk factors, include chronic inflammation, increased levels of CRP and homocysteine, autoantibodies, deranged lipid function and profile, corticosteroid treatment, increasing age and disease duration [40, 65, 66, 81]. Beside these factors, there is also association with the dysfunction of the coagulation and fibrinolytic system and increased production of adhesion molecules [82–86]. Specifically, corticosteroids and immunosuppression seem not to be associated with the risk of CAD [76].

Results from studies on lipids are contradictory. Lipid metabolism seems to be altered and accompanied by lower levels of high-density lipoprotein (HDL) [87] or significantly elevated lipoprotein(a) (LpA) without any significant difference in other cholesterol parameters [88]. High levels of LpA in SSc are usually associated with increased CV risk [88]. In addition, high levels of LpA adversely affect the effect of thrombosis, due to reduced fibrinolysis [88, 89]. Of interest, the presence of anti-centromere antibodies (ACA) is associated with decreased levels of HDL [87]. SSc patients may have some higher detected pro-inflammatory-HDL levels (representing an increased risk for ATS) [74]. Of note, increased IgG autoantibody against the lipoprotein lipase (anti-LPL) in SSc (detected in 24% of SSc patients) may cause elevation of triglyceride (TG) levels [90]. On the other hand, some studies have not described any alteration of the components of the lipid profile in SSc patients [88].

Some novel CV risk factors have been reported to be elevated in SSc, such as oxidized low-density lipoprotein (oxLDL) and endothelin [7]. In terms of pro-thrombotic state in SSc, the coagulation system can be activated, and fibrinolysis can be impaired [89].

4.3. Pathogenesis and risk factors specific for SSc

Pathogenesis of SSc is characterized by inflammatory, vascular, and fibrotic events. It primarily affects the microvessels (e.g. Raynaud's phenomenon); however, macrovascular obliterative disease has also been described in SSc [40, 42, 70, 82, 83, 91].

Endothelial dysfunction, one of the earliest events in the pathogenesis of SSc and vasculopathy, is critical in the development of ATS, and represents a loss in vasodilatory function, together with increased platelet aggregation and leukocyte adhesion due to decreased nitric oxide (NO) as a key vasodilator [92]. Endothelial injury results in lumen occlusion and tissue hypoxia. The histopathological picture of scleroderma includes intima proliferation, the proliferation of endothelial and smooth muscle cells, destruction of internal elastic lamina and transmural lympho-plasmocytic infiltration of the vessel wall. Thus, vasculopathy in SSc does not represent the classical ATS but rather an obliterative vasculopathy [40, 82]. This has been documented by reports of very severe clinical cases of obliterative peripheral artery disease (PAD) despite the lack of traditional risk factors for ATS. About 15–20% of scleroderma patients exert multiple vascular abnormalities including the combination of CVD, stroke and PAD [2, 70, 82].

In addition, ischemia, oxidative stress, and oxLDL may trigger inflammation in the vessel wall. Homocysteine levels correlate with the development of macrovascular disease and PAH, and decreased vitamin B12 release in SSc [83].

Regarding vascular pathogenesis, the possible role of methylene-tetrahydrofolate reductase (MTHFR) gene C677T polymorphism was described in the development of macrovascular manifestations of SSc [83].

4.4. Mechanisms of endothelial damage

Vascular endothelium as a functionally remarkable organ regulates coagulation, fibrinolysis, permeability, vasomotion, and inflammation. Clinical and pathological features of vascular damage and endothelial cell activation represent an important hallmark of SSc vasculopathy, even in the absence of other concomitant risk factors [10]. Endothelial dysfunction is a component of the pathophysiology of both SSc and ATS. In SSc, the initiating injury is unknown [72].

Endothelial cell damage leads to enhanced expression of adhesion molecules and elevated levels of circulating soluble adhesion molecules, such as soluble E-selectin, intercellular adhesion molecule-1 (ICAM-1), and vascular cell adhesion molecule-1 (VCAM-1), which are all significantly increased in SSc, reflecting endothelial activation [93]. This results into adhesion of inflammatory cells, trans-migration across the vessel wall, and infiltration of the extracellular matrix.

Different mechanisms may induce and perpetuate endothelial dysfunction, which contributes to the pathogenesis of atherosclerotic risk, and progressive vasculopathy in SSc. The main pathogenic mechanisms underlying endothelial damage have been proposed: (1) dysregulation of vascular tone, as a consequence of an imbalance between vasoconstrictor and vasodilator mediators; (2) defective angiogenesis; (3) injury/activation elicited by the activation of innate and adaptive immune response; and (4) functional defects of endothelial progenitor cells (EPCs) [94, 95].

1) The important component of endothelial dysfunction in SSc is derangement of vasoactive mediators, with an increase in vasoconstrictive endothelin and a decrease in the vasodilator nitric oxide (NO) [93]. In addition, increased levels of endothelin, the most potent vasoconstrictive peptide released from the endothelial layer, play a pivotal role in endothelial dysfunction in both SSc and ATS [96]. An impairment of endothelium-dependent vasodilation occurs before the onset of clinical ATS in SSc [40].

2) Although there is an increased circulation of angiogenic factors, such as vascular endothelial growth factor (VEGF) [97], a reduction in the density of blood vessels is one of the hallmarks of vascular disease in SSc [97]. Abnormal angiogenesis results from increased VEGF, which is stimulated particularly by severe tissue hypoxia associated with chronic blood flow reduction in SSc. This leads to a condition of defective vascularization. There is also a reduction in circulating EPCs [98–100]. Moreover, the up-regulation of VEGF also

contributes to the development of fibrosis in both inflammatory and non-inflammatory stages of the disease [101].

3) In the early stage of scleroderma, the endothelial cell layer of microcirculation is activated and/or injured by unknown and various mechanisms, including infection-induced apoptosis, immune mediated cytotoxicity, anti-endothelial antibodies, or ischemia-reperfusion injury [96].

4) In particular, new blood vessels may form as a consequence of endothelial sprouting from pre-existing endothelial cells (angiogenesis) or as peripheral recruitment of bone marrow-derived circulating EPCs. EPCs contribute, at least in the early stage of the disease, to vascular healing by homing in the damaged endothelium [102].

5. Components involved in the atherogenesis in SSc

5.1. Endothelial progenitor cells

The elevation of endothelial progenitor cells (EPCs) in early disease is followed by its decrease during the disease duration [103], suggesting a probable exhaustion of the precursor endothelial pool during disease course. A decreased number of EPCs in the peripheral circulation has been shown to be predictive of recurrent acute coronary artery events [104]. Moreover, a low number of circulating EPCs seems to characterize a more active disease phenotype, identified by a higher risk of digital vascular lesions and higher severity score. Scleroderma circulating EPCs are characterized by a defective functional phenotype with consequent defective migratory activity and impaired recruitment to ischemic damaged tissue [100, 105–107].

The true significance of EPCs as a potential biomarker of both CV risk and SSc disease activity is not determined. It is not clear whether the cells are true progenitor cells [99] that incorporate into new blood vessels or rather cells of hematopoietic lineage, which have a paracrine effect on blood vessel formation [108]. Assessment of EPCs levels in SSc may be conflicting mainly because of the different methods of detection [109, 110].

5.2. Circulating endothelial cells

Circulating endothelial cells (CECs) are released into the systemic circulation after detachment of cells from basement membrane in response to endothelial injury. Increased number of CECs, a novel marker of endothelial damage, has been demonstrated not only in patients with myocardial infarction (MI), unstable angina, peripheral vascular disease (PAD), but also in SSc, suggesting their role as a marker of chronic endothelial damage [111, 112].

5.3. Antibodies against the anti-oxidized low-density lipoproteins (anti-oxLDL)

Patients with diffuse cutaneous SSc (dcSSc) were found to have higher levels of anti-oxidized LDL (oxLDL) antibodies [113], the titer of which correlates with the severity of ATS as well as with CV complications [114]. In addition, higher levels of circulating complexes of anti-beta-2-glycoprotein I (anti-oxLDL/β2GPI), considered as pro-atherogenic, were demonstrated in SSc as well [115, 116].

5.4. Antiphospholipid antibodies

Anti-β2-glycoprotein I (anti-β2GPI) in the presence of anticardiolipin (aCL) antibodies could be independently predictive of incident ischemic stroke and MI over 20 years of follow-up [117]. The prevalence of aCL and anti-β2GPI antibodies occurring in the absence of typical clinical manifestations of antiphospholipid syndrome (APS) has been demonstrated to be increased in patients with SSc compared to controls [118]. Anti-β2GPI is associated with both higher mortality and vascular disease, including digital ischemia and PAH, in SSc [119].

5.5. Anti-endothelial cell antibodies

Elevated anti-endothelial cell antibodies (AECA) correlate with increased subclinical ATS in non-rheumatic patients [120], SLE patients [121], and may contribute to an increased risk of early ATS in SSc, similarly as elevated levels of ICAM-1 [122]. However, in general the levels of AECA do not always have to be increased in all cases of chest pain and atherosclerotic involvement of the coronary arteries (compared with patients with chest pain and normal coronary angiography) [123]. The presence of circulating antibodies with anti-endothelial activity in scleroderma patients may be considered as an adjunctive mechanism associated with chronic endothelial damage [109, 110].

5.6. Angiotensin converting enzyme gene polymorphism

Polymorphism (insertion or deletion, I/D) of the angiotensin converting enzyme (ACE) gene can be another factor possibly influencing ATS. The highest levels of plasma ACE are associated with the DD genotype and the lowest levels are associated with the II genotype [124]. The D allele of the ACE gene, associated with ATS severity [125], has an increased frequency in SSc [2]. The risk of MI in patients with the DD genotype is higher compared with those with either the II or ID genotype [126, 127]. The presence of a D allele in SSc correlates with increased carotid intima-media thickness (CIMT) [128].

5.7. Microparticles

Microparticles (MPs), small circulating membrane-coated vesicles, are important mediators of intercellular signaling arising from a variety of cell types. MPs contribute to the immunopathogenesis of various thrombotic and rheumatic diseases via their role in the regulation of inflammation, thrombosis, and angiogenesis. MPs have been suggested as a biomarker of CAD. High levels result in severe endothelial dysfunction by selectively impairing the production of NO and are found in patients with acute MI [129].

MPs levels are also elevated in patients with SSc and correlate with the presence of ILD [130].

6. Types of damage

The main clinical features of atherosclerotic disease in SSc patients are represented by an involvement of peripheral, cerebrovascular, carotid, and coronary arteries with consequent high risk of peripheral vascular disease, stroke, and coronary heart disease, in particular in late disease [131]. SSc is associated with about a twofold increased risk of developing MI and stroke, and a fourfold increased risk for peripheral vascular disease, even after adjustment for CV risk factors (BMI, smoking, hypertension, diabetes, and hyperlipidaemia). This fact suggests that the increased risk of CV events in SSc may depend on both ATS and non-atherosclerotic factors, such as vasospasm, SSc specific vasculopathy, vasculitis, and thrombosis [73].

Presence of plaques and ischemic arterial events positively correlates with the positivity of ACA, while anti-topoisomerase I antibodies (ATA) positivity in SSc is rather associated with fewer ischemic events. The antibody profile and different disease subsets are supposed to contribute to macrovascular involvement [76].

6.1. Coronary arteries

Even though cardiac disease is a major cause of death in SSc patients, clinical signs of cardiac disease are apparent in only 10% [71], mostly appearing late in the course of disease [132], and predicting an adverse prognosis [133]. Up to 80% of postmortem evaluation of SSc patients' hearts may reveal a form of cardiac involvement [134].

The prevalence of ATS involving coronary vessels and its clinical manifestation, including angina, MI, and sudden death, is difficult to evaluate in SSc, because of the primary cardiac involvement possibly depending on myocardial damage secondary to microvascular alterations, myocardial fibrosis, arrhythmias resulting from the conduction system involvement, and last but not least, pericardial and valvular disease [135]. Myocardial fibrosis in SSc patients is considered a hallmark cardiac manifestation [133]. Foci of fibrosis not corresponding to coronary artery distribution were reported in 50% of autopsies conducted on SSc patients [136].

Moreover, secondary heart disease due to renal vasculopathy, ILD, and PAH could adversely influence cardiac function. Thus, symptoms of cardiac complications could be nonspecific, and could overlap with those of other comorbidities. Furthermore, hypertension, obesity, diabetes, and other comorbidities may contribute to adverse influence on cardiac function, mainly in older SSc patients [135].

The risk of acute MI may be 2.45x greater in SSc than in population of the same age, sex, and comorbidities [78]. In addition, the impact of SSc on acute MI risk may be even greater than that of hypertension (increasing the risk 2.08x), and diabetes (2.14x), while immunosuppressant drugs probably do not reduce this risk of MI [78].

Of note, MI has been described in SSc patients with unaffected coronary arteries. In this setting, microvascular disease leading to ischemic events and contraction band necrosis, resulting from both occlusive vascular disease and intermittent vasospasm (the so called "myocardial

Raynaud's phenomenon"), has been demonstrated to be the main mechanism associated with myocardial ischemic events in these patients [136]. In addition, epicardial coronary arteries in SSc patients have been reported to be free of significant lesions even in the setting of MI, congestive heart failure, and sudden cardiac death [137].

On the other hand, while the frequency of epicardial coronary vessel ATS appeared to be similar in SSc and general population (48% *vs.* 43%), the atherosclerotic lesions of the small coronary arteries or arterioles occurred significantly more often in SSc patients, compared with controls [138].

The coronary vessel involvement was ascertained invasively by coronarography with the conclusion, that the prevalence of CAD in SSc patients with suspected CAD was similar to that detected in controls [71]. Angiographic abnormalities may be higher than previously thought in asymptomatic patients with SSc, including significant coronary artery stenosis, coronary artery ectasia, slow flow, tortuosity, calcification, and spasm, and must not be related to traditional CV risk factors [132]. These abnormalities (demonstrated in asymptomatic female SSc patients free from CV risk factors) suggest that coronary artery vasculopathy is common even in the absence of classic CV risk factors, supporting the role of SSc as a relevant risk factor for CAD [132].

The presence of coronary calcified plaques in SSc patients asymptomatic for angina evaluated by computed tomography (CT) coronary angiography confirms the subclinical ATS as a common one in SSc [139]. In addition, SSc seems to be an independent risk factor for increased coronary artery calcium deposition [75].

6.2. Peripheral macrovascular abnormalities in SSc

Macrovascular complications (involving the arms and legs) may be detected even in SSc patients with minimal underlying CV risk factors [140]. Peripheral vascular disease (PAD) in patients with SSc has been reported to be significantly increased, with use of techniques such as the ankle brachial pressure index (ABPI), lower-limb Doppler ultrasound, and angiography [140–143]. Similarly, evaluation of the PAD using the WHO questionnaire for intermittent claudication may reveal more frequent impairment in SSc (almost 22%) than in general population (4.5%) [65]. PAD diagnosed by the ABPI may reach 17% of patients with SSc (in contrast to no healthy control), while there is no difference in the traditional CV risk factor profile [66].

Studies have showed a six times increased prevalence of PAD, detected by angiography, Doppler ultrasound, or physical examination in patients with limited cutaneous SSc (lcSSc) compared to healthy controls [141], and almost five times greater presence of intermittent lower limb claudication in SSc, detected by Edinburgh Claudication questionnaire, than the prevalence of symptomatic PAD in the general population, as reported by a similar WHO claudication questionnaire [65]. According to one study, approximately 4.2% of SSc patients (including the ones treated with vasodilators) suffer from clinical intermittent claudication, and even may develop ischemic stroke [143]. However, other studies failed to prove the increased prevalence of stroke in SSc [7].

The traditional CV risk factors seem to contribute to proximal, but not distal, vascular disease in the lower limb, as demonstrated in angiograms performed in a single SSc cohort [142]. In at least some cases, peripheral vascular disease in SSc is not atherosclerotic but related to the vasculopathy of SSc itself, which is supported by finding of chronic obliterative thromboangiitis on histological examination of an amputated limb [141]. Involvement of the vasa vasorum has been suggested as a potential cause of macrovascular disease in SSc [144].

Macrovascular disease, defined as an involvement of blood vessels with an internal diameter >100 microns, is probably associated with the more distal small vessel pathology [96]. Morphology and blood flow of the proper palmar digital arteries correlate with nailfold capillary morphology, and progression of microvascular disease (detected by capillaroscopy—from early capillaroscopy pattern to an active and late capillaroscopy pattern) is linked to macrovascular disease. ATA may represent an independent predictive factor for macrovascular damage [145].

6.3. Cerebrovascular disease

Literature data aimed to estimate the prevalence of cerebrovascular disease in SSc and the relationship between disease and risk of ischemic stroke is inconclusive [146]. Several studies suggested that cerebral disease may be underestimated [147–149]. The prevalence of cerebrovascular disease (transient ischemic attack, stroke, carotid or vertebral artery bruits, Doppler evidence of carotid or vertebral artery disease, or angiographic evidence of carotid artery stenosis) in SSc patients was found to be 1.3-times higher compared to controls [141].

The increased ischemic stroke risk in SSc may be due to different pathogenic mechanisms such as vascular injury, chronic inflammation, and vasospasm [146]. SSc may be independently associated with a 43% increase in ischemic stroke risk compared to healthy controls [73]. This risk is not even modified by commonly employed medications (such as calcium channel blockers, angiotensin converting enzyme inhibitors, oral corticosteroids, or immunosuppressant drugs) [146].

Cerebral vascular involvement may be caused by endothelial dysfunction, as well as by ATS [150]. The role of inflammatory or immune mechanisms can be declared by the apparent efficacy of immunosuppressive drugs in stroke treatment [151]. Finally, cerebral vasospasm ("Raynaud's phenomenon-like") may be associated with transient ischemic attacks or focal neurological defects and it is evidenced by reversibility of arterial lesions and absence of specific histologic findings [152].

Stenosis of carotid arteries, a predictive factor of stroke, is more often found in SSc patients with respect to general population with no difference in the traditional CV risk factor profile, supporting the increased risk of stroke in SSc [66]. Moreover, intracerebral vascular calcifications, an independent risk factor of ischemic stroke in the general population [153], are significantly more prevalent in asymptomatic SSc patients compared to the controls investigated by non-contrast CT scan [154]. Similarly, white matter hyperintensities on brain magnetic resonance imaging (MRI), a known risk factor for future symptomatic stroke [155], are more common in asymptomatic SSc patients than in population without autoimmune diseases [156, 157].

Another tool for examining cerebral artery involvement, a single photon emission computed tomography (SPECT), showed focal or diffuse hypoperfusion in mainly neurologically asymptomatic SSc patients, probably caused by the microangiopathic damage of brain vessels [158].

Of note, central nervous system may be affected by microvascular damage as a complication of systemic involvement [159]. A higher risk for developing neurological complications is associated with circulating anti-U1 RNP (ribonucleoprotein) and ATA [160].

6.4. Carotid arteries

Regarding vascular morphology and function, carotid ATS has been detected in more than 60% of scleroderma patients [40, 64, 161–163]. In line with this finding, the prevalence of carotid plaque, carotid wall thickening, and carotid artery stenosis has been showed to be significantly higher in SSc compared to the general population of the same age and gender [66].

Some studies found no difference in CIMT values between scleroderma patients and controls [161, 164, 165], while others depicted increased CIMT in SSc patients [64, 166]. Nevertheless, significantly higher CIMT values in SSc demonstrating increased risk of ATS were found in less than half of the studies [8, 167]. The data interpretation may be hampered by small size of the cohorts enrolled and by variability of CIMT ultrasonographic measurement among studies [7].

CIMT values seem to directly correlate with disease duration, similarly to the observations in patients with RA, diabetes mellitus, or familial hypercholesterolemia [8]. High CIMT was variably associated with age, oxLDL [166], corticosteroid treatment [168], ACE gene polymorphism, and antibodies against human heat shock protein (HSP)-60, and mycobacterial HSP-65 [166]. Increase in CIMT (≥0.10 mm) correlates with age- and sex-adjusted relative risk of 1.15 for MI, and 1.18 for stroke [131].

SSc patients with plaques are characterized by increased concentration of serum proteins implicated in both vasculopathy, and fibrosis in comparison to patients without plaques [169].

7. Methods of detection

To elucidate the prevalence of PAD in SSc, several techniques, beside the physical examination (history of claudication or absence of pulses), have been employed. In particular, surrogate markers of atherosclerotic damage have been demonstrated to be useful indicators of atherosclerotic wall damage. These include ankle brachial pressure index (ABPI) for arterial involvement of the lower extremities, blood pressure interarm difference (systolic/diastolic interarm difference) for proximal arterial disease of the upper extremities, and pulse wave velocity (PWV) and pulse wave analysis (PWA) to evaluate arterial stiffness. A novel non-invasive tool to evaluate subclinical coronary ATS, a multidetector CT, generates a coronary calcium score, a surrogate marker for coronary ATS [170, 171].

7.1. Intima-media thickness in SSc

Vessel intima-media thickness (IMT) is calculated by measuring the average thickness of the intima-media complex, the distance between the first and the second echogenic lines from the lumen [40, 64]. Carotid intima-media thickness (CIMT) as measured by high-resolution ultrasound is a well-validated marker of subclinical ATS. Increased CIMT has been shown to correlate with traditional CV risk factors, and to independently predict future vascular events in general population [64, 131].

A meta-analysis of CIMT in rheumatic diseases, including RA, SLE, and SSc, found significantly increased values of CIMT in this population compared with healthy, age- and sex-matched controls [167]. The pooled result of the SSc studies demonstrated a greater CIMT in SSc than in controls, suggesting an increased prevalence of subclinical ATS in both dcSSc and lcSSc [166, 172, 173]. The effect size seen in SSc was also greater than those in RA and SLE. Higher CIMT values are associated with increased age, but probably not with disease type, duration, or clinical characteristics [166].

In contrast to these findings, a number of individual studies have found no increase in CIMT in patients with SSc [40, 79, 161, 164, 165, 174]. Interestingly, there is also an anecdotal report of significantly lower CIMT in 10 SSc patients than in an age- and sex-matched control group without coronary risk factors [175].

7.2. Ultrasonographic evaluation and duplex scanning

SSc patients may have more severe, as well as more frequent, carotid disease (evaluating common carotid and its branches as well as the vertebral arteries) than the general population with similar rates of CV risk factors [66]. Carotid plaques are present in SSc, but probably not significantly more when compared to controls [161]. Evaluating other arteries using the ultrasonographic examination, the most impaired arteries in SSc are ulnar arteries, which are significantly narrower than those of the healthy controls. Other arteries are not significantly altered [176].

7.3. Flow-mediated dilation

Flow-mediated vasodilation (FMD) is usually evaluated by ultrasonographic measurement of artery diameter at baseline and maximal vasodilation following periodic ischemia, achieved by external cuff inflation [64]. FMD is calculated as a change in percentage following cuff release divided by baseline diameter [64]. The dilation is dependent on the endothelium function following the release of endogenous substance from endothelial cells, such as NO [70, 163, 177]. Endothelial dysfunction (as reflected by abnormally lower FMD values) is a key mechanism in predicting ATS involvement [63, 74].

Impaired FMD is associated with the presence of traditional CV risk factors [178], and is independently predictive of incident CV events [179].

Many, but not all, studies have found FMD to be decreased in SSc compared with controls [8, 40, 64, 162, 163, 165, 172, 177, 180–182]. The results were independent of SSc type, disease duration, clinical findings, and traditional CV risk factors [64]. On the other hand, unchanged FMD in SSc patients was reported as well [163].

It was suggested that increased levels of LpA in SSc patients cause impaired FMD, since LpA is capable of inhibiting inducible NO synthase [88].

7.4. Nitroglycerin-mediated dilation in SSc

Nitroglycerin-mediated dilation (NMD) is measured by evaluating the percentage of change of the arterial diameter from baseline following administration of 25–400 μg of sublingual nitroglycerin [40, 162]. Unlike FMD, the NMD value is independent of endothelium function [163].

Several studies have reported abnormally low NMD values in SSc patients. However, an impaired FMD was also demonstrated in SSc, while NMD was preserved [40, 70].

NMD values appear to be reduced in dsSSc with Raynaud's phenomenon compared to controls [172, 180]. However, some studies did not find abnormal NMD in SSc patients [40, 163, 165, 183].

Impaired NMD was found to correlate with increased age in SSc patients [40]. Reduced nitrate-mediated dilation [172, 180, 184] could suggest a coexisting functional or structural abnormality of arterial smooth muscle, adventitia, or both.

7.5. Ankle Brachial Pressure Index in SSc

Ankle Brachial Pressure Index (ABPI) is a validated diagnostic tool for PAD of the lower extremity. It is calculated by dividing the posterior tibial artery systolic pressure by the brachial systolic pressure (both in mmHg) [66]. Normally ABPI equals 1.0, whereas abnormal ABPI is defined as a continuous variable less than 0.90 (American College of Cardiologist/American Heart Association Practice Guidelines for Management of Patients with PAD). Increasingly lower values reflect an increased rate of arterial disease [66, 80]. According to the American Diabetes Association consensus paper, values lower than 0.9 are only mildly abnormal, and a ratio lower than 0.4 reflects a severe disease [185].

Several studies found that ABPI was more commonly abnormal in SSc patients.

Values of ABPI of 0.9–1.0 are described in about 60% of SSc patients, compared to 0–10% of general population with the same rate of CV risk factors [66]. When comparing the subsets of SSc, dcSSc may rather tend to have altered ABPI than lcSSc [143]. ABPI values remain stable in most SSc patients over time [186].

7.6. Arterial stiffness

Arterial stiffness is increased in the presence of CV risk factors [187], and is an independent predictor of CV events and CV and all-cause mortality across a wide range of patient populations [188]. This parameter performs as a well-validated surrogate marker of subclinical ATS, and an independent predictor of CV events and mortality [188].

Arterial stiffness has been examined in SSc but with varying results [122, 162–165, 177, 189]. This parameter is measured by the techniques of pulse wave analysis (PWA), and pulse wave velocity (PWV). Carotid-femoral PWV is considered the current "gold-standard" measurement of arterial stiffness [190]. PWA, expressed as the augmentation index (AI), reflects the stiffness of the aorta, whereas carotid-femoral PWV reflects the velocity of the pulse wave along the aortic and aortoiliac pathways. Increased arterial stiffness results in premature return of reflected waves in late systole, causing increased load on the left ventricle and increased myocardial oxygen demand [72].

Elevated values of PWA and PWV have been described in patients with dcSSc [162] and even more increased in patients with lcSSc. Moreover, PWV correlates positively with disease duration. Thus, it could be postulated that PWV may be a better measure of arterial stiffness than AI in SSc [122].

Arterial stiffness elevated in patients with SSc may correlate with elevated levels of soluble markers of endothelial activation, including plasma nitrate, soluble E-selectin, and soluble VCAM-1 [163].

However, microvascular disease or myocardial dysfunction may also contribute to the observed abnormality in AI [191]. SSc patients free from CVD were demonstrated to have higher AI, with respect to healthy controls. PWV, however, was not significantly increased. Interestingly, there was a paradoxical association between calcium channel blocker therapy and higher AI. This correlation may reflect generalized vasculopathy rather than atherosclerotic disease [192].

Significantly increased stiffness parameters (evaluating the macrovascular disease and subclinical ATS) may correlate positively with ATA serum levels and inversely with ACA [193].

7.7. Angiography examination

Angiographic findings of the lower and upper extremity in SSc patients showed a correlation between CV risk factors and proximal, but not distal, PAD. The microvasculopathy related to disease pathogenesis may be considered the leading mechanism of peripheral vascular abnormalities in SSc according to a retrospective study of angiograms, when compared to atherosclerotic damage [142].

Taken together, these data suggest that SSc patients are more likely to develop PAD and scleroderma may be considered a risk factor of PAD.

8. Cardiac evaluation in SSc

8.1. Coronary artery evaluation

Angiographic evaluating of SSc patients with suspected coronary artery disease can reveal coronary artery disease, which seems to affect 22% of SSc patients. However, comparing the findings with the calculated standardized prevalence ratios according to Diamond and http://dx.doi.org/10.5772/67495

Forrester's probability analysis, the prevalence of coronary artery disease in SSc patients seems not to be larger than expected in patients without SSc [71].

A novel method of assessing coronary artery disease is the coronary calcium score, as determined by multidetector computed tomography. This technique measures coronary artery calcification that occurs in atherosclerotic plaque and has a good negative predictive value for CAD in the general population [194]. There is an evidence of higher presence of coronary calcification and higher coronary calcium score in patients with SSc compared to the healthy controls. Nevertheless, the correlation of coronary calcification with the angiographic findings in SSc is unknown [74].

Coronary artery calcifications may represent the same process as the process of subcutaneous calcinosis in SSc. However, in SSc patients, who did not have any subcutaneous calcinosis, coronary artery calcifications can be often detected as well [74]. Hence, subcutaneous calcinosis in SSc does not necessarily need to be associated with increased risk of coronary artery calcification.

8.2. Coronary flow reserve in SSc

Coronary flow reserve (CFR) is calculated by dividing the peak diastolic velocity during adenosine infusion, with the peak diastolic velocity at rest, and with a resting velocity time integral [195]. Abnormal CFR may reflect coronary artery disease or the incapability of microcirculation to supply the heart in cases of increased demand [134].

Several reports have found abnormal CFR in SSc patients. Reduced CFR alone cannot differentiate vasospasm from anatomic arterial stenosis. Therefore, abnormal CFR in SSc does not necessarily imply the presence of atherosclerotic plaque [134]. Examination by myocardial multidetector CT may elucidate the relationship between CFR and coronary anatomy [196].

Assessing CFR in the left anterior descending coronary artery using contrast enhanced transthoracic Doppler during adenosine infusion, even severe reduction can be detected in 50% of SSc patients, who have no heart disease symptoms [134, 195, 197].

Patients with dcSSc seem to have more severe reduction of CFR than lcSSc. Even younger dcSSc than lsSSc may suffer from worse damage of coronary arteries [195, 197].

8.3. Assessment of myocardial perfusion in SSc patients

Using 99m-Tc sestamibi gated myocardial perfusion SPECT with a stress-rest protocol reveals perfusion defects reported in 38% of SSc patients, which are probably not associated with age, sex, SSc subset or duration of Raynaud's phenomenon [198]. On the other hand, this perfusion defects may be associated with severe skin thickness, digital ulcers, and esophageal involvement [198].

Stress perfusion defects in cardiac MRI are common in asymptomatic SSc patients. There can be a non-segmental perfusion defect too, not corresponding to epicardial coronary artery distribution, which suggests microvascular impairment [199]. Most of SSc patients have at least one segmental MRI perfusion defect (e.g. reduced signal intensity or delayed wash-in) at baseline [200]. Nifedipine can cause a significant increase in myocardial perfusion, according to an increased MRI perfusion index [200].

9. Prevention, management, and treatment of ATS in SSc

In general, early CV screening is mandatory in order to prevent and early treat vascular disease. A European League Against Rheumatism (EULAR) task force has published recommendations for screening, prevention and treatment of CVD in arthritis [47]. Similar recommendations regarding SLE and scleroderma are to follow soon [26]. According to the EULAR recommendations for inflammatory arthritis, CV risk assessment should follow the national guidelines, or in case of absence of such guidelines, Systemic Coronary Risk Evaluation (SCORE) function mode should be used [47]. Detection of CV risk includes laboratory screening, physical examination (blood pressure, body composition, and body mass index), and non-invasive imaging methods [171].

9.1. Laboratory markers

Laboratory markers include: (1) the parameters of lipid metabolism: total cholesterol (TC), LDL, HDL, TC/HDL ratio, TG or LpA and oxLDL, both associated with ATS in autoimmune diseases [171]; (2) glucose metabolism alteration and insulin resistance: fasting glucose or oral glucose tolerance test [171, 201]; (3) acute phase reactants, hsCRP, and erythrocyte sedimentation rate (ESR), which are associated with the presence of subclinical ATS, CV events, and CV mortality [202–204].

The association of specific biomarkers of endothelial activation, markers of inflammatory pathways, and specific genes with ATS and increased CV risk have been described, for example: cytokines (TNF superfamily and receptors for TNF, interferon gamma (IFNγ), interleukin 6 (IL-6), IL-1, transforming growth factor beta 1 (TGF-β1)), chemokines, and adipokines [205].

Biologic markers of possible cardiac dysfunction such as brain natriuretic peptide (BNP) or N-terminal pro-BNP (NT-proBNP) are often elevated in patients with SSc [133]. Troponin has not been found to be elevated in SSc, so its elevated levels are suspected from non-scleroderma CVD or myopericarditis [206].

9.2. Non-invasive imaging methods

Screening non-invasive and imaging techniques include a broad spectrum of methods for detection of ATS: US of peripheral arteries, and especially of common carotid arteries to provide CIMT measurement and plaque detection, assessment of subclinical ATS (using ABPI, FMD, NMD, PWA, PVW, AI), assessment of cardiac disease (using coronary calcium score detected by CT, SPECT or PET, MRI, etc.), all of which were mentioned above [170].

9.3. Therapy

Beside the administration of vasculoprotective pharmacological agents, such as aspirin, statins, ACE inhibitors, and angiotensin II receptor blockers [47, 207–209], tight control over the disease activity and inflammatory activity is needed, using low-dose corticosteroids, immunosuppressive agents, or biologics [43, 207, 208, 210, 211].

There are no specific recommendations for management of traditional risk factors, such as dyslipidemia, diabetes mellitus, or smoking in SSc patients. Their treatment mostly follows the national guidelines. According to the EULAR recommendations, statins, ACE inhibitors, and angiotensin II (AT-II) blockers are considered as preferred treatment options [47, 212].

Statins significantly reduce the risk of CV disease by lipid lowering effect and modulation of inflammatory pathways [213, 214]. Aspirin is used in general population to prevent the risk of CVD. Glitazones (peroxisome proliferator-activated receptor gamma, PPARγ agonists) are preferred in treatment of insulin resistance because of their potential vasculoprotective and anti-inflammatory effects [215].

The most severe complications (e.g. PAH and SRC) are treated according to the EULAR recommendations for SSc, with use of calcium channel blockers in case of PAH, and ACE inhibitors in case of SRC [216]. Both of them, similarly as endothelin receptor antagonist (ERA) bosentan [217], have been demonstrated to have beneficial effects on myocardial perfusion, and on limiting further progression of life-threatening complications [200, 218, 219].

Nonsteroidal anti-inflammatory drugs (NSAIDs), administrated in pericarditis in SSc [216], are not recommended for long-term use with respect to the CV perspective [220].

To control the disease activity and inflammation, proper anti-inflammatory therapy should be administered. Corticosteroids and disease modifying antirheumatic drugs (DMARDs), used in some SSc manifestations according to the EULAR recommendation [216], may influence the CV risk.

Corticosteroids (used e.g. for treatment of myocarditis) may reduce vascular risk by effectively suppressing systemic inflammation [47]. On the other hand, they are pro-atherogenic and lead to dyslipidaemia, diabetes and hypertension [220, 221]. A daily threshold dose of 8 mg of prednisone was established, above which the number of deaths increases in a dose-dependent manner [222]. Corticosteroids should be used at the lowest doses possible for the shortest period of time possible [47].

Methotrexate (MTX), recommended particularly to treat the skin manifestations, exerts bimodal effects on the vasculature. It increases the production of pro-atherogenic homocysteine, which can promote endothelial injury, and increases LDL oxidation [223, 224]. On the other hand, hyperhomocysteinemia can be reversed by folate supplementation [225]. However, MTX may also be atheroprotective by inhibiting foam cell formation and modifying reverse cholesterol transport [226]. In the EULAR cardiovascular recommendations for inflammatory arthritis, administration of MTX to the adequate control of disease activity is preferred to the possible negative CV effects of treatment [47].

Cyclophosphamide (CPA), used in treatment of ILD, induces cardiac damage and heart failure by its influence on the myocardial cells metabolism and induction of apoptosis [227]. According to experimental studies, CPA may influence the lipid metabolism [228], for example, via the cholesterol transfer activity enhancement [229].

Regarding the biologics, studies in CV effects are almost exclusively in RA, and these drugs are not commonly used in patients with SSc. Numerous recent studies concluded, that infliximab, etanercept, adalimumab and rituximab may improve endothelial function and decrease CIMT and arterial stiffness in arthritis patients [208, 210, 211].

There may be differences among anti-TNF agents in terms of their effects on CV risk. There are controversial results on the effects of TNF blockers on lipid profiles, while infliximab may worsen the atherogenic index [211, 230]. On the other hand, biologics may also improve insulin sensitivity, decrease resistin, and increase adiponectin production [211, 231]. Rituximab may also exert vasculoprotective effects [232–234].

10. Conclusion

Systemic sclerosis is a chronic, progressive, potentially lethal rheumatic disease. The management and treatment of life-threating disease manifestations, such as pulmonary arterial hypertension or scleroderma renal crisis, have improved over the last decades. Other causes, which increase the morbidity and mortality, have arisen, including the cardiovascular diseases in the first place. Similar to other rheumatic diseases, and based on many above-mentioned studies on pathogenesis of atherosclerosis in autoimmune conditions, cardiovascular risk in scleroderma is believed to be increased compared to the general population. The rate of this risk is not clear to date. Angiographic, sonographic, and computed tomography studies have provided conflicting data regarding the presence of macrovascular coronary lesions and accelerated atherosclerosis in scleroderma. Screening for subclinical cardiac involvement provides an opportunity for early diagnosis and treatment, which is crucial for positive outcome and prognosis. Thus, patients with systemic sclerosis should be closely observed, followed, and modifiable risk factors should be treated in the early stage. Moreover, future studies assessing larger cohorts of patients using standardized tools are needed to elucidate the cardiovascular risk in scleroderma patients.

Acknowledgements

This chapter was supported by grant projects AZV 16-33542A, AZV 16-33574A, SVV 260263, PRVOUK, and the Ministry of Health of the Czech Republic [Research Project No. 00023728].

Author details

Sabina Oreska and Michal Tomcik*

*Address all correspondence to: michaltomcik@yahoo.com

Department of Rheumatology, First Faculty of Medicine, Institute of Rheumatology, Prague, Czech Republic

References

[1] Krause I, Shoenfeld Y. Intravenous immunoglobulin treatment for fibrosis, atherosclerosis, and malignant conditions. Methods in Molecular Medicine. 2005;109:403-8.

[2] Shoenfeld Y, Gerli R, Doria A, Matsuura E, Cerinic MM, Ronda N, et al. Accelerated atherosclerosis in autoimmune rheumatic diseases. Circulation. 2005;112(21):3337-47.

[3] Zinger H, Sherer Y, Shoenfeld Y. Atherosclerosis in autoimmune rheumatic diseases-mechanisms and clinical findings. Clinical Reviews in Allergy & Immunology. 2009;37(1):20-8.

[4] Gargiulo P, Marsico F, Parente A, Paolillo S, Cecere M, Casaretti L, et al. Ischemic heart disease in systemic inflammatory diseases. An appraisal. International Journal of Cardiology. 2014;170(3):286-90.

[5] Hesselstrand R, Scheja A, Akesson A. Mortality and causes of death in a Swedish series of systemic sclerosis patients. Annals of the Rheumatic Diseases. 1998;57(11):682-6.

[6] Jacobsen S, Halberg P, Ullman S. Mortality and causes of death of 344 Danish patients with systemic sclerosis (scleroderma). British Journal of Rheumatology. 1998;37(7):750-5.

[7] Hettema ME, Bootsma H, Kallenberg CG. Macrovascular disease and atherosclerosis in SSc. Rheumatology. 2008;47(5):578-83.

[8] Au K, Singh MK, Bodukam V, Bae S, Maranian P, Ogawa R, et al. Atherosclerosis in systemic sclerosis: A systematic review and meta-analysis. Arthritis and Rheumatism. 2011;63(7):2078-90.

[9] Soriano A, Afeltra A, Shoenfeld Y. Is atherosclerosis accelerated in systemic sclerosis? Novel insights. Current Opinion in Rheumatology. 2014;26(6):653-7.

[10] Cannarile F, Valentini V, Mirabelli G, Alunno A, Terenzi R, Luccioli F, et al. Cardiovascular disease in systemic sclerosis. Annals of Translational Medicine. 2015;3(1):8.

[11] Libby P, Ridker PM, Hansson GK. Progress and challenges in translating the biology of atherosclerosis. Nature. 2011;473(7347):317-25.

[12] Ross R. Atherosclerosis: An inflammatory disease. The New England Journal of Medicine. 1999;340(2):115-26.

[13] Danesh J, Wheeler JG, Hirschfield GM, Eda S, Eiriksdottir G, Rumley A, et al. C-reactive protein and other circulating markers of inflammation in the prediction of coronary heart disease. The New England Journal of Medicine. 2004;350(14):1387-97.

[14] Murray CJ, Vos T, Lozano R, Naghavi M, Flaxman AD, Michaud C, et al. Disability-adjusted life years (DALYs) for 291 diseases and injuries in 21 regions, 1990-2010: A systematic analysis for the Global Burden of Disease Study 2010. Lancet. 2012;380(9859):2197-223.

[15] Libby P. Mechanisms of acute coronary syndromes and their implications for therapy. The New England Journal of Medicine. 2013;368(21):2004-13.

[16] Alkaabi JK, Ho M, Levison R, Pullar T, Belch JJ. Rheumatoid arthritis and macrovascular disease. Rheumatology. 2003;42(2):292-7.

[17] de Leeuw K, Freire B, Smit AJ, Bootsma H, Kallenberg CG, Bijl M. Traditional and non-traditional risk factors contribute to the development of accelerated atherosclerosis in patients with systemic lupus erythematosus. Lupus. 2006;15(10):675-82.

[18] Hak AE, Karlson EW, Feskanich D, Stampfer MJ, Costenbader KH. Systemic lupus erythematosus and the risk of cardiovascular disease: Results from the nurses' health study. Arthritis and Rheumatism. 2009;61(10):1396-402.

[19] Roman MJ, Shanker BA, Davis A, Lockshin MD, Sammaritano L, Simantov R, et al. Prevalence and correlates of accelerated atherosclerosis in systemic lupus erythematosus. The New England Journal of Medicine. 2003;349(25):2399-406.

[20] Sherer Y, Shoenfeld Y. Mechanisms of disease: Atherosclerosis in autoimmune diseases. Nature Clinical Practice Rheumatology. 2006;2(2):99-106.

[21] Hansson GK. Immune mechanisms in atherosclerosis. Arteriosclerosis, Thrombosis, and Vascular Biology. 2001;21(12):1876-90.

[22] Hansson GK. Inflammatory mechanisms in atherosclerosis. Journal of Thrombosis and Haemostasis. 2009;7(Suppl 1):328-31.

[23] Libby P, Ridker PM, Hansson GK, Leducq Transatlantic Network on Atherothrombosis. Inflammation in atherosclerosis: From pathophysiology to practice. Journal of the American College of Cardiology. 2009;54(23):2129-38.

[24] Soltesz P, Prohaszka Z, Fust G, Der H, Kerekes G, Szodoray P, et al. Vasculopathiak autoimmun vonatkozasai [The autoimmune features of vasculopathies]. Orvosi Hetilap. 2007;148(Suppl 1):53-7.

[25] Szekanecz Z. Pro-inflammatory cytokines in atherosclerosis. The Israel Medical Association Journal. 2008;10(7):529-30.

[26] Soltesz P, Kerekes G, Der H, Szucs G, Szanto S, Kiss E, et al. Comparative assessment of vascular function in autoimmune rheumatic diseases: Considerations of prevention and treatment. Autoimmunity Reviews. 2011;10(7):416-25.

[27] Hansson GK, Jonasson L, Seifert PS, Stemme S. Immune mechanisms in atherosclerosis. Arteriosclerosis. 1989;9(5):567-78.

[28] Tervaert JW. Translational mini-review series on immunology of vascular disease: Accelerated atherosclerosis in vasculitis. Clinical and Experimental Immunology. 2009;156(3):377-85.

[29] Abusamieh M, Ash J. Atherosclerosis and systemic lupus erythematosus. Cardiology in Review. 2004;12(5):267-75.

[30] Alexandroff AB, Pauriah M, Camp RD, Lang CC, Struthers AD, Armstrong DJ. More than skin deep: Atherosclerosis as a systemic manifestation of psoriasis. The British Journal of Dermatology. 2009;161(1):1-7.

[31] Ames PR. Antiphospholipid antibodies, thrombosis and atherosclerosis in systemic lupus erythematosus: A unifying 'membrane stress syndrome' hypothesis. Lupus. 1994;3(5):371-7.

[32] Belizna CC, Richard V, Thuillez C, Levesque H, Shoenfeld Y. Insights into atherosclerosis therapy in antiphospholipid syndrome. Autoimmunity Reviews. 2007;7(1):46-51.

[33] Bruce IN, Gladman DD, Urowitz MB. Premature atherosclerosis in systemic lupus erythematosus. Rheumatic Diseases Clinics of North America. 2000;26(2):257-78.

[34] Gerli R, Sherer Y, Bocci EB, Vaudo G, Moscatelli S, Shoenfeld Y. Precocious atherosclerosis in rheumatoid arthritis: Role of traditional and disease-related cardiovascular risk factors. Annals of the New York Academy of Sciences. 2007;1108:372-81.

[35] Jara LJ, Medina G, Vera-Lastra O, Shoenfeld Y. Atherosclerosis and antiphospholipid syndrome. Clinical Reviews in Allergy & Immunology. 2003;25(1):79-88.

[36] Matsuura E, Kobayashi K, Yasuda T, Koike T. Antiphospholipid antibodies and atherosclerosis. Lupus. 1998;7(Suppl 2):S135-9.

[37] Merrill JT. The antiphospholipid syndrome and atherosclerosis: Clue to pathogenesis. Current Rheumatology Reports. 2003;5(5):401-6.

[38] Sherer Y, Shoenfeld Y. Antiphospholipid syndrome, antiphospholipid antibodies, and atherosclerosis. Current Atherosclerosis Reports. 2001;3(4):328-33.

[39] Shoenfeld Y, Harats D, George J. Atherosclerosis and the antiphospholipid syndrome: A link unravelled? Lupus. 1998;7(Suppl 2):S140-3.

[40] Szucs G, Timar O, Szekanecz Z, Der H, Kerekes G, Szamosi S, et al. Endothelial dysfunction precedes atherosclerosis in systemic sclerosis: Relevance for prevention of vascular complications. Rheumatology. 2007;46(5):759-62.

[41] Kerekes G, Szekanecz Z, Der H, Sandor Z, Lakos G, Muszbek L, et al. Endothelial dysfunction and atherosclerosis in rheumatoid arthritis: A multiparametric analysis using imaging techniques and laboratory markers of inflammation and autoimmunity. The Journal of Rheumatology. 2008;35(3):398-406.

[42] Soltesz P, Der H, Kerekes G, Szodoray P, Szucs G, Danko K, et al. A comparative study of arterial stiffness, flow-mediated vasodilation of the brachial artery, and the thickness of the carotid artery intima-media in patients with systemic autoimmune diseases. Clinical Rheumatology. 2009;28(6):655-62.

[43] Szekanecz Z, Kerekes G, Der H, Sandor Z, Szabo Z, Vegvari A, et al. Accelerated atherosclerosis in rheumatoid arthritis. Annals of the New York Academy of Sciences. 2007;1108:349-58.

[44] Szekanecz Z, Koch AE. Vascular involvement in rheumatic diseases: 'Vascular rheumatology'. Arthritis Research & Therapy. 2008;10(5):224.

[45] Gonzalez-Juanatey C, Vazquez-Rodriguez TR, Miranda-Filloy JA, Dierssen T, Vaqueiro I, Blanco R, et al. The high prevalence of subclinical atherosclerosis in patients with ankylosing spondylitis without clinically evident cardiovascular disease. Medicine. 2009;88(6):358-65.

[46] Heeneman S, Daemen MJ. Cardiovascular risks in spondyloarthritides. Current Opinion in Rheumatology. 2007;19(4):358-62.

[47] Peters MJ, Symmons DP, McCarey D, Dijkmans BA, Nicola P, Kvien TK, et al. EULAR evidence-based recommendations for cardiovascular risk management in patients with rheumatoid arthritis and other forms of inflammatory arthritis. Annals of the Rheumatic Diseases. 2010;69(2):325-31.

[48] Gladman DD, Ang M, Su L, Tom BD, Schentag CT, Farewell VT. Cardiovascular morbidity in psoriatic arthritis. Annals of the Rheumatic Diseases. 2009;68(7):1131-5.

[49] Gonzalez-Juanatey C, Llorca J, Miranda-Filloy JA, Amigo-Diaz E, Testa A, Garcia-Porrua C, et al. Endothelial dysfunction in psoriatic arthritis patients without clinically evident cardiovascular disease or classic atherosclerosis risk factors. Arthritis and Rheumatism. 2007;57(2):287-93.

[50] Vegh J, Soos G, Csipo I, Demeter N, Ben T, Dezso B, et al. Pulmonary arterial hypertension in mixed connective tissue disease: Successful treatment with Iloprost. Rheumatology International. 2006;26(3):264-9.

[51] Numano F. Vasa vasoritis, vasculitis and atherosclerosis. International Journal of Cardiology. 2000;75(Suppl 1):S1-8; discussion S17-9.

[52] Gerli R, Vaudo G, Bocci EB, Schillaci G, Alunno A, Luccioli F, et al. Functional impairment of the arterial wall in primary Sjogren's syndrome: Combined action of immunologic and inflammatory factors. Arthritis Care & Research. 2010;62(5):712-8.

[53] Sarzi-Puttini P, Atzeni F, Gerli R, Bartoloni E, Doria A, Barskova T, et al. Cardiac involvement in systemic rheumatic diseases: An update. Autoimmunity Reviews. 2010;9(12):849-52.

[54] Sitia S, Atzeni F, Sarzi-Puttini P, Di Bello V, Tomasoni L, Delfino L, et al. Cardiovascular involvement in systemic autoimmune diseases. Autoimmunity Reviews. 2009;8(4):281-6.

[55] Zardi EM, Afeltra A. Endothelial dysfunction and vascular stiffness in systemic lupus erythematosus: Are they early markers of subclinical atherosclerosis? Autoimmunity Reviews. 2010;9(10):684-6.

[56] Turiel M, Sitia S, Atzeni F, Tomasoni L, Gianturco L, Giuffrida M, et al. The heart in rheumatoid arthritis. Autoimmunity Reviews. 2010;9(6):414-8.

[57] Dumoitier N, Lofek S, Mouthon L. Pathophysiology of systemic sclerosis: State of the art in 2014. Presse Medicale. 2014;43(10 Pt 2):e267-78.

[58] Papagoras C, Achenbach K, Tsifetaki N, Tsiouris S, Fotopoulos A, Drosos AA. Heart involvement in systemic sclerosis: A combined echocardiographic and scintigraphic study. Clinical Rheumatology. 2014;33(8):1105-11.

[59] Bartoloni Bocci E, Luccioli F, Angrisani C, Moscatelli S, Alunno A, Gerli R. Accelerated atherosclerosis in systemic lupus erythematosus and other connective tissue diseases. Expert Review of Clinical Immunology. 2007;3(4):531-41.

[60] Bartoloni E, Alunno A, Bistoni O, Gerli R. How early is the atherosclerotic risk in rheumatoid arthritis? Autoimmunity Reviews. 2010;9(10):701-7.

[61] Bartoloni E, Shoenfeld Y, Gerli R. Inflammatory and autoimmune mechanisms in the induction of atherosclerotic damage in systemic rheumatic diseases: Two faces of the same coin. Arthritis Care & Research. 2011;63(2):178-83.

[62] Baraut J, Michel L, Verrecchia F, Farge D. Relationship between cytokine profiles and clinical outcomes in patients with systemic sclerosis. Autoimmunity Reviews. 2010;10(2):65-73.

[63] Belch JJ, McSwiggan S, Lau C. Macrovascular disease in systemic sclerosis: The tip of an iceberg? Rheumatology. 2008;47(Suppl 5):v16-7.

[64] Bartoli F, Blagojevic J, Bacci M, Fiori G, Tempestini A, Conforti ML, et al. Flow-mediated vasodilation and carotid intima-media thickness in systemic sclerosis. Annals of the New York Academy of Sciences. 2007;1108:283-90.

[65] Veale DJ, Collidge TA, Belch JJ. Increased prevalence of symptomatic macrovascular disease in systemic sclerosis. Annals of the Rheumatic Diseases. 1995;54(10):853-5.

[66] Ho M, Veale D, Eastmond C, Nuki G, Belch J. Macrovascular disease and systemic sclerosis. Annals of the Rheumatic Diseases. 2000;59(1):39-43.

[67] Rubio-Rivas M, Royo C, Simeon CP, Corbella X, Fonollosa V. Mortality and survival in systemic sclerosis: Systematic review and meta-analysis. Seminars in Arthritis and Rheumatism. 2014;44(2):208-19.

[68] Steen VD, Medsger TA. Changes in causes of death in systemic sclerosis, 1972-2002. Annals of the Rheumatic Diseases. 2007;66(7):940-4.

[69] Tyndall AJ, Bannert B, Vonk M, Airo P, Cozzi F, Carreira PE, et al. Causes and risk factors for death in systemic sclerosis: A study from the EULAR Scleroderma Trials and Research (EUSTAR) database. Annals of the Rheumatic Diseases. 2010;69(10):1809-15.

[70] Nussinovitch U, Shoenfeld Y. Atherosclerosis and macrovascular involvement in systemic sclerosis: Myth or reality. Autoimmunity Reviews. 2011;10(5):259-66.

[71] Akram MR, Handler CE, Williams M, Carulli MT, Andron M, Black CM, et al. Angiographically proven coronary artery disease in scleroderma. Rheumatology. 2006;45(11):1395-8.

[72] Ngian GS, Sahhar J, Wicks IP, Van Doornum S. Cardiovascular disease in systemic sclerosis: An emerging association? Arthritis Research & Therapy. 2011;13(4):237.

[73] Man A, Zhu Y, Zhang Y, Dubreuil M, Rho YH, Peloquin C, et al. The risk of cardiovascular disease in systemic sclerosis: A population-based cohort study. Annals of the Rheumatic Diseases. 2013;72(7):1188-93.

[74] Khurma V, Meyer C, Park GS, McMahon M, Lin J, Singh RR, et al. A pilot study of subclinical coronary atherosclerosis in systemic sclerosis: Coronary artery calcification in cases and controls. Arthritis and Rheumatism. 2008;59(4):591-7.

[75] Mok MY, Lau CS, Chiu SS, Tso AW, Lo Y, Law LS, et al. Systemic sclerosis is an independent risk factor for increased coronary artery calcium deposition. Arthritis and Rheumatism. 2011;63(5):1387-95.

[76] Nordin A, Jensen-Urstad K, Bjornadal L, Pettersson S, Larsson A, Svenungsson E. Ischemic arterial events and atherosclerosis in patients with systemic sclerosis: A population-based case-control study. Arthritis Research & Therapy. 2013;15(4):R87.

[77] Ngian GS, Sahhar J, Proudman SM, Stevens W, Wicks IP, Van Doornum S. Prevalence of coronary heart disease and cardiovascular risk factors in a national cross-sectional cohort study of systemic sclerosis. Annals of the Rheumatic Diseases. 2012;71(12):1980-3.

[78] Chu SY, Chen YJ, Liu CJ, Tseng WC, Lin MW, Hwang CY, et al. Increased risk of acute myocardial infarction in systemic sclerosis: A nationwide population-based study. The American Journal of Medicine. 2013;126(11):982-8.

[79] Zakopoulos NA, Kotsis VT, Gialafos EJ, Papamichael CM, Pitiriga V, Mitsibounas DN, et al. Systemic sclerosis is not associated with clinical or ambulatory blood pressure. Clinical and Experimental Rheumatology. 2003;21(2):199-204.

[80] Zeng Y, Li M, Xu D, Hou Y, Wang Q, Fang Q, et al. Macrovascular involvement in systemic sclerosis: Evidence of correlation with disease activity. Clinical and Experimental Rheumatology. 2012;30(2 Suppl 71):S76-80.

[81] Blagojevic J, Matucci Cerinic M. Macrovascular involvement in systemic sclerosis: Comorbidity or accelerated atherosclerosis? Current Rheumatology Reports. 2007;9(3):–2.

[82] Muller-Ladner U, Distler O, Ibba-Manneschi L, Neumann E, Gay S. Mechanisms of vascular damage in systemic sclerosis. Autoimmunity. 2009;42(7):587-95.

[83] Szamosi S, Csiki Z, Szomjak E, Szolnoki E, Szoke G, Szekanecz Z, et al. Plasma homocysteine levels, the prevalence of methylenetetrahydrofolate reductase gene C677T polymorphism and macrovascular disorders in systemic sclerosis: Risk factors for accelerated macrovascular damage? Clinical Reviews in Allergy & Immunology. 2009;36(2-3):145-9.

[84] Pignone A, Scaletti C, Matucci-Cerinic M, Vazquez-Abad D, Meroni PL, Del Papa N, et al. Anti-endothelial cell antibodies in systemic sclerosis: Significant association with vascular involvement and alveolo-capillary impairment. Clinical and Experimental Rheumatology. 1998;16(5):527-32.

[85] Koch AE, Kronfeld-Harrington LB, Szekanecz Z, Cho MM, Haines GK, Harlow LA, et al. In situ expression of cytokines and cellular adhesion molecules in the skin of patients with systemic sclerosis. Their role in early and late disease. Pathobiology: Journal of Immunopathology, Molecular and Cellular Biology. 1993;61(5-6):239-46.

[86] Gruschwitz M, von den Driesch P, Kellner I, Hornstein OP, Sterry W. Expression of adhesion proteins involved in cell-cell and cell-matrix interactions in the skin of patients with progressive systemic sclerosis. Journal of the American Academy of Dermatology. 1992;27(2 Pt 1):169-77.

[87] Borba EF, Borges CT, Bonfa E. Lipoprotein profile in limited systemic sclerosis. Rheumatology International. 2005;25(5):379-83.

[88] Lippi G, Caramaschi P, Montagnana M, Salvagno GL, Volpe A, Guidi G. Lipoprotein[a] and the lipid profile in patients with systemic sclerosis. Clinica Chimica Acta; International Journal of Clinical Chemistry. 2006;364(1-2):345-8.

[89] Cerinic MM, Valentini G, Sorano GG, D'Angelo S, Cuomo G, Fenu L, et al. Blood coagulation, fibrinolysis, and markers of endothelial dysfunction in systemic sclerosis. Seminars in Arthritis and Rheumatism. 2003;32(5):285-95.

[90] Kodera M, Hayakawa I, Komura K, Yanaba K, Hasegawa M, Takehara K, et al. Anti-lipoprotein lipase antibody in systemic sclerosis: Association with elevated serum triglyceride concentrations. The Journal of Rheumatology. 2005;32(4):629-36.

[91] Czirjak L, Kumanovics G, Varju C, Nagy Z, Pakozdi A, Szekanecz Z, et al. Survival and causes of death in 366 Hungarian patients with systemic sclerosis. Annals of the Rheumatic Diseases. 2008;67(1):59-63.

[92] Munzel T, Sinning C, Post F, Warnholtz A, Schulz E. Pathophysiology, diagnosis and prognostic implications of endothelial dysfunction. Annals of Medicine. 2008;40(3):180-96.

[93] Andersen GN, Caidahl K, Kazzam E, Petersson AS, Waldenstrom A, Mincheva-Nilsson L, et al. Correlation between increased nitric oxide production and markers of endothelial activation in systemic sclerosis: Findings with the soluble adhesion molecules E-selectin, intercellular adhesion molecule 1, and vascular cell adhesion molecule 1. Arthritis and Rheumatism. 2000;43(5):1085-93.

[94] Altorok N, Wang Y, Kahaleh B. Endothelial dysfunction in systemic sclerosis. Current Opinion in Rheumatology. 2014;26(6):615-20.

[95] Fleming JN, Nash RA, Mahoney WM, Jr., Schwartz SM. Is scleroderma a vasculopathy? Current Rheumatology Reports. 2009;11(2):103-10.

[96] Matucci-Cerinic M, Kahaleh B, Wigley FM. Review: Evidence that systemic sclerosis is a vascular disease. Arthritis and Rheumatism. 2013;65(8):1953-62.

[97] Distler O, Distler JH, Scheid A, Acker T, Hirth A, Rethage J, et al. Uncontrolled expression of vascular endothelial growth factor and its receptors leads to insufficient skin angiogenesis in patients with systemic sclerosis. Circulation Research. 2004;95(1):109-16.

[98] Farouk HM, Hamza SH, El Bakry SA, Youssef SS, Aly IM, Moustafa AA, et al. Dysregulation of angiogenic homeostasis in systemic sclerosis. International Journal of Rheumatic Diseases. 2013;16(4):448-54.

[99] Asahara T, Murohara T, Sullivan A, Silver M, van der Zee R, Li T, et al. Isolation of putative progenitor endothelial cells for angiogenesis. Science. 1997;275(5302):964-7.

[100] Kuwana M, Okazaki Y, Yasuoka H, Kawakami Y, Ikeda Y. Defective vasculogenesis in systemic sclerosis. Lancet. 2004;364(9434):603-10.

[101] Maurer B, Distler A, Suliman YA, Gay RE, Michel BA, Gay S, et al. Vascular endothelial growth factor aggravates fibrosis and vasculopathy in experimental models of systemic sclerosis. Annals of the Rheumatic Diseases. 2014;73(10):1880-7.

[102] Bartoloni E, Alunno A, Bistoni O, Caterbi S, Luccioli F, Santoboni G, et al. Characterization of circulating endothelial microparticles and endothelial progenitor cells in primary Sjogren's syndrome: New markers of chronic endothelial damage? Rheumatology. 2015;54(3):536-44.

[103] Del Papa N, Cortiana M, Comina DP, Maglione W, Silvestri I, Maronetti Mazzeo L, et al. Progenitori delle cellule endoteliali di origine midollare in corso di sclerosi sistemica: possibile ruolo nell'angiogenesi [Endothelial progenitor cells in systemic sclerosis: Their possible role in angiogenesis]. Reumatismo. 2005;57(3):174-9.

[104] Werner N, Kosiol S, Schiegl T, Ahlers P, Walenta K, Link A, et al. Circulating endothelial progenitor cells and cardiovascular outcomes. The New England Journal of Medicine. 2005;353(10):999-1007.

[105] Del Papa N, Quirici N, Soligo D, Scavullo C, Cortiana M, Borsotti C, et al. Bone marrow endothelial progenitors are defective in systemic sclerosis. Arthritis and Rheumatism. 2006;54(8):2605-15.

[106] Avouac J, Juin F, Wipff J, Couraud PO, Chiocchia G, Kahan A, et al. Circulating endothelial progenitor cells in systemic sclerosis: Association with disease severity. Annals of the Rheumatic Diseases. 2008;67(10):1455-60.

[107] Allanore Y, Batteux F, Avouac J, Assous N, Weill B, Kahan A. Levels of circulating endothelial progenitor cells in systemic sclerosis. Clinical and Experimental Rheumatology. 2007;25(1):60-6.

[108] Yoder MC, Mead LE, Prater D, Krier TR, Mroueh KN, Li F, et al. Redefining endothelial progenitor cells via clonal analysis and hematopoietic stem/progenitor cell principals. Blood. 2007;109(5):1801-9.

[109] Kuwana M, Okazaki Y. Brief report: Impaired in vivo neovascularization capacity of endothelial progenitor cells in patients with systemic sclerosis. Arthritis & Rheumatology. 2014;66(5):1300-5.

[110] Del Papa N, Quirici N, Scavullo C, Gianelli U, Corti L, Vitali C, et al. Antiendothelial cell antibodies induce apoptosis of bone marrow endothelial progenitors in systemic sclerosis. The Journal of Rheumatology. 2010;37(10):2053-63.

[111] Erdbruegger U, Haubitz M, Woywodt A. Circulating endothelial cells: A novel marker of endothelial damage. Clinica Chimica Acta; International Journal of Clinical Chemistry. 2006;373(1-2):17-26.

[112] Del Papa N, Colombo G, Fracchiolla N, Moronetti LM, Ingegnoli F, Maglione W, et al. Circulating endothelial cells as a marker of ongoing vascular disease in systemic sclerosis. Arthritis and Rheumatism. 2004;50(4):1296-304.

[113] Herrick AL, Illingworth KJ, Hollis S, Gomez-Zumaquero JM, Tinahones FJ. Antibodies against oxidized low-density lipoproteins in systemic sclerosis. Rheumatology. 2001;40(4):401-5.

[114] Nussinovitch U, Shoenfeld Y. Autoimmunity and heart diseases: Pathogenesis and diagnostic criteria. Archivum Immunologiae et Therapiae Experimentalis. 2009;57(2):95-104.

[115] Lopez LR, Simpson DF, Hurley BL, Matsuura E. OxLDL/beta2GPI complexes and autoantibodies in patients with systemic lupus erythematosus, systemic sclerosis, and antiphospholipid syndrome: Pathogenic implications for vascular involvement. Annals of the New York Academy of Sciences. 2005;1051:313-22.

[116] Matsuura E, Kobayashi K, Inoue K, Lopez LR, Shoenfeld Y. Oxidized LDL/beta2-glycoprotein I complexes: New aspects in atherosclerosis. Lupus. 2005;14(9):736-41.

[117] Brey RL, Abbott RD, Curb JD, Sharp DS, Ross GW, Stallworth CL, et al. Beta(2)-glycoprotein 1-dependent anticardiolipin antibodies and risk of ischemic stroke and myocardial infarction: The Honolulu heart program. Stroke; A Journal of Cerebral Circulation. 2001;32(8):1701-6.

[118] Sanna G, Bertolaccini ML, Mameli A, Hughes GR, Khamashta MA, Mathieu A. Antiphospholipid antibodies in patients with scleroderma: Prevalence and clinical significance. Annals of the Rheumatic Diseases. 2005;64(12):1795-6.

[119] Boin F, Franchini S, Colantuoni E, Rosen A, Wigley FM, Casciola-Rosen L. Independent association of anti-beta(2)-glycoprotein I antibodies with macrovascular disease and mortality in scleroderma patients. Arthritis and Rheumatism. 2009;60(8):2480-9.

[120] van Haelst PL, Kobold AC, van Doormaal JJ, Tervaert JW. AECA and ANCA in patients with premature atherosclerosis. International Reviews of Immunology. 2002;21(1):19-26.

[121] Fischer K, Brzosko M, Walecka A, Ostanek L, Sawicki M. Przeciwciala przeciw komorkom endotelialnym--czynnik ryzyka miazdzycy u chorych na toczen rumieniowaty ukladowy [Antiendothelial cell antibodies as a risk factor of atherosclerosis in systemic lupus erythematosus]. Annales Academiae Medicae Stetinensis. 2006;52(Suppl 2):95-9.

[122] Timar O, Soltesz P, Szamosi S, Der H, Szanto S, Szekanecz Z, et al. Increased arterial stiffness as the marker of vascular involvement in systemic sclerosis. The Journal of Rheumatology. 2008;35(7):1329-33.

[123] George J, Meroni PL, Gilburd B, Raschi E, Harats D, Shoenfeld Y. Anti-endothelial cell antibodies in patients with coronary atherosclerosis. Immunology Letters. 2000;73(1):23-7.

[124] Rigat B, Hubert C, Alhenc-Gelas F, Cambien F, Corvol P, Soubrier F. An insertion/deletion polymorphism in the angiotensin I-converting enzyme gene accounting for half the variance of serum enzyme levels. The Journal of Clinical Investigation. 1990;86(4):1343-6.

[125] Niemiec P, Zak I, Wita K. The D allele of angiotensin I-converting enzyme gene insertion/deletion polymorphism is associated with the severity of atherosclerosis. Clinical Chemistry and Laboratory Medicine. 2008;46(4):446-52.

[126] Cambien F, Poirier O, Lecerf L, Evans A, Cambou JP, Arveiler D, et al. Deletion polymorphism in the gene for angiotensin-converting enzyme is a potent risk factor for myocardial infarction. Nature. 1992;359(6396):641-4.

[127] Keavney B, McKenzie C, Parish S, Palmer A, Clark S, Youngman L, et al. Large-scale test of hypothesised associations between the angiotensin-converting-enzyme insertion/deletion polymorphism and myocardial infarction in about 5000 cases and 6000 controls. International Studies of Infarct Survival (ISIS) Collaborators. Lancet. 2000;355(9202):434-42.

[128] Bartoli F, Angotti C, Fatini C, Conforti ML, Guiducci S, Blagojevic J, et al. Angiotensin-converting enzyme I/D polymorphism and macrovascular disease in systemic sclerosis. Rheumatology. 2007;46(5):772-5.

[129] Boulanger CM, Scoazec A, Ebrahimian T, Henry P, Mathieu E, Tedgui A, et al. Circulating microparticles from patients with myocardial infarction cause endothelial dysfunction. Circulation. 2001;104(22):2649-52.

[130] Nomura S, Inami N, Ozaki Y, Kagawa H, Fukuhara S. Significance of microparticles in progressive systemic sclerosis with interstitial pneumonia. Platelets. 2008;19(3):192-8.

[131] Lorenz MW, Markus HS, Bots ML, Rosvall M, Sitzer M. Prediction of clinical cardiovascular events with carotid intima-media thickness: A systematic review and meta-analysis. Circulation. 2007;115(4):459-67.

[132] Tarek el G, Yasser AE, Gheita T. Coronary angiographic findings in asymptomatic systemic sclerosis. Clinical Rheumatology. 2006;25(4):487-90.

[133] Kahan A, Coghlan G, McLaughlin V. Cardiac complications of systemic sclerosis. Rheumatology. 2009;48(Suppl 3):iii45-8.

[134] Montisci R, Vacca A, Garau P, Colonna P, Ruscazio M, Passiu G, et al. Detection of early impairment of coronary flow reserve in patients with systemic sclerosis. Annals of the Rheumatic Diseases. 2003;62(9):890-3.

[135] Ferri C, Giuggioli D, Sebastiani M, Colaci M, Emdin M. Heart involvement and systemic sclerosis. Lupus. 2005;14(9):702-7.

[136] Bulkley BH, Ridolfi RL, Salyer WR, Hutchins GM. Myocardial lesions of progressive systemic sclerosis. A cause of cardiac dysfunction. Circulation. 1976;53(3):483-90.

[137] Derk CT, Jimenez SA. Acute myocardial infarction in systemic sclerosis patients: A case series. Clinical Rheumatology. 2007;26(6):965-8.

[138] D'Angelo WA, Fries JF, Masi AT, Shulman LE. Pathologic observations in systemic sclerosis (scleroderma). A study of fifty-eight autopsy cases and fifty-eight matched controls. The American Journal of Medicine. 1969;46(3):428-40.

[139] Mok MY, Chiu SS, Lo Y, Mak HK, Wong WS, Khong PL, et al. Coronary atherosclerosis using computed tomography coronary angiography in patients with systemic sclerosis. Scandinavian Journal of Rheumatology. 2009;38(5):381-5.

[140] Youssef P, Englert H, Bertouch J. Large vessel occlusive disease associated with CREST syndrome and scleroderma. Annals of the Rheumatic Diseases. 1993;52(6):464-6.

[141] Youssef P, Brama T, Englert H, Bertouch J. Limited scleroderma is associated with increased prevalence of macrovascular disease. The Journal of Rheumatology. 1995;22(3):469-72.

[142] Dick EA, Aviv R, Francis I, Hamilton G, Baker D, Black C, et al. Catheter angiography and angioplasty in patients with scleroderma. The British Journal of Radiology. 2001;74(888):1091-6.

[143] Wan MC, Moore T, Hollis S, Herrick AL. Ankle brachial pressure index in systemic sclerosis: Influence of disease subtype and anticentromere antibody. Rheumatology. 2001;40(10):1102-5.

[144] Kahaleh MB, LeRoy EC. Autoimmunity and vascular involvement in systemic sclerosis (SSc). Autoimmunity. 1999;31(3):195-214.

[145] Rosato E, Gigante A, Barbano B, Cianci R, Molinaro I, Pisarri S, et al. In systemic sclerosis macrovascular damage of hands digital arteries correlates with microvascular damage. Microvascular Research. 2011;82(3):410-5.

[146] Chiang CH, Liu CJ, Huang CC, Chan WL, Huang PH, Chen TJ, et al. Systemic sclerosis and risk of ischaemic stroke: A nationwide cohort study. Rheumatology. 2013;52(1):161-5.

[147] Schedel J, Kuchenbuch S, Schoelmerich J, Feuerbach S, Geissler A, Mueller-Ladner U. Cerebral lesions in patients with connective tissue diseases and systemic vasculitides: Are there specific patterns? Annals of the New York Academy of Sciences. 2010;1193:167-75.

[148] Terrier B, Charbonneau F, Touze E, Berezne A, Pagnoux C, Silvera S, et al. Cerebral vasculopathy is associated with severe vascular manifestations in systemic sclerosis. The Journal of Rheumatology. 2009;36(7):1486-94.

[149] Bertinotti L, Mortilla M, Conforti ML, Colangelo N, Nacci F, Del Rosso A, et al. Proton magnetic resonance spectroscopy reveals central neuroaxonal impairment in systemic sclerosis. The Journal of Rheumatology. 2006;33(3):546-51.

[150] Roquer J, Segura T, Serena J, Castillo J. Endothelial dysfunction, vascular disease and stroke: The ARTICO study. Cerebrovascular Diseases. 2009;27(Suppl 1):25-37.

[151] Faucher B, Granel B, Nicoli F. Acute cerebral vasculopathy in systemic sclerosis. Rheumatology International. 2013;33(12):3073-7.

[152] Heron E, Fornes P, Rance A, Emmerich J, Bayle O, Fiessinger JN. Brain involvement in scleroderma: Two autopsy cases. Stroke; A Journal of Cerebral Circulation. 1998;29(3):719-21.

[153] Chen XY, Lam WW, Ng HK, Fan YH, Wong KS. Intracranial artery calcification: A newly identified risk factor of ischemic stroke. Journal of Neuroimaging: Official Journal of the American Society of Neuroimaging. 2007;17(4):300-3.

[154] Heron E, Hernigou A, Chatellier G, Fornes P, Emmerich J, Fiessinger JN. Intracerebral calcification in systemic sclerosis. Stroke; A Journal of Cerebral Circulation. 1999;30(10):2183-5.

[155] Tanabe J. White matter hyperintensities are associated with an increased risk of stroke, dementia and mortality. Evidence-Based Mental Health. 2011;14(1):1.

[156] Sardanelli F, Iozzelli A, Cotticelli B, Losacco C, Cutolo M, Sulli A, et al. White matter hyperintensities on brain magnetic resonance in systemic sclerosis. Annals of the Rheumatic Diseases. 2005;64(5):777-9.

[157] Mohamed RH, Nassef AA. Brain magnetic resonance imaging findings in patients with systemic sclerosis. International Journal of Rheumatic Diseases. 2010;13(1):61-7.

[158] Nobili F, Cutolo M, Sulli A, Vitali P, Vignola S, Rodriguez G. Brain functional involvement by perfusion SPECT in systemic sclerosis and Behcet's disease. Annals of the New York Academy of Sciences. 2002;966:409-14.

[159] Pathak R, Gabor AJ. Scleroderma and central nervous system vasculitis. Stroke; A Journal of Cerebral Circulation. 1991;22(3):410-3.

[160] Hietarinta M, Lassila O, Hietaharju A. Association of anti-U1RNP- and anti-Scl-70-antibodies with neurological manifestations in systemic sclerosis (scleroderma). Scandinavian Journal of Rheumatology. 1994;23(2):64-7.

[161] Hettema ME, Zhang D, de Leeuw K, Stienstra Y, Smit AJ, Kallenberg CG, et al. Early atherosclerosis in systemic sclerosis and its relation to disease or traditional risk factors. Arthritis Research & Therapy. 2008;10(2):R49.

[162] Cypiene A, Laucevicius A, Venalis A, Dadoniene J, Ryliskyte L, Petrulioniene Z, et al. The impact of systemic sclerosis on arterial wall stiffness parameters and endothelial function. Clinical Rheumatology. 2008;27(12):1517-22.

[163] Andersen GN, Mincheva-Nilsson L, Kazzam E, Nyberg G, Klintland N, Petersson AS, et al. Assessment of vascular function in systemic sclerosis: Indications of the development of nitrate tolerance as a result of enhanced endothelial nitric oxide production. Arthritis and Rheumatism. 2002;46(5):1324-32.

[164] Liu J, Zhang Y, Cao TS, Duan YY, Yuan LJ, Yang YL, et al. Preferential macrovasculopathy in systemic sclerosis detected by regional pulse wave velocity from wave intensity analysis: Comparisons of local and regional arterial stiffness parameters in cases and controls. Arthritis Care & Research. 2011;63(4):579-87.

[165] Roustit M, Simmons GH, Baguet JP, Carpentier P, Cracowski JL. Discrepancy between simultaneous digital skin microvascular and brachial artery macrovascular post-occlusive hyperemia in systemic sclerosis. The Journal of Rheumatology. 2008;35(8):1576-83.

[166] Sherer Y, Cerinic MM, Bartoli F, Blagojevic J, Conforti ML, Gilburd B, et al. Early atherosclerosis and autoantibodies to heat-shock proteins and oxidized LDL in systemic sclerosis. Annals of the New York Academy of Sciences. 2007;1108:259-67.

[167] Tyrrell PN, Beyene J, Feldman BM, McCrindle BW, Silverman ED, Bradley TJ. Rheumatic disease and carotid intima-media thickness: A systematic review and meta-analysis. Arteriosclerosis, Thrombosis, and Vascular Biology. 2010;30(5):1014-26.

[168] Vettori S, Maresca L, Cuomo G, Abbadessa S, Leonardo G, Valentini G. Clinical and subclinical atherosclerosis in systemic sclerosis: Consequences of previous corticosteroid treatment. Scandinavian Journal of Rheumatology. 2010;39(6):485-9.

[169] Schiopu E, Au KM, McMahon MA, Kaplan MJ, Divekar A, Singh RR, et al. Prevalence of subclinical atherosclerosis is increased in systemic sclerosis and is associated with serum proteins: A cross-sectional, controlled study of carotid ultrasound. Rheumatology. 2014;53(4):704-13.

[170] Kerekes G, Soltesz P, Nurmohamed MT, Gonzalez-Gay MA, Turiel M, Vegh E, et al. Validated methods for assessment of subclinical atherosclerosis in rheumatology. Nature Reviews Rheumatology. 2012;8(4):224-34.

[171] Szekanecz Z, Kerekes G, Vegh E, Kardos Z, Barath Z, Tamasi L, et al. Autoimmune atherosclerosis in 3D: How it develops, how to diagnose and what to do. Autoimmunity Reviews. 2016;15(7):756-69.

[172] Lekakis J, Mavrikakis M, Papamichael C, Papazoglou S, Economou O, Scotiniotis I, et al. Short-term estrogen administration improves abnormal endothelial function in women with systemic sclerosis and Raynaud's phenomenon. American Heart Journal. 1998;136(5):905-12.

[173] Kaloudi O, Basta G, Perfetto F, Bartoli F, Del Rosso A, Miniati I, et al. Circulating levels of Nepsilon-(carboxymethyl)lysine are increased in systemic sclerosis. Rheumatology. 2007;46(3):412-6.

[174] Cheng KS, Tiwari A, Boutin A, Denton CP, Black CM, Morris R, et al. Carotid and femoral arterial wall mechanics in scleroderma. Rheumatology. 2003;42(11):1299-305.

[175] Kawasaki M, Ito Y, Yokoyama H, Arai M, Takemura G, Hara A, et al. Assessment of arterial medial characteristics in human carotid arteries using integrated backscatter ultrasound and its histological implications. Atherosclerosis. 2005;180(1):145-54.

[176] Stafford L, Englert H, Gover J, Bertouch J. Distribution of macrovascular disease in scleroderma. Annals of the Rheumatic Diseases. 1998;57(8):476-9.

[177] Sfikakis PP, Papamichael C, Stamatelopoulos KS, Tousoulis D, Fragiadaki KG, Katsichti P, et al. Improvement of vascular endothelial function using the oral endothelin receptor antagonist bosentan in patients with systemic sclerosis. Arthritis and Rheumatism. 2007;56(6):1985-93.

[178] Celermajer DS, Sorensen KE, Bull C, Robinson J, Deanfield JE. Endothelium-dependent dilation in the systemic arteries of asymptomatic subjects relates to coronary risk factors and their interaction. Journal of the American College of Cardiology. 1994;24(6):1468-74.

[179] Yeboah J, Crouse JR, Hsu FC, Burke GL, Herrington DM. Brachial flow-mediated dilation predicts incident cardiovascular events in older adults: The Cardiovascular Health Study. Circulation. 2007;115(18):2390-7.

[180] Lekakis J, Papamichael C, Mavrikakis M, Voutsas A, Stamatelopoulos S. Effect of long-term estrogen therapy on brachial arterial endothelium-dependent vasodilation in women with Raynaud's phenomenon secondary to systemic sclerosis. The American Journal of Cardiology. 1998;82(12):1555-7, A8.

[181] D'Andrea A, Stisi S, Caso P, Uccio FS, Bellissimo S, Salerno G, et al. Associations between left ventricular myocardial involvement and endothelial dysfunction in systemic sclerosis: Noninvasive assessment in asymptomatic patients. Echocardiography. 2007;24(6):587-97.

[182] Rollando D, Bezante GP, Sulli A, Balbi M, Panico N, Pizzorni C, et al. Brachial artery endothelial-dependent flow-mediated dilation identifies early-stage endothelial dysfunction in systemic sclerosis and correlates with nailfold microvascular impairment. The Journal of Rheumatology. 2010;37(6):1168-73.

[183] D'Andrea A, Caso P, Cuomo S, Scotto di Uccio F, Scarafile R, Salerno G, et al. Myocardial and vascular dysfunction in systemic sclerosis: The potential role of noninvasive assessment in asymptomatic patients. International Journal of Cardiology. 2007;121(3):298-301.

[184] Rossi P, Granel B, Marziale D, Le Mee F, Frances Y. Endothelial function and hemodynamics in systemic sclerosis. Clinical Physiology and Functional Imaging. 2010;30(6):453-9.

[185] Al-Qaisi M, Nott DM, King DH, Kaddoura S. Ankle brachial pressure index (ABPI): An update for practitioners. Vascular Health and Risk Management. 2009;5:833-41.

[186] Wig S, Wilkinson J, Moore T, Manning J, Chevance A, Vail A, et al. A longitudinal study of ankle brachial pressure indices in a cohort of patients with systemic sclerosis. Rheumatology. 2014;53(11):2009-13.

[187] Oliver JJ, Webb DJ. Noninvasive assessment of arterial stiffness and risk of atherosclerotic events. Arteriosclerosis, Thrombosis, and Vascular Biology. 2003;23(4):554-66.

[188] Vlachopoulos C, Aznaouridis K, Stefanadis C. Prediction of cardiovascular events and all-cause mortality with arterial stiffness: A systematic review and meta-analysis. Journal of the American College of Cardiology. 2010;55(13):1318-27.

[189] Peled N, Shitrit D, Fox BD, Shlomi D, Amital A, Bendayan D, et al. Peripheral arterial stiffness and endothelial dysfunction in idiopathic and scleroderma associated pulmonary arterial hypertension. The Journal of Rheumatology. 2009;36(5):970-5.

[190] Laurent S, Cockcroft J, Van Bortel L, Boutouyrie P, Giannattasio C, Hayoz D, et al. Expert consensus document on arterial stiffness: Methodological issues and clinical applications. European Heart Journal. 2006;27(21):2588-605.

[191] Mahmud A, Feely J. Arterial stiffness is related to systemic inflammation in essential hypertension. Hypertension. 2005;46(5):1118-22.

[192] Ngian GS, Sahhar J, Wicks IP, Van Doornum S. Arterial stiffness is increased in systemic sclerosis: A cross-sectional comparison with matched controls. Clinical and Experimental Rheumatology. 2014;32(6 Suppl 86):S-161-6.

[193] Piccione MC, Bagnato G, Zito C, Di Bella G, Caliri A, Catalano M, et al. Early identification of vascular damage in patients with systemic sclerosis. Angiology. 2011;62(4):338-43.

[194] Sarwar A, Shaw LJ, Shapiro MD, Blankstein R, Hoffmann U, Cury RC, et al. Diagnostic and prognostic value of absence of coronary artery calcification. JACC Cardiovascular Imaging. 2009;2(6):675-88.

[195] Sulli A, Ghio M, Bezante GP, Deferrari L, Craviotto C, Sebastiani V, et al. Blunted coronary flow reserve in systemic sclerosis. Rheumatology. 2004;43(4):505-9.

[196] Vacca A, Siotto P, Cauli A, Montisci R, Garau P, Ibba V, et al. Absence of epicardial coronary stenosis in patients with systemic sclerosis with severe impairment of coronary flow reserve. Annals of the Rheumatic Diseases. 2006;65(2):274-5.

[197] Sulli A, Ghio M, Bezante GP, Deferrari L, Craviotto C, Sebastiani V, et al. Blunted coronary flow reserve in systemic sclerosis: A sign of cardiac involvement in asymptomatic patients. Annals of the Rheumatic Diseases. 2004;63(2):210-1.

[198] Belloli L, Carlo-Stella N, Ciocia G, Chiti A, Massarotti M, Marasini B. Myocardial involvement in systemic sclerosis. Rheumatology. 2008;47(7):1070-2.

[199] Kobayashi H, Yokoe I, Hirano M, Nakamura T, Nakajima Y, Fontaine KR, et al. Cardiac magnetic resonance imaging with pharmacological stress perfusion and delayed enhancement in asymptomatic patients with systemic sclerosis. The Journal of Rheumatology. 2009;36(1):106-12.

[200] Vignaux O, Allanore Y, Meune C, Pascal O, Duboc D, Weber S, et al. Evaluation of the effect of nifedipine upon myocardial perfusion and contractility using cardiac magnetic resonance imaging and tissue Doppler echocardiography in systemic sclerosis. Annals of the Rheumatic Diseases. 2005;64(9):1268-73.

[201] Montecucco F, Mach F. Common inflammatory mediators orchestrate pathophysiological processes in rheumatoid arthritis and atherosclerosis. Rheumatology. 2009;48(1):11-22.

[202] Gonzalez-Gay MA, Gonzalez-Juanatey C, Pineiro A, Garcia-Porrua C, Testa A, Llorca J. High-grade C-reactive protein elevation correlates with accelerated atherogenesis in patients with rheumatoid arthritis. The Journal of Rheumatology. 2005;32(7):1219-23.

[203] Gonzalez-Gay MA, Gonzalez-Juanatey C, Lopez-Diaz MJ, Pineiro A, Garcia-Porrua C, Miranda-Filloy JA, et al. HLA-DRB1 and persistent chronic inflammation contribute to cardiovascular events and cardiovascular mortality in patients with rheumatoid arthritis. Arthritis and Rheumatism. 2007;57(1):125-32.

[204] Book C, Saxne T, Jacobsson LT. Prediction of mortality in rheumatoid arthritis based on disease activity markers. The Journal of Rheumatology. 2005;32(3):430-4.

[205] Lopez-Mejias R, Castaneda S, Gonzalez-Juanatey C, Corrales A, Ferraz-Amaro I, Genre F, et al. Cardiovascular risk assessment in patients with rheumatoid arthritis: The relevance of clinical, genetic and serological markers. Autoimmun Rev. 2016 Nov;15(11):1013-1030

[206] Montagnana M, Lippi G, Volpe A, Salvagno GL, Biasi D, Caramaschi P, et al. Evaluation of cardiac laboratory markers in patients with systemic sclerosis. Clinical Biochemistry. 2006;39(9):913-7.

[207] Tomasoni L, Sitia S, Borghi C, Cicero AF, Ceconi C, Cecaro F, et al. Effects of treatment strategy on endothelial function. Autoimmunity Reviews. 2010;9(12):840-4.

[208] Atzeni F, Turiel M, Caporali R, Cavagna L, Tomasoni L, Sitia S, et al. The effect of pharmacological therapy on the cardiovascular system of patients with systemic rheumatic diseases. Autoimmunity Reviews. 2010;9(12):835-9.

[209] Bruce IN. Cardiovascular disease in lupus patients: Should all patients be treated with statins and aspirin? Best Practice & Research Clinical Rheumatology. 2005;19(5):823-38.

[210] Kerekes G, Soltesz P, Der H, Veres K, Szabo Z, Vegvari A, et al. Effects of biologics on vascular function and atherosclerosis associated with rheumatoid arthritis. Annals of the New York Academy of Sciences. 2009;1173:814-21.

[211] Szekanecz Z, Kerekes G, Soltesz P. Vascular effects of biologic agents in RA and spondyloarthropathies. Nature Reviews Rheumatology. 2009;5(12):677-84.

[212] Giles JT, Post W, Blumenthal RS, Bathon JM. Therapy insight: Managing cardiovascular risk in patients with rheumatoid arthritis. Nature Clinical Practice Rheumatology. 2006;2(6):320-9.

[213] Costenbader KH, Coblyn JS. Statin therapy in rheumatoid arthritis. Southern Medical Journal. 2005;98(5):534-40; quiz 41, 72.

[214] Timar O, Szekanecz Z, Kerekes G, Vegh J, Olah AV, Nagy G, et al. Rosuvastatin improves impaired endothelial function, lowers high sensitivity CRP, complement and immuncomplex production in patients with systemic sclerosis: A prospective case-series study. Arthritis Research & Therapy. 2013;15(5):R105.

[215] Ormseth MJ, Oeser AM, Cunningham A, Bian A, Shintani A, Solus J, et al. Reversing vascular dysfunction in rheumatoid arthritis: Improved augmentation index but not endothelial function with peroxisome proliferator-activated receptor gamma agonist therapy. Arthritis & Rheumatology. 2014;66(9):2331-8.

[216] Kowal-Bielecka O, Landewe R, Avouac J, Chwiesko S, Miniati I, Czirjak L, et al. EULAR recommendations for the treatment of systemic sclerosis: A report from the EULAR Scleroderma Trials and Research group (EUSTAR). Annals of the Rheumatic Diseases. 2009;68(5):620-8.

[217] Allanore Y, Meune C, Vignaux O, Weber S, Legmann P, Kahan A. Bosentan increases myocardial perfusion and function in systemic sclerosis: A magnetic resonance imaging and tissue-Doppler echography study. The Journal of Rheumatology. 2006;33(12):2464-9.

[218] Kahan A, Devaux JY, Amor B, Menkes CJ, Weber S, Guerin F, et al. Pharmacodynamic effect of nicardipine on left ventricular function in systemic sclerosis. Journal of Cardiovascular Pharmacology. 1990;15(2):249-53.

[219] Allanore Y, Avouac J, Kahan A. Systemic sclerosis: An update in 2008. Joint, Bone, Spine: Revue du Rhumatisme. 2008;75(6):650-5.

[220] Nurmohamed MT, van Halm VP, Dijkmans BA. Cardiovascular risk profile of anti-rheumatic agents in patients with osteoarthritis and rheumatoid arthritis. Drugs. 2002;62(11):1599-609.

[221] Kerekes G, Nurmohamed MT, Gonzalez-Gay MA, Seres I, Paragh G, Kardos Z, et al. Rheumatoid arthritis and metabolic syndrome. Nature Reviews Rheumatology. 2014;10(11):691-6.

[222] del Rincon I, Battafarano DF, Restrepo JF, Erikson JM, Escalante A. Glucocorticoid dose thresholds associated with all-cause and cardiovascular mortality in rheumatoid arthritis. Arthritis & Rheumatology. 2014;66(2):264-72.

[223] Suissa S, Bernatsky S, Hudson M. Antirheumatic drug use and the risk of acute myocardial infarction. Arthritis and Rheumatism. 2006;55(4):531-6.

[224] van Halm VP, Nurmohamed MT, Twisk JW, Dijkmans BA, Voskuyl AE. Disease-modifying antirheumatic drugs are associated with a reduced risk for cardiovascular disease in patients with rheumatoid arthritis: A case control study. Arthritis Research & Therapy. 2006;8(5):R151.

[225] van Ede AE, Laan RF, Blom HJ, Boers GH, Haagsma CJ, Thomas CM, et al. Homocysteine and folate status in methotrexate-treated patients with rheumatoid arthritis. Rheumatology. 2002;41(6):658-65.

[226] Reiss AB, Carsons SE, Anwar K, Rao S, Edelman SD, Zhang H, et al. Atheroprotective effects of methotrexate on reverse cholesterol transport proteins and foam cell transformation in human THP-1 monocyte/macrophages. Arthritis and Rheumatism. 2008;58(12):3675-83.

[227] Finsterer J, Ohnsorge P. Influence of mitochondrion-toxic agents on the cardiovascular system. Regulatory Toxicology and Pharmacology: RTP. 2013;67(3):434-45.

[228] Loudet AM, Dousset N, Carton M, Douste-Blazy L. Effects of an antimitotic agent (cyclophosphamide) on plasma lipoproteins. Biochemical Pharmacology. 1984;33(19):2961-5.

[229] Loudet AM, Dousset N, Perret B, Ierides M, Carton M, Douste-Blazy L. Triacylglycerol increase in plasma very low density lipoproteins in cyclophosphamide-treated rabbit: Relationship with cholesteryl ester transfer activity. Biochimica et Biophysica Acta. 1985;836(3):376-84.

[230] Garces SP, Parreira Santos MJ, Vinagre FM, Roque RM, da Silva JA. Anti-tumour necrosis factor agents and lipid profile: A class effect? Annals of the Rheumatic Diseases. 2008;67(6):895-6.

[231] Gonzalez-Gay MA, De Matias JM, Gonzalez-Juanatey C, Garcia-Porrua C, Sanchez-Andrade A, Martin J, et al. Anti-tumor necrosis factor-alpha blockade improves insulin resistance in patients with rheumatoid arthritis. Clinical and Experimental Rheumatology. 2006;24(1):83-6.

[232] Kerekes G, Soltesz P, Der H, Veres K, Szabo Z, Vegvari A, et al. Effects of rituximab treatment on endothelial dysfunction, carotid atherosclerosis, and lipid profile in rheumatoid arthritis. Clinical Rheumatology. 2009;28(6):705-10.

[233] Gonzalez-Juanatey C, Llorca J, Vazquez-Rodriguez TR, Diaz-Varela N, Garcia-Quiroga H, Gonzalez-Gay MA. Short-term improvement of endothelial function in rituximab-treated rheumatoid arthritis patients refractory to tumor necrosis factor alpha blocker therapy. Arthritis and Rheumatism. 2008;59(12):1821-4.

[234] van Leeuwen M, Damoiseaux J, Duijvestijn A, Tervaert JW. The therapeutic potential of targeting B cells and anti-oxLDL antibodies in atherosclerosis. Autoimmunity Reviews. 2009;9(1):53-7.

Chapter 3

Survival, Mortality, Causes of Death and Risk Factors of Poor Outcome

Manuel Rubio-Rivas

Additional information is available at the end of the chapter

http://dx.doi.org/10.5772/intechopen.68549

Abstract

Systemic sclerosis is a rare autoimmune disorder with a historically bad prognosis. Survival has been improving over time and we can currently estimate a 1-year survival, 94.9; a 5-year survival, 84.4; a 10-year survival, 70.9 and a 20-year survival, 44.9%, from the time of diagnosis. Accordingly, mortality has been decreasing over time, being the overall standardized mortality ratio (SMR) 2.72 (1.90–3.83), SMR 2.4 after 1990. Among the SSc-related causes of death, the lung death is the most important cause and its relative percentage is increasing over time since the introduction of ACE inhibitors for the treatment of scleroderma renal crisis (SRC) in early 1990s. Among the SSc-non-related causes of death, cancer, infection and cardiovascular disorders are the leading causes of death. Risk factor predictors of poor outcomes are an elder age at diagnosis, the male gender, diffuse subset, visceral involvement and non-Raynaud's phenomenon onset.

Keywords: systemic sclerosis, survival, mortality, death, prognosis

1. Introduction

Systemic sclerosis (SSc) represents one of the autoimmune systemic diseases with worse prognosis. It was actually a devastating scenario until it became well advanced in the twentieth century in terms of survival and mortality, but since late 1980s, the knowledge and course of scleroderma have been progressively improving. Nowadays, more risk factors are recognized and allow physicians to focus on patients with worse prognosis. As traditional SSc-related involvements improved, secondary involvements or SSc-non-related diseases have gained prominence.

2. Survival

Scleroderma was a devastating disease for ages. Physicians were short of proper tools to change significantly the prognosis of the disease since late 1980s–early 1990s due to the introduction of new therapies, firstly angiotensin converting enzyme (ACE) inhibitors for the treatment of the scleroderma renal crisis (SRC) and, in late 1990s-early 2000s, due to the implementation of pulmonary arterial hypertension (PAH) treatment with new drugs such as phosphodiesterase five (PDE5) inhibitors and antagonists of the receptor of endothelin (AREs). Survival has improved over time, measured at any time of the follow-up, from onset (in most studies described in the form of Raynaud's phenomenon) as well as from diagnosis and what is more important is that it keeps improving. This is true that survival in all stages has improved but especially 1-year and 5-year survival. Since late death is related the most to SSc-non-related causes, it might be reflecting the fact that physicians are improving significantly the prognosis of SSc-related involvements but not that much in other SSc-non-related diseases. Thus, just like in other autoimmune diseases, scleroderma is becoming step-by-step a chronic disease and not a terminal and deleterious diagnosis.

Prior to the assessment of survival of any cohort, we must pay attention to the methodology of the study because there is a huge variability among them, sometimes assessing survival from diagnosis and sometimes from the onset of disease. These last data are obviously a more imprecise data but certainly more real. Several survival and mortality studies from single cohorts and reviews have been published from the last mid-century, reporting data about cumulative survival at different times of follow-up and measured sometimes from the onset of disease and sometimes from the time of diagnosis (**Table 1**) [1–42].

We show data previously released in Seminars in Arthritis and Rheumatism in the last and more precise meta-analysis, so that we can currently predict at the time of diagnosis: a 1-year survival, 94.9; a 5-year survival, 84.4; a 10-year survival, 70.9 and a 20-year survival, 44.9% (**Table 2** and **Figure 1**) [43].

Study	Country	Years (mid-cohort)	1-year survival	5-year survival	10-year survival	20-year survival	From onset/ diagnosis
Tuffanelli [1]	The USA	1935–1958(46)	NA	70.3%	69%	NA	Diagnosis
Farmer [2]	The USA	1945–1952(48)	NA	53%	NA	NA	Diagnosis
Bennet [3]	The UK	1947–1970(58)	94%	73%	50%	NA	Diagnosis
Medsger [4]	The USA	1955–1970(62)	78%	48%	NA	NA	Diagnosis
Zarafonetis [5]	The USA	1948–1980(64)	NA	81.4%	69.4%	NA	Diagnosis
Medsger [6]	The USA	1963–1970(66)	70%	44%	NA	NA	Diagnosis
Rowell [7]	The UK	1960–1975(67)	NA	NA	74%	NA	Onset (first Raynaud)
Barnett [8]	AUS	1953–1983(68)	NA	83.6%	59.3%	27.1%	Onset (first Raynaud)
Gouet [9]	FR	1960–1984(72)	88%	62.5%	50.5%	NA	Diagnosis

Study	Country	Years (mid-cohort)	1-year survival	5-year survival	10-year survival	20-year survival	From onset/diagnosis
Giordano [10]	ITA	1965–1983(74)	NA	72%	32%	NA	Diagnosis
Altman [11]	The USA	1973–1977(75)	NA	63%	42%	NA	Diagnosis
Eason [12]	NZ	1970–1980(75)	85%	60%	42%	NA	Diagnosis
Wynn [13]	The USA	1970–1980(75)	98.4%	68.9%	51.2%	31.7%	Diagnosis
Peters-Golden [14]	The USA	1972–1983(77)	84%	66%	60%	NA	Diagnosis
Ferri [15]	ITA	1955–1999(77)	NA	83%	69.2%	45.5%	Diagnosis
Lally [16]	The USA	1972–1984(78)	NA	77%	NA	NA	Diagnosis
Jacobsen [17]	DEN	1960–1996(78)	NA	81%	71%	42%	Onset (first non-Raynaud's symptom)
Kuwana [18]	JAP	1971–1990(80)	NA	NA	NA	NA	Diagnosis
Geirsson [19]	ICE	1975–1990(82)	NA	100%	81%	NA	Diagnosis
Kaburaki [20]	JAP	1976–1991(83)	NA	78%	68.2%	NA	Diagnosis
Nishioka [21]	JAP	1974–1994(84)	NA	93.7%	82%	56.7%	Onset (first Raynaud)
Simeón [22]	SPA	1976–1996(86)	NA	71%	64%	62%	Onset (first Raynaud)
Bulpitt [23]	The USA	1982–1992(87)	92%	68%	NA	NA	Onset (first non-Raynaud's symptom)
Bryan [24]	The UK	1982–1992(87)	NA	87%	75%	NA	Onset (first non-Raynaud's symptom)
Nagy [25]	HUN	1982–1993(87)	NA	82.9%	70.4%	NA	Onset (first non-Raynaud's symptom)
Hesselstrand [26]	SWE	1983–1995(89)	NA	92%	78%	NA	Onset (first non-Raynaud's symptom)
			NA	86%	69%	NA	Diagnosis
Kim [27]	KOR	1972–2007(89)	NA	85.4%	80.1%	NA	Diagnosis
Mayes [28]	The USA	1989–1991(90)	NA	77.9%	55.1%	26.8%	Diagnosis
Hashimoto [29]	JAP	1973–2008(90)	NA	NA	88%	77.4%	Onset (first Raynaud)
Pérez-Bocanegra [30]	SPA	1976–2007(91)	NA	89%	81%	63%	Diagnosis
Alamanos [31]	GRE	1981–2002(91)	NA	83%	70%	NA	Diagnosis

Study	Country	Years (mid-cohort)	1-year survival	5-year survival	10-year survival	20-year survival	From onset/ diagnosis
Nihtyanova [32]	The UK	1990–1993(91)	NA	84.2%	NA	NA	Diagnosis
		2000–2003(01)	NA	89.9%	NA	NA	Onset (first non-Raynaud's symptom)
Joven [33]	SPA	1980–2006(93)	95%	85%	75%	55%	Onset (first non-Raynaud's symptom)
Ruangjutipopan [34]	THAI	1987–2001(94)	NA	73%	67.4%	NA	Onset (no definition)
Czirják [35]	HUN	1983–2005(94)	NA	84%	72.6%	NA	Diagnosis
Arias-Núñez [36]	SPA	1988–2006(97)	NA	83.9%	64.9%	NA	Diagnosis
Alba [37]	SPA	1986–2010(98)	NA	90.7%	NA	NA	Diagnosis
Al-Dhaher [38]	CAN	1994–2004(99)	NA	90%	82%	NA	Diagnosis
Sampaio-Barros [39]	BRA	1991–2010(00)	NA	90%	84%	NA	Onset (no definition)
Hoffmann-Vold [40]	NOR	1999–2009(04)	NA	95%	86%	NA	Onset (first non-Raynaud's symptom)
Vettori [41]	ITA	2000–2008(04)	NA	94.8	NA	NA	Onset (first Raynaud)
Kuo [42]	TAIW	2002–2007(05)	94.9%	83.2%	NA	NA	Diagnosis

NA: non-available. Reprinted from Rubio-Rivas et al. [43], with permission from Elsevier.

Table 1. Survival studies on scleroderma [43].

	Survival from onset (first Raynaud)			Survival from onset (first non-Raynaud's symptom)			Survival from diagnosis		
	Before 1990 (five studies)	**After 1990 (three studies)**	**p**	**Before 1990 (four studies)**	**After 1990 (three studies)**	**p**	**Before 1990 (18 studies)**	**After 1990 (eight studies)**	**p**
Number of patients	840	1693		846	802		4365	3476	
1-year survival% mean (SD)	–	–	–	92 (NA)	95 (NA)	–	85.3(9.5)	94.9(NA)	0.384
5-year survival% mean (SD)	85.1(10.4)	92.8(2.9)	0.385	79.7 (8.2)	90 (5.0)	0.118	70.6(14.3)	84.4(3.8)	0.001
10-year survival% mean (SD)	71.5(9.5)	88(NA)	0.189	72.1 (2.5)	80.5 (7.8)	0.358	58.8(14.8)	70.9(10.1)	0.086

http://dx.doi.org/10.5772/intechopen.68549

	Survival from onset (first Raynaud)			Survival from onset (first non-Raynaud's symptom)			Survival from diagnosis		
	Before 1990 (five studies)	**After 1990 (three studies)**	**p**	**Before 1990 (four studies)**	**After 1990 (three studies)**	**p**	**Before 1990 (18 studies)**	**After 1990 (eight studies)**	**p**
20-year survival% mean (SD)	48.6(18.8)	77.4(NA)	0.316	42 (NA)	55 (NA)	–	38.6(9.8)	44.9(25.6)	0.790

T-test for independent groups among studies before and after 1990 (mid-cohort year). NA: non-available. Reprinted from Rubio-Rivas et al. [43], with permission from Elsevier.

Table 2. Survival studies on scleroderma [43].

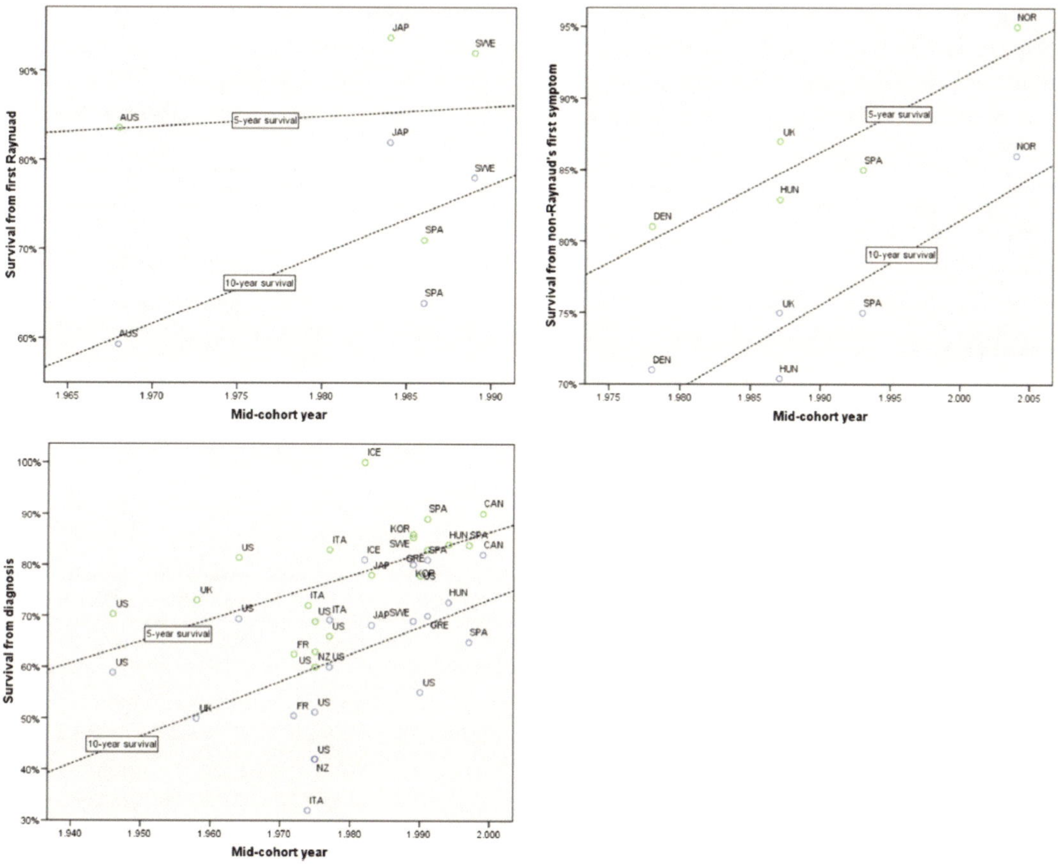

Figure 1. Survival evolution over time. Meta-regression. Five-year survival (coefficient b = 0.308 and p = 0.402) and 10-year survival (coefficient b = 0.595 and p = 0.237) from the onset (first Raynaud). Five-year survival (coefficient b = 0.612 and p = 0.113) and 10-year survival (coefficient b = 0.590 and p = 0.037) from the onset (first non-Raynaud's symptom). Five-year survival (coefficient b = 0.595 and p < 0.001) and 10-year survival (coefficient b = 0.536 and p = 0.025) from diagnosis. Reprinted from Rubio-Rivas et al., with permission from Elsevier [43].

3. Mortality

SSc is an autoimmune disease with a broad spectrum of severity, ranging from a mild disease to a devastating one. The most valuable parameter in order to compare mortality (instead of a crude mortality rate) is the assessment of the SMR, a fundamental tool in the only five mortality meta-analyses reported so far in SSc (**Table 3**). The SMR is the ratio between observed mortality and expected mortality in sex- and age-matched general population. These five meta-analyses are based on the assessment of the SMR: Elhai et al. {nine studies, overall SMR is 3.53 (3.03–4.11)} [45], Loannidis et al. {seven studies} [44], Toledano et al. {seven studies, overall SMR 3.51 (2.74–4.50)} [46], Komócsi et al. {10 studies, overall SMR 3.24} [47] and Rubio-Rivas et al. {17 studies, overall SMR 2.72 (1.90–3.83)} [43]. In base of this last study based on 17 studies, we could state that mortality is over 2.7-fold compared to the general population (**Table 4** and **Figure 2**) [5, 17, 24, 26, 29, 30, 31, 33, 37, 40, 42, 48–53]. Mortality has been decreasing over time and notoriously after 1990, being more reasonable to accept nowadays an SMR over 2.4-fold in a patient diagnosed today (**Figure 2**). Obviously, prognosis should be individualized since different risk factors present at diagnosis or during the follow-up can modify this predicted SMR. For instance, SMR in males and dcSSc subset is expected to be worse compared to SMR in females or lcSSc subset (**Figure 3**).

Study	Year of publication	Number of studies included	SMR (95% CI)
Ioannidis et al. [44]	2005	7	–
Elhai et al. [45]	2012	9	3.53 (3.03–4.11)
Toledano et al. [46]	2012	7	3.51 (2.74–4.50)
Komócsi et al. [47]	2012	10	3.24 (NA)
Rubio-Rivas et al. [43]	2014	17	2.72 (1.93–3.83)
NA: non-available.			

Table 3. Meta-analyses on scleroderma and mortality.

Study	Country	Years (mid-cohort year)	Death	Overall SMR (95%CI)	dcSSc SMR (95%CI)	lcSSc SMR (95%CI)	Male SMR (95%CI)	Female SMR (95%CI)
Zarafonetis [5]	US	1948–1980 (64)	142	5.40 (3.17-7.63)	NA	NA	NA	NA
Jacobsen [17]	DEN	1960–1996 (78)	160	2.90 (2.50-3.40)	4.50 (3.50-5.70)	2.30 (1.80-2.80)	3.70 (2.70-5.10)	2.70 (2.30-3.30)
Abu-Shakra [48]	CAN	1976–1990 (83)	61	4.69 (3.73-5.65)	6.18 (4.17-8.81)	3.80 (2.58-5.39)	4.18 (2.09-7.48)	4.81 (3.65-6.44)
Walsh [49]	US	1981–1990 (85)	2123	1.05 (1.01-1.1)	NA	NA	NA	NA
Bryan [24]	UK	1982–1992 (87)	55	4.05 (3.03-5.22)	NA	NA	3.22 (1.85-4.97)	4.59 (3.22-6.19)
Hesselstrand [26]	SWE	1983–1995 (89)	49	4.59 (3.48-6.07)	6.06 (4.09-9.02)	3.72 (2.41-532)	4.77 (3.21-7.09)	4.44 (2.87-6.34)
Hashimoto [29]	JAP	1973–1908 (90)	86	2.76 (2.18-3.35)	5.90 (4.20-7.61)	1.71 (1.18-2.24)	3.31 (1.15-5.47)	2.71 (2.10-3.32)

Study	Country	Years (mid-cohort year)	Death	Overall SMR (95%CI)	dcSSc SMR (95%CI)	lcSSc SMR (95%CI)	Male SMR (95%CI)	Female SMR (95%CI)
Alamanos [31]	GRE	1981–2002 (91)	36	2.0 (1.2-2.8)	NA	NA	NA	NA
Scussel-Lonzetti [50]	CAN	1984–1999 (91)	66	2.69 (2.10-3.40)	6.17 (2.80-11.70)	2.71 (1.85-3.80)	1.76 (0.80-3.30)	2.55 (1.90-3.30)
Pérez-Bocanegra [30]	SPA	1976–2007 (91)	73	1.90 (1.50-2.30)	6.50 (4.10-9.80)	1.70 (1.20-2.20)	1.80 (0.80-3.40)	2.50 (1.90-3.20)
Joven [33]	SPA	1980–2006 (93)	44	3.10 (1.60-6.10)	NA	NA	NA	NA
Alba [37]	SPA	1986–2010 (98)	151	3.80 (3.18-4.43)	NA	NA	NA	NA
Hissaria [51]	AUS	1993–2007 (00)	331	1.46 (1.28-1.69)	2.92 (2.20-3.89)	1.30 (1.11-1.53)	NA	NA
Mok [52]	CHI	1999–2008 (03)	110	3.94 (3.20-4.68)	NA	NA	2.59 (1.32-3.87)	4.32 (3.45-5.20)
Hoffmann-Vold [40]	NOR	1999–2009 (04)	43	2.03 (1.40-2.60)	5.33 (3.90-10.30)	1.62 (1.10-2.50)	2.61 (1.40-3.90)	1.80 (1.20-2.70)
Strickland [53]	UK	1999–2010 (04)	53	1.34 (0.95-1.74)	1.66 (0.83-2.97)	1.27 (0.92-1.72)	1.54 (0.67-3.04)	1.30 (0.95-1.74)
Kuo [42]	TAIW	2002–2007 (05)	204	3.24 (2.82-3.71)	NA	NA	3.53 (2.97-4.16)	2.92 (2.29-3.66)

NA: non-available, SMR: standardized mortality ratio, dcSSc: diffuse cutaneous systemic sclerosis and lcSSc: limited cutaneous systemic sclerosis. Reprinted from Rubio-Rivas et al. [43], with permission from Elsevier.

Table 4. Studies included in the SMR meta-analysis by Rubio-Rivas et al [43].

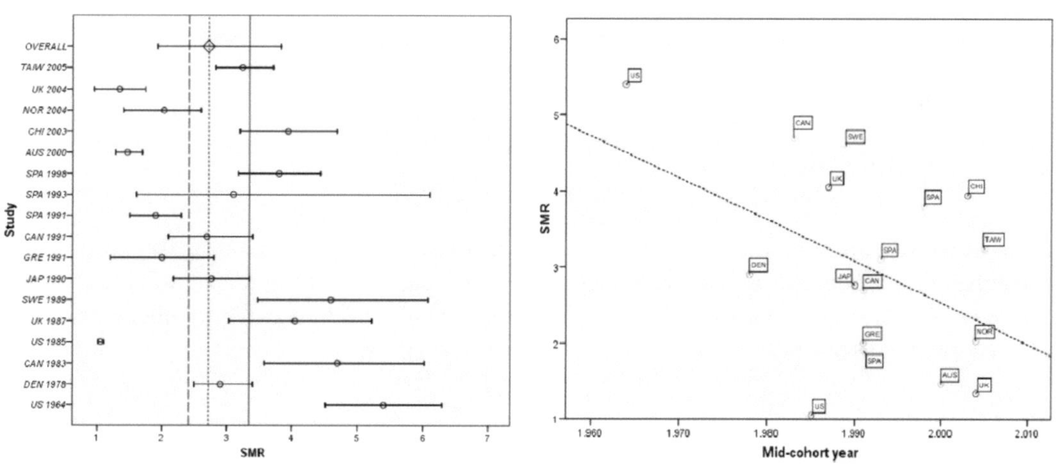

Figure 2. SMR meta-analysis. The overall SMR (discontinuous points) is 2.71 (1.95–3.75). SMR before 1990 (continuous line) is 3.33 (1.64–6.75). SMR after 1990 (discontinuous lines) is 2.42 (1.89–3.11). Forest plot. Meta-regression of change in SMR (lnSMR) with mid-cohort year (Coefficient b = –0.055 and p = 0.064). Reprinted from Rubio-Rivas et al., with permission from Elsevier [43].

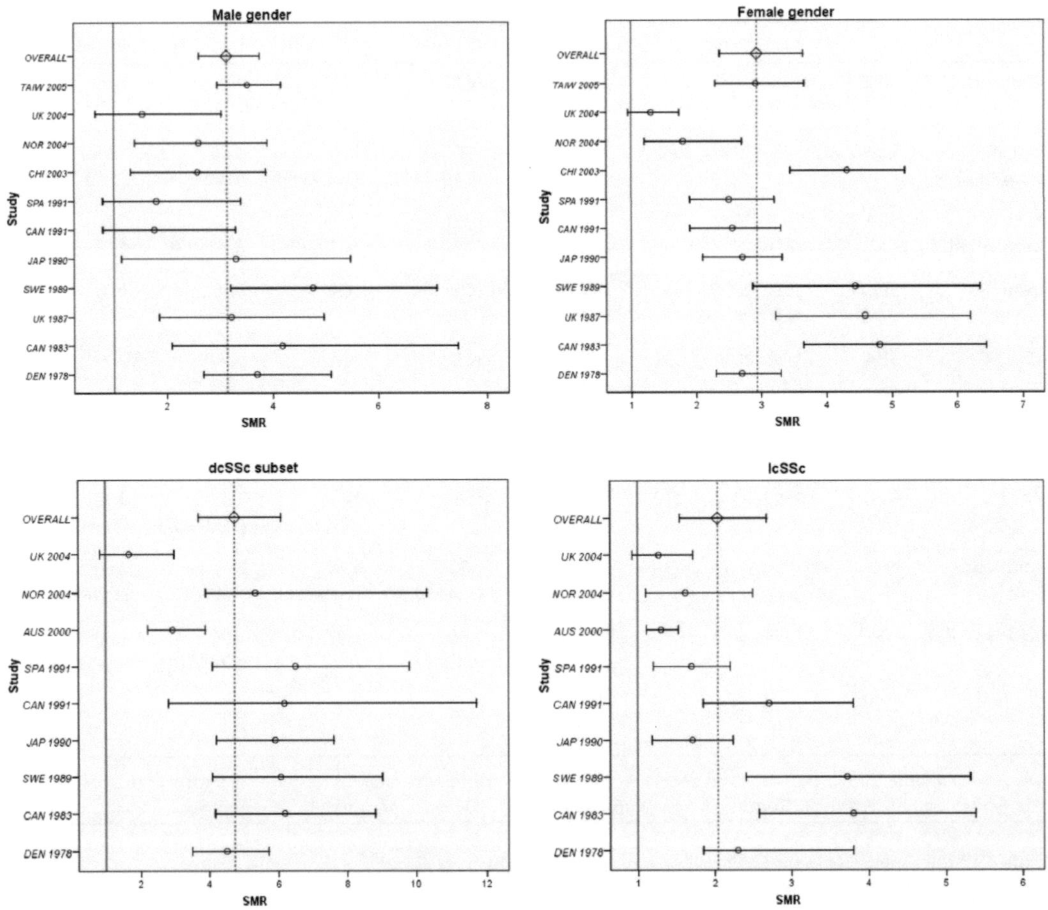

Figure 3. SMR meta-analysis. For the male gender, overall SMR is 3.18 (2.62–3.85) and for the female gender, overall SMR is 2.81 (2.25–3.50); for dcSSc subtype, the overall SMR is 4.73 (3.69–6.07) and for lcSSc subtype, overall SMR is 2.04 (1.55–2.68). Forest plot. Reprinted from Rubio-Rivas et al., with permission from Elsevier [43].

4. Causes of death

As in other autoimmune diseases, the pattern of mortality has been changing over time since the autoimmune disease by itself has been the main cause of death in these patients for ages but the more physicians control the disease, the more likely it is to die due to other causes not directly related to SSc [43, 54–56].

4.1. SSc-related causes of death

Among the SSc-related causes, there are four major organs potentially involved: the lungs, heart, kidneys and gastrointestinal tract. Among them, lung and renal involvement were the most important as a cause of death during the twentieth century (**Table 5**) [2, 3, 7, 8, 11–13, 15, 17–19, 21–24, 26, 29, 31, 33–42, 48, 50–53, 56, 57, 59–62].

4.1.1. Lung involvement

In the case of lung involvement, death can be due to the progression towards respiratory failure due to PAH or interstitial lung disease (ILD).

In the case of PAH, evidence suggests that SSc-PAH patients have a worse response to therapy when compared to idiopathic PAH. New therapies (phosphodiesterase type 5 inhibitors and endothelin receptor antagonists) have improved its prognosis but not that much and thus, this is still a severe manifestation of the disease and a frequent cause of death. An early combination schedule of treatment has been suggested to be better in terms of prognosis. However, more studies are required to demonstrate and standardize this strategy of treatment [63].

Interstitial lung disease constitutes the most severe manifestation of the disease and is in fact the first cause of death in these patients (**Figure 4**). Therefore, it is crucial to perform a regular screening of this involvement and an early treatment when diagnosed. Patients showing the following criteria would warrant an immunosuppressive treatment: (1) either an extent of lung disease >20% on High-resolution computed tomography (HRCT) or an indeterminate extent (disease extent not readily classifiable as minimal or severe; HRCT extent is 10–30%) of disease plus an FVC < 70%, (2) patients experiencing a significant decrease in pulmonary functional assessment during the follow-up (FVC > 10% or DLco >15% or both, whatever the extent of lung involvement is for 12 months). Currently, the management of SSc–ILD is largely confined to immunomodulvation. Non-selective immunosuppressants such as cyclophosphamide followed by mycophenolate mofetil and azathioprine are still the most widely used medications in SSc-ILD. Several alternative approaches may be considered, including B cell depletion therapies (rituximab), anti-TGF-β antibody, tyrosine kinase inhibitors (imatinib, dasatinib), anti-IL-6 antibody, anti-IL-13 antibody, pirfenidone and haematopoietic stem cell transplantation (HSCT). Finally, lung transplantation may be limited to those patients, with severe SSc-ILD, unresponsive to pharmacologic therapy [64]. It is important to remember that, although often used, during the first stages of treatment, prednisone doses over 15 mg a day can be dangerous in order to trigger a scleroderma renal crisis.

4.1.2. Renal involvement

Scleroderma renal crisis occurs during the rapid progression of skin thickening in the early stages of dcSSc (<5 years after disease onset). Several case series published during the past 20 years and a 2013 systematic literature review has estimated that SRC develops in 5–15 and 15% of patients with dcSSc, respectively. Interestingly, the incidence and prevalence of SRC seem to be decreasing over time, possibly as a result of early recognition and management of SRC risk factors and early signs and symptoms in patients with dcSSc [65]. The introduction of ACE inhibitors (captopril) reduced dramatically its frequency as the cause of death since early 1990s of the past century (**Figure 4**). Besides, its incidence is decreasing but due to unknown reasons. The extended use of ACE inhibitors prescribed for other reasons (i.e. arterial hypertension or heart failure) has not been found as the cause of this decreasing incidence.

	Country	Years (mid-cohort year)	Deads/n	SSc-related death	Lung death	Heart death	Kidney death	GI death
Farmer [2]	US	1945–1952 (48)	115/271 (49%)	17 (14.8%)	5 (29.4%)	6 (35.3%)	1 (5.9%)	1 (5.9%)
Bennet [3]	UK	1947–1970 (58)	26/67 (38.8%)	1 (9.1%)	0 (0%)	1 (9.1%)	0 (0%)	0 (0%)
Rowell [7]	UK	1960–1975 (67)	22/84 (26.2%)	NA	NA	NA	NA	NA
Barnett [8]	AUS	1953–1983 (68)	86/177 (48.6%)	42 (48.8%)	8 (19%)	10 (11.6%)	16 (38.1%)	8 (9.3%)
Altman [11]	US	1973–1977 (75)	131/264 (49.6%)	89 (68%)	19 (21.3%)	19 (21.3%)	35 (39.3%)	13 (14.6%)
Eason [12]	NZ	1970–1980 (75)	24/47 (51%)	18 (75%)	7 (38.9%)	4 (22.2%)	5 (27.8%)	2 (11.1%)
Wynn [13]	US	1970–1980 (75)	25/64 (39.1%)	17 (68%)	7 (41.2%)	6 (35.3%)	4 (23.5%)	0 (0%)
Ferri [15]	ITA	1955–1999 (77)	279/1012 (27.6%)	61 (35.9%)	NA	NA	NA	NA
Lally [16]	US	1972–1984 (78)	17/91 (18.7%)	14 (82.4%)	0 (0%)	8 (57.1%)	6 (42.9%)	0 (0%)
Jacobsen [17]	DEN	1960–1996 (78)	160/344 (46.5%)	41 (25.6%)	13 (31.7%)	1 (2.4%)	17 (41.5%)	9 (22%)
Kuwana [18]	JAP	1971–1990 (80)	51/275 (18.5%)	32 (62.7%)	23 (71.9%)	4 (12.5%)	5 (15.6%)	0 (0%)
Geirsson [19]	ICE	1975–1990 (82)	5/23 (21.7%)	2 (40%)	0 (0%)	1 (50%)	1 (50%)	0 (0%)
Abu-Shakra [48]	CAN	1976–1990 (83)	61/237 (25.7%)	44 (77.1%)	13 (29.5%)	5 (11.4%)	5 (11.4%)	0 (0%)
Nishioka [21]	JAP	1974–1994 (84)	90/496 (18.1%)	64 (71.1%)	44 (68.8%)	31 (48.4%)	12 (18.8%)	13 (20.3%)
Steen [56]	US	1972–1996 (84)	364/1508 (24.1%)	182 (50%)	NA	NA	NA	NA
Simeón [22]	SPA	1976–1996 (86)	12/79 (15.2%)	11 (91.7%)	4 (36.4%)	0 (0%)	7 (63.6%)	0 (0%)
Bulpitt [23]	US	1982–1992 (87)	15/48 (31.3%)	9 (60%)	4 (44.4%)	1 (11.1%)	4 (44.4%)	0 (0%)
Bryan [24]	UK	1982–1992 (87)	55/283 (19.4%)	34 (61.8%)	15 (44.1%)	5 (14.7%)	5 (14.7%)	3 (8.8%)
Geirsson [57]	SWE	1982–1995 (88)	30/100 (30%)	10 (33.3%)	5 (50%)	4 (40%)	1 (10%)	0 (0%)
Hesselstrand [26]	SWE	1983–1995 (89)	49/249 (19.7%)	15 (30.6%)	10 (66.7%)	1 (6.7%)	1 (6.7%)	3 (20%)
Bond [58]	AUS	1983–1996 (89)	123/123 (100%)	43 (35%)	13 (30.2%)	14 (32.6%)	6 (14%)	NA

	Country	Years (mid-cohort year)	Deads/n	SSc-related death	Lung death	Heart death	Kidney death	GI death
Vlachoyiannopoulos [59]	GRE	1982–1996 (89)	7/254 (2.8%)	6 (85.7%)	2 (33.3%)	2 (33.3%)	2 (33.3%)	0 (0%)
Hashimoto [29]	JAP	1973–1908 (90)	86/405 (21.2%)	NA	NA	NA	NA	NA
Scussel-Lonzetti [50]	CAN	1984–1999 (91)	66/309 (21.4%)	35 (53%)	6 (17.1%)	4 (11.4%)	7 (20%)	3 (8.6%)
Alamanos [31]	GRE	1981–2002 (91)	36/109 (33%)	23 (63.9%)	21 (58.3%)	21 (58.3%)	2 (5.6%)	0 (0%)
Joven [33]	SPA	1980–1906 (93)	44/204 (21.6%)	36 (82%)	20 (55.6%)	8 (22.2%)	1 (2.8%)	3 (8.3%)
Ruangjutipopan [34]	THAI	1987–2001 (94)	31/222 (26.7%)	18 (58.1%)	NA	NA	NA	0 (0%)
Czirják [35]	HUN	1983–2005 (94)	93/366 (25.4%)	86 (92.5%)	30 (34.9%)	29 (33.7%)	16 (18.6%)	8 (9.3%)
Derk [60]	US	1985–2007 (96)	87/87 (100%)	67 (77%)	65 (97%)	55 (82.1%)	2 (3%)	0 (0%)
Arias-Núñez [36]	SPA	1988–2006 (97)	20/78 (25.6%)	11 (55%)	10 (90.9%)	1 (9.1%)	0 (0%)	0 (0%)
Alba [37]	SPA	1986–2010 (98)	151/1037 (14.6%)	61 (78.2%)	NA	13 (16.7%)	0 (0%)	5 (4.1%)
Al-Dhaher [38]	CAN	1994–2004 (99)	42/185 (23%)	NA	15 (45.5%)	9 (27.3%)	9 (27.3%)	0 (0%)
Sampaio-Barros [39]	BRA	1991–2010 (00)	168/947 (17.7%)	110 (65.5%)	53 (48.2%)	27 (24.5%)	12 (10.9%)	5 (4.5%)
Assassi [61]	US	1998–2008 (03)	52/250 (20.8%)	29 (55.8%)	10 (34.5%)	4 (13.8%)	NA	2 (6.9%)
Mok [52]	CHI	1999–2008 (03)	110/449 (24.5%)	26 (24%)	11 (42.3%)	NA	5 (19.2%)	2 (7.7%)
Hoffmann-Vold [40]	NOR	1999–2009 (04)	43/312 (13.8%)	13 (54.2%)	0 (0%)	5 (20.8%)	6 (25%)	2 (4.7%)
Vettori [41]	ITA	2000–2008 (04)	20/251 (8%)	12 (60%)	5 (41.7%)	4 (33.3%)	1 (8.3%)	2 (16.7%)
Hachulla [62]	FR	2002–2006 (04)	47/546 (8.6%)	24 (51.1%)	19 (79.2%)	0 (0%)	3 (12.5%)	2 (8.3%)
Strickland [53]	UK	1999–2010 (04)	53/204 (26%)	19 (35.9%)	9 (47.4%)	4 (21.1%)	0 (0%)	1 (5.3%)
Kuo [42]	TAIW	2002–2007 (05)	204/1479 (13.8%)	57 (27.9%)	9 (4.4%)	29 (0.1%)	14 (6.9%)	10 (5%)

Lung, heart, kidney and GI are deaths related to SSc. NA: non-available; GI: gastrointestinal. Reprinted from Rubio-Rivas et al. [43], with permission from Elsevier.

Table 5. SSc-related causes of death in medical literature [43].

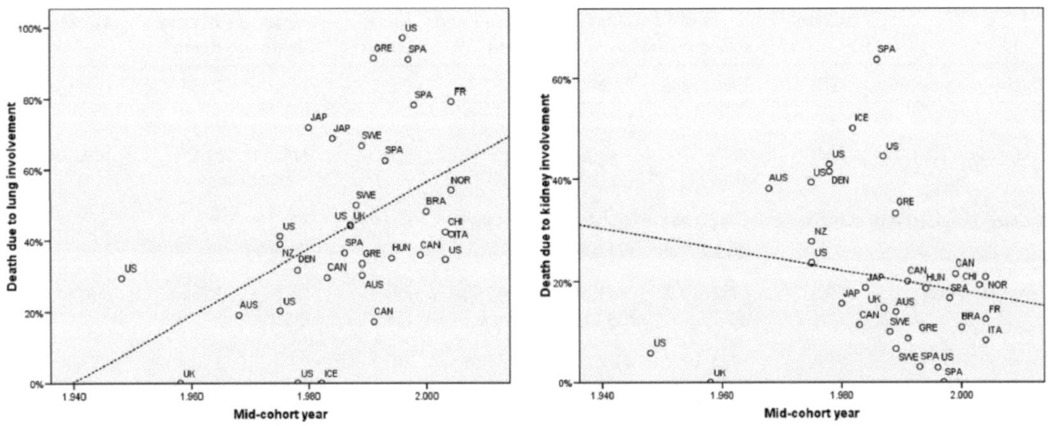

Figure 4. Meta-regression of deaths due to lung over time (coefficient b = 0.935 and p = 0.005) and renal (coefficient b=−0.206 and p = 0.352). Reprinted from Rubio-Rivas et al., with permission from Elsevier [43].

4.1.3. Heart involvement

Despite the fact that definite SSc for cardiac involvement does not exist, we could categorize its involvement in five major groups: pericarditis with or without cardiac tamponade, ischemic cardiopathy (documented myocardial infarction, angina, ischemic alterations in myocardial perfusion SPECT or requirement of coronary revascularization, surgical or percutaneous), pacemaker bearing regardless of the time of arrhythmia, sudden death and congestive heart failure [66]. As it is more recognized nowadays, its ratio is increasing, but the real challenge in the years to come shall be to distinguish the real scleroderma involvement from a cardiac SSc-non-related involvement. Anyway, we can hypothesize today that this is related to SSc in younger patients without classical cardiovascular risk factors.

4.1.4. Gastrointestinal involvement

The gastrointestinal tract is the most affected organ after the skin and can be affected from the oral cavity to the anus. About 90% of all patients will be affected during follow-up. This involvement can result in a decreased quality of life more often than a direct cause of death. In fact, it has been a rare cause of death over time. The few fatal cases have been related to those with severe intestinal involvement leading to malabsorption and secondary starvation. We cannot forget the possible role of the oesophageal involvement in the development of interstitial lung disease [67].

4.2. SSc-non-related causes of death

Among SSc-non-related causes of death, we can find three major diseases: cancer, infections and cardiovascular diseases (**Table 6**) [2, 3, 7, 8, 11–13, 15, 17–19, 21–24, 26, 29, 31, 33–42, 48, 50–53, 56, 57, 59–62].

http://dx.doi.org/10.5772/intechopen.68549

	Country	Years (mid-cohort)	Deads/n	Cancer death	Infection death	Atherosclerosis death
Farmer [2]	US	1945–1952 (48)	115/271 (49%)	6 (5.2%)	4 (3.5%)	20 (17.4%)
Bennet [3]	UK	1947–1970 (58)	26/67 (38.8%)	2 (18.2%)	3 (27.3%)	5 (45.5%)
Rowell [7]	UK	1960–1975 (67)	22/84 (26.2%)	0 (0%)	NA	1 (4.5%)
Barnett [8]	AUS	1953–1983 (68)	86/177 (48.6%)	NA	NA	NA
Altman [11]	US	1973–1977 (75)	131/264 (49.6%)	9 (6.9%)	3 (2.3%)	17 (13%)
Eason [12]	NZ	1970–1980 (75)	24/47 (51%)	2 (8.3%)	2 (8.3%)	2 (8.3%)
Wynn [13]	US	1970–1980 (75)	25/64 (39.1%)	3 (12%)	0 (0%)	3 (12%)
Ferri [15]	ITA	1955–1999 (77)	279/1012 (27.6%)	25 (14.7%)	NA	
Lally [16]	US	1972–1984 (78)	17/91 (18.7%)	1 (5.9%)	2 (11.8%)	0 (0%)
Jacobsen [17]	DEN	1960–1996 (78)	160/344 (46.5%)	30 (18.8%)	19 (11.9 %)	43/160
Kuwana [18]	JAP	1971–1990 (80)	51/275 (18.5%)	5 (9.8%)	1 (2%)	5 (9.8%)
Geirsson [19]	ICE	1975–1990 (82)	5/23 (21.7%)	1 (20%)	0 (0%)	2 (40%)
Abu-Shakra [48]	CAN	1976–1990 (83)	61/237 (25.7%)	6 (9.8%)	0 (0%)	NA
Nishioka [21]	JAP	1974–1994 (84)	90/496 (18.1%)	21 (23.3%)	5 (5.6%)	NA
Steen [56]	US	1972–1996 (84)	364/1508 (24.1%)	63 (17.3%)	32 (8.8%)	30 (8.2%)
Simeón [22]	SPA	1976–1996 (86)	12/79 (15.2%)	1 (8.3%)	0 (0%)	0 (0%)
Bulpitt [23]	US	1982–1992 (87)	15/48 (31.3%)	1 (6.7%)	1 (6.7%)	0 (0%)
Bryan [24]	UK	1982–1992 (87)	55/283 (19.4%)	1 (1.8%)	4 (7.3%)	11 (20%)
Geirsson [57]	SWE	1982–1995 (88)	30/100 (30%)	9 (30%)	6 (20%)	3 (10%)
Hesselstrand [26]	SWE	1983–1995 (89)	49/249 (19.7%)	12 (24.5%)	9 (18.4%)	9 (18.4%)
Bond [58]	AUS	1983–1996 (89)	123/123 (100%)	10 (8.1%)	6 (4.9%)	17 (13.8%)
Vlachoyiannopoulos [59]	GRE	1982–1996 (89)	7/254 (2.8%)	0 (0%)	0 (0%)	0 (0%)
Hashimoto [29]	JAP	1973–2008 (90)	86/405 (21.2%)	19 (22.1%)	14 (16.3%)	NA
Scussel-Lonzetti [50]	CAN	1984–1999 (91)	66/309 (21.4%)	13 (19.7%)	NA	10 (15.2%)
Alamanos [31]	GRE	1981–2002 (91)	36/109 (33%)	4 (11.1%)	1 (0.2%)	6 (16.7%)
Joven [33]	SPA	1980–2006 (93)	44/204 (21.6%)	3 (6.8%)	2 (4.5%)	5 (11.4%)
Ruangjutipopan [34]	THAI	1987–2001 (94)	31/222 (26.7%)	0 (0%)	13 (42%)	0 (0%)
Czirják [35]	HUN	1983–2005 (94)	93/366 (25.4%)	12 (12.9%)	2 (2.2%)	NA
Derk [60]	US	1985–2007 (96)	87/87 (100%)	3 (4.5%)	4.6%	0 (0%)
Arias-Núñez [36]	SPA	1988–2006 (97)	20/78 (25.6%)	1 (5%)	3 (15%)	2 (10%)
Alba [37]	SPA	1986–2010 (98)	151/1037 (14.6%)	61 (78.2%)	18 (14.8%)	NA
Al-Dhaher [38]	CAN	1994–2004 (99)	42/185 (23%)	NA	NA	NA
Sampaio-Barros [39]	BRA	1991–2010 (00)	168/947 (17.7%)	8 (4.8%)	24 (14.3%)	8 (4.8%)

	Country	Years (mid-cohort)	Deads/n	Cancer death	Infection death	Atherosclerosis death
Assassi [61]	US	1998–2008 (03)	52/250 (20.8%)	NA	NA	NA
Mok [52]	CHI	1999–2008 (03)	110/449 (24.5%)	11 (10%)	19 (17.3%)	NA
Hoffmann-Vold [40]	NOR	1999–2009 (04)	43/312 (13.8%)	13 (54.2%)	6 (14%)	4 (9.3%)
Vettori [41]	ITA	2000–2008 (04)	20/251 (8%)	2 (10%)	1 (5%)	2 (10%)
Hachulla [63]	FR	2002–2006 (04)	47/546 (8.6%)	8 (17%)	4 (8.5%)	2 (4.3%)
Strickland [53]	UK	1999–2010 (04)	53/204 (26%)	10 (18.9%)	13(24.5%)	12 (22.6%)
Kuo [42]	TAIW	2002–2007 (05)	204/1479 (13.8%)	30 (14.7%)	12 (5.9%)	29 (14.2%)

Reprinted from Rubio-Rivas et al. [43], with permission from Elsevier.

Table 6. SSc-non-related causes of death in medical literature [43].

4.2.1. Cancer

A higher standardized incidence ratio (SIR) of cancer in these patients not only compared to the general population that could be related to immunosuppressive treatment but also to the self-nature of the disease has been described [68]. In fact, those cancers diagnosed within the first 3 years after the diagnosis of scleroderma have been suggested to be classified as SSc-related causes. Cancer among SSc patients with RNA polymerase III antibodies has been reported to be in a close temporal relationship to the onset of SSc (first 36 months after the onset of SSc), which supports the paraneoplastic phenomenon in this subset of patients [69]. Thus, it is recommended to rule out this possibility at the time of the diagnosis, although protocol for this purpose has not been standardized so far. Cancers most frequently found in SSc patients are those from breast, blood, lung, gastrointestinal tract, genitourinary tract and skin and, out of these, those most related to the presence of RNAp III antibodies were breast cancer, skin cancer and genitourinary cancer [69].

4.2.2. Infections

Risk factors associated with infections in patients diagnosed with scleroderma include oesophageal (increased risk for aspiration pneumonia) and interstitial lung disease (increased risk for pneumonia), severe Raynaud's phenomenon or calcinosis (risk for localized super-infections) and the use of specific treatments for the management of the disease. Bacterial infections due to Gram-positive bacilli have been described, especially in patients with severe Raynaud or calcinosis. In patients receiving immunosuppressive treatment, especially corticosteroids, *Nocardia* sp. and *Mycobacteria* sp. must be taken into account. A few viruses such as *Epstein-Barr virus* and *CMV* have been described as triggering the onset of scleroderma, and *Parvovirus B19* DNA has been detected in patients who have scleroderma, but the clinical correlate of this finding is unclear. Finally, among fungi, *Pneumocystis jirovecii* pneumonia has been reported in some patients who have scleroderma [70]. *Aspergillus* sp. has been rarely reported in scleroderma, but in any patient under cellular immunosuppression has to be taken into account as well [71].

4.2.3. Cardiovascular disease

Scleroderma, as other autoimmune diseases, shows up as an inflammatory background that leads to the fibroblast activation. This background is more visual in the first stages of the skin or lung involvement, but it is thought to happen elsewhere. Thus, scleroderma itself can be understood as a new cardiovascular risk factor not only involved in the development of microvascular disease but also of macrovascular disease [72]. Atherosclerosis has been found to be increased in patients with SSc in all territories: coronary arteries, carotid arteries, cerebrovascular vessels and peripheral arteries [72]. This is the most controversial group of diseases in terms of classification since it is a challenge to differentiate whether it is an SSc-related or a SSc-non-related event. Although sometimes undistinguishable, currently, the clinical context has been hypothesized to aid for this purpose. Thus, in young patients without other classical cardiovascular risk factors (smoking behaviour, diabetes mellitus, arterial hypertension, hyperlipidaemia, obesity), we state that a particular event should be classified as SSc-related.

According to the latest studies [43], the big picture when talking about causes of death should be that SSc-related death is estimated nowadays in 56.7% of all deaths. Among them, representing lung death 57%, heart death 28.2%, renal death 11.7% and gastrointestinal death 6.4% (**Table 7**). In contrast, SSc-non-related death is estimated in 43.3% of all patients and among them being cancer, infections and cardiovascular disease the leading cause of SSc-non-related death.

4.3. A temporary pattern of SSc-related causes of death

In general, we could state that early death within the first years after the diagnosis of scleroderma is primarily due to the autoimmune disease itself, and late death is due to SSc-non directly related causes. Besides, this progression is currently even more notorious since data from the Spanish Registry show the fact that beyond 10 years after diagnosis, 83% of all deaths are due to SSc-non-related causes, supporting the idea that by struggling with the disease in the first years could save quite a few deaths due to the self-disease [54, 55].

	Before 1990 (22 studies)	After 1990 (18 studies)	p
SSc-related deaths % mean (SD)	52.5 (24.7)	56.7 (17.4)	0.544
Lung	34.5 (21.3)	57.0 (24.7)	0.008
Heart	29.3 (23.8)	28.2 (28.1)	0.905
Kidney	26.4 (17.6)	11.7 (7.9)	0.003
GI	6.8 (8.7)	6.4 (7.0)	0.881

T-test for independent groups among studies before and after 1990 (mid-cohort year). GI: gastrointestinal. Reprinted from Rubio-Rivas et al. [43], with permission from Elsevier.

Table 7. SSc-related causes of death [43].

Among these SSc-related causes, pulmonary death (due to ILD or PAH) has been and still currently is the leading SSc-related cause of death in all stages of the disease. In contrast, renal death was the second cause of the death in the past and most of all in the dcSSc subset and within the first 5 years after SSc diagnosis, but, in the last years, we have been witnesses of an important decrease of renal death rate. Heart death is at first sight more present nowadays and within the early stages of the disease but possibly due to a better understanding and knowledge of this involvement. Gastrointestinal death has been the cause of death only inisolated cases over time (**Table 8**).

Thus, it is expected to see an increasing rate of SSc-non-related causes in the years to come, mainly cancer and cardiovascular causes. Among the SSc-related causes, cardiovascular causes will be the cornerstone and the challenge will be to distinguish SSc-related and SSc-non-related cardiovascular events.

	Cause of death	1990–1999	2000–2009	p
Early	**SSc-non-related**	3 (17.6%)	23 (48.9%)	**0.042**
	Pulmonary	8 (47.1%)	16 (34.0%)	0.390
	Renal	6 (35.3%)	1 (2.1%)	**< 0.001**
	Cardiac	0 (0.0%)	7 (14.9%)	0.175
	Gastrointestinal	0 (0.0%)	0 (0.0%)	–
Intermediate	**SSc-non-related**	5 (23.8%)	11 (50.0%)	0.116
	Pulmonary	13 (61.9%)	6 (27.3%)	**0.033**
	Renal	1 (4.8%)	1 (4.5%)	1.000
	Cardiac	2 (9.5%)	4 (18.2%)	0.664
	Gastrointestinal	0 (0.0%)	0 (0.0%)	–
Late	**SSc-non-related**	10 (37.0%)	5 (83.3%)	**0.070**
	Pulmonary	11 (40.7%)	1 (16.7%)	0.379
	Renal	1 (3.7%)	0 (0.0%)	1.000
	Cardiac	4 (14.8%)	0 (0.0%)	1.000
	Gastrointestinal	1 (3.7%)	0 (0.0%)	1.000

Early (first 5 years after diagnosis), intermediate (5–10 years after diagnosis) and late death (>10 years after diagnosis) from the Spanish Scleroderma Network. Reprinted from Rubio-Rivas [54].

Table 8. SSc-non-related and SSc-related (lung, heart, renal and gastrointestinal) causes of death. In bold, p-values reaching statistical significance or close to significance.

5. Risk factors of poor outcome

To date, several risk factors have been identified related to poor prognosis, sometimes reported as a result of univariate analysis and sometimes as a result of multivariate analysis [43].

Taking into account the number of citations from the different studies (**Figure 5**), more cited risk factors would be an older age at diagnosis, dcSSc subset, male gender and visceral involvement (most of all lung, heart and renal involvement).

It is not easy to quantify the overall risk attributed to any of these factors since they have been described in different ways, but by meta-analysing those described homogeneously (**Figure 6**), we could state a hazard ratio for kidney involvement 4.22 (3.42–5.19), for heart involvement 3.43 (1.35–8.70), for ILD 2.89 (2.24–3.72), for high eritrosedimentation rate 2.77 (2.06–3.71), for PAH 2.62 (1.64–4.17), for dcSSc 2.28 (1.69–3.08), for male gender 1.88 (1.48–2.38) and age/year 1.05 (1.04–1.06) [43].

New risk factors are required in order to identify those patients with worse prognosis who could get some benefits in terms of a more aggressive therapy and/or closer follow-up. Recently, the mode of onset has been evaluated as a potential risk factor, finding a worse prognosis in those patients with an onset in the form of non-Raynaud's phenomenon, with the only exception of arthralgia (data not yet released).

Anyway, the risk should be individualized and accordingly lead to the decision-making for every patient. Thus, it should be our aim to create prognosis scales based on these known risk factors.

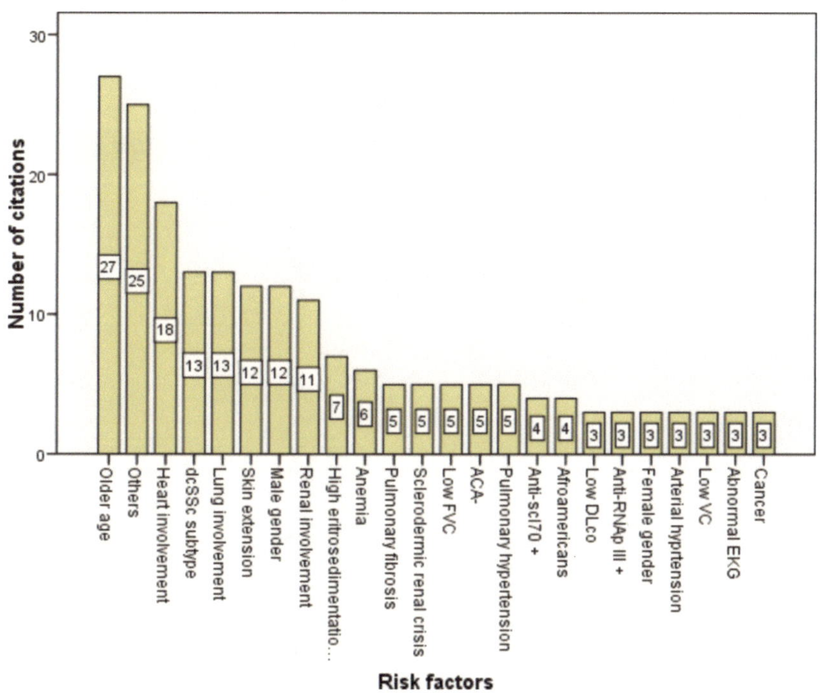

Figure 5. Risk factors for poor outcomes (number of citations in the different studies). Into "others" are included proteinuria, gastrointestinal and osteoarticular involvement, high BUN, hypo/hyperpigmentation, digital ulcers, HLADQA1 and HLA DRB1, low body mass index, hands deformity, low STC and low total lung compliance, myositis, anti-RNP +, S3 heart gallop, corticosteroid treatment, longer time from first Raynaud, no CREST, tobacco and alcohol uptake and hypoproteinaemia. Reprinted from Rubio-Rivas et al., with permission from Elsevier [43].

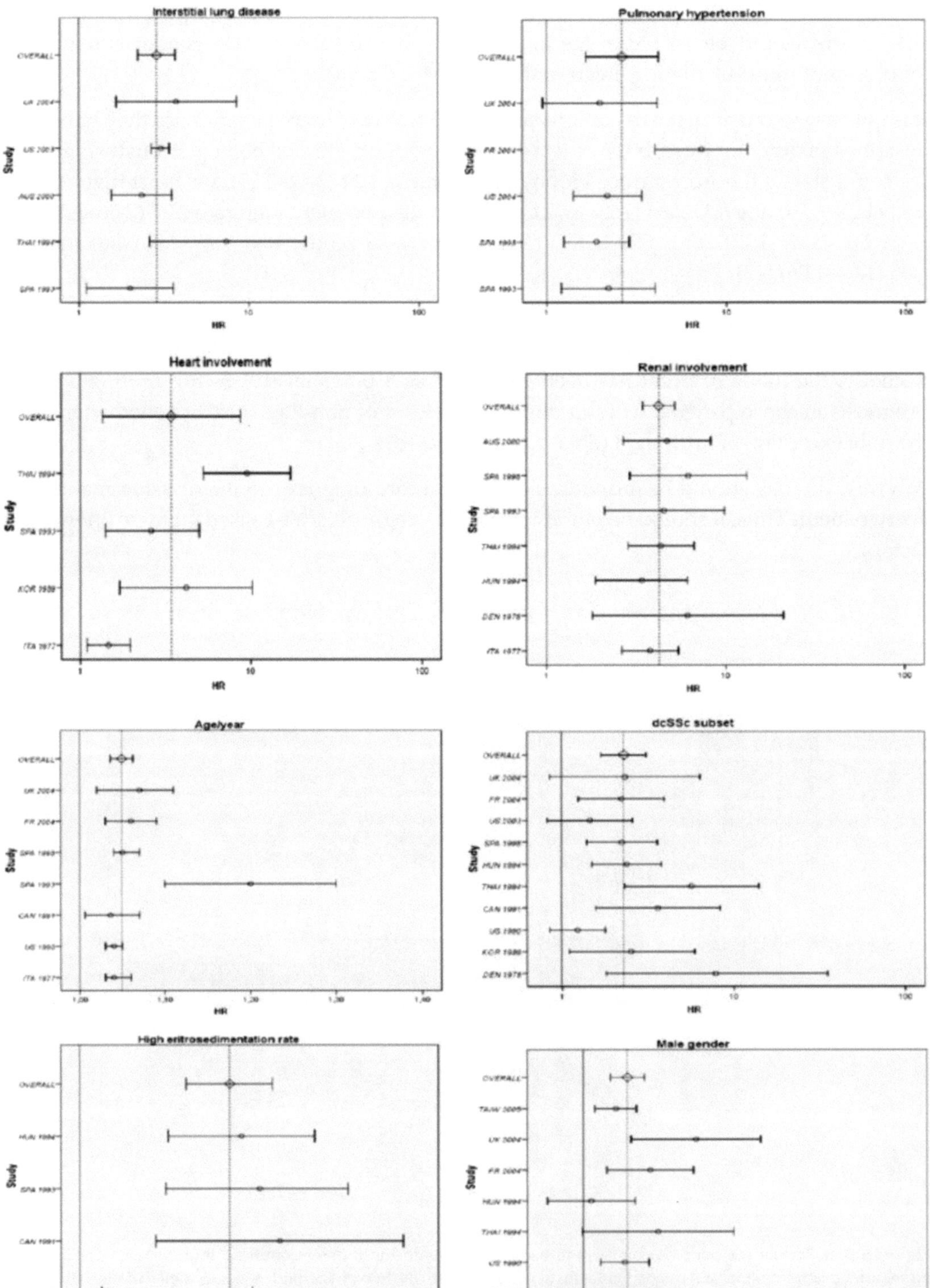

Figure 6. A quantitative meta-analysis of the main risk factors related to mortality. Reprinted from Rubio-Rivas et al., with permission from Elsevier [43].

Author details

Manuel Rubio-Rivas

Address all correspondence to: mrubio@bellvitgehospital.cat

Autoimmune Diseases Unit, Department of Internal Medicine, Bellvitge University Hospital-IDIBELL. L'Hospitalet de Llobregat, Barcelona, Spain

References

[1] Tuffanelli DL, Winkelmann RK. Systemic scleroderma. A clinical study of 727 cases. Archives of Dermatology. 1961;**84**(3):359-71

[2] Farmer RG, Gifford RW, Hines EA. Prognostic significance of Raynaud's phenomenon and other clinical characteristics of systemic scleroderma: A study of 271 cases. Circulation. 1960;**21**:1088-1095

[3] Bennet R, Bluestone R, Holt PJL. Survival in scleroderma. Annals of the Rheumatic Disease. 1971;**30**:581-588

[4] Medsger TA, Masi AT. The epidemiology of systemic sclerosis (scleroderma) among male U.S. veterans. International Journal of Chronic Obstructive Pulmonary Disease. 1978;**31**:73-85

[5] Zarafonetis C, Dabich L, Negri D, Skovronski JJ, DeVol EB, Wolfe R. Retrospective studies in scleroderma: effect of potassium para-aminobenzoate on survival. Journal of Clinical Epidemiology. 1988;**41**(2):193-205

[6] Medsger TA, Masi AT. Survival with scleroderma. A life-table analysis of clinical and demographic factors in 358 male U.S. veteran patients. International Journal of Chronic Obstructive Pulmonary Disease. 1973;**26**:647-660

[7] Rowell NR. The prognosis of systemic sclerosis. British Journal of Dermatology. 1976;**95**:57-60

[8] Barnett AJ, Miller MH, Littlejohn GO. A survival study of patients with scleroderma diagnosed over 30 years (1953-1983): The value of a simple cutaneous classification in the early stages of the disease. The Journal of Rheumatology. 1988;**15**:276-283

[9] Gouet D, Azais I, Marechaud R, Alcalay M, Barriere H, Bontoux D. Pronostic de la sclérodermie generalise. Étude retrospective de 78 observations. Rev Med Interne. 1986;**7**:233-41

[10] Giordano M, Valentini G, Migliaresi S, Picillo U, Vatti M. Different antibody patterns and different prognoses in patients with scleroderma with various extent of skin sclerosis. The Journal of Rheumatology. 1986;**13**:911-916

[11] Altman RD, Medsger TA, Bloch DA, Michel BA. Predictors of survival in systemic sclerosis (scleroderma). Arthritis & Rheumatology. 1991;**34**(4):403-413

[12] Eason RJ, Tan PL, Gow PJ. Progressive systemic sclerosis in Auckland: A ten year review with emphasis on prognostic features. Australian and New Zealand Journal of Medicine. 1981;**11**(6):657-662

[13] Wynn J, Fineberg N, Matzer L, Cortada X, Armstrong W, Dillon JC. et al. Prediction of survival in progressive systemic sclerosis by multivariate analysis of clinical features. American Heart Journal. 1985;**110**:123-127

[14] Peters-Golden M, Wise RA, Hochberg MC, Stevens MB, Wigley FM. Carbon monoxide diffusing capacity as predictor of outcome in systemic sclerosis. American Journal of Medicine. 1984;**77**:1027-1033

[15] Ferri C, Valentini G, Cozzi F, Sebastiani M, Michelassi C, La Montagna G. Systemic sclerosis. Demographic, clinical and serologic features and survival in 1012 Italian patients. Medicine. 2002;**81**:139-53

[16] Lally EV, Jiménez SA, Kaplan SR. Progressive systemic sclerosis: mode of presentation, rapidly progressive disease course, and mortality based on an analysis of 91 patients. Seminars in Arthritis and Rheumatism. 1988;**18**(1):1-13

[17] Jacobsen S, Halberg P, Ullman S. Mortality and causes of death of 344 Danish patients with systemic sclerosis (scleroderma). British Journal of Rheumatology. 1998;**37**:750-755

[18] Kuwana M, Kaburaki J, Okano Y, Tojo T, Homma M. Clinical and prognostic associations based on serum antinuclear antibodies in Japanese patients with systemic sclerosis. Arthritis & Rheumatology. 1994;**37**(1):75-83

[19] Geirsson AJ, Steinsson K, Gudmundsson S, Sigurdsson V. Systemic sclerosis in Iceland. A nationwide epidemiological study. Annals of Rheumatic Disease. 1994;**53**:502-505

[20] Kaburaki J, Lee CC, Kuwana M, Tojo T, Ikeda Y, Takano M et al. Initial predictors of survival in Systemic Sclerosis. The Keio Journal of Medicine. 1992;**41**(3):141-145

[21] Nishioka K, Katayama I, Kondo H, Shinkai H, Ueki H, Tamaki K et al. Epidemiological analysis of prognosis of 496 Japanese patients with progressive systemic sclerosis. The Journal of Dermatology. 1996;**23**:677-682

[22] Simeón CP, Armadans L, Fonollosa V, Vilardell M, Candell J, Tolosa C. et al. Survival prognostic factors and markers of morbidity in Spanish patients with systemic sclerosis. Annals of Rheumatic Disease. 1997;**56**:723-728

[23] Bulpitt KJ, Clements PJ, Lachenbruch PA, Paulus HE, Peter JB, Agopian MS et al. Early undifferentiated connective tissue disease:III. Outcome and prognostic indicators in early scleroderma (systemic sclerosis). Annals of Internal Medicine. 1993;**118**:602-609

[24] Bryan C, Howard Y, Brennan P, Black C, Silman A. Survival following the onset of scleroderma: results from a retrospective inception cohort study of the UK patient population. British Journal of Rheumatology. 1996;**35**:1122-1126

[25] Nagy Z, Czirják L. Predictors of survival in 171 patients with systemic sclerosis (Sclero derma). Clinical Rheumatology. 1997;**16**(5):454-460

[26] Hesselstrand R, Scheja A, Akesson A. Mortality and causes of death in a Swedish series of systemic sclerosis patients. Annals of Rheumatic Diseases. 1998;**57**:682-686

[27] Kim J, Park SK, Moon KW, Lee EY, Lee YJ, Song YW et al. The prognostic factors of systemic sclerosis for survival among Koreans. Clinical Rheumatology. 2010;**29**:297-302

[28] Mayes MD, Lacey JV, Beebe-Dimmer J, Gillespie BW, Cooper B, Laing TJ et al. Prevalence, incidence, survival, and disease characteristics of systemic sclerosis in a large US population. Arthritis & Rheumatology. 2003;**48**(8):2246-2255

[29] Hashimoto A, Tejima S, Tono T, Suzuki M, Tanaka S, Matsui T et al. Predictors of survival and causes of death in Japanese patients with systemic sclerosis. The Journal of Rheumatology. 2011;**38**:1-9

[30] Pérez-Bocanegra C, Solans-Laqué R, Simeón-Aznar CP, Campillo M, Fonollosa V, Vilardell M. Age-related survival and clinical features in systemic sclerosis patients older or younger than 65 at diagnosis. Rheumatology. 2010;**49**:1112-1117

[31] Alamanos Y, Tsifetaki N, Voulgari PV, Siozos C, Tsamandouraki K, Alexiou GA et al. Epidemiology of systemic sclerosis in Northwest Greece 1981 to 2002. Seminars in Arthritis and Rheumatism. 2005;**34**:714-720

[32] Nihtyanova SI, Tang EC, Coghlan JG, Wells AU, Black CM. Improved survival in systemic sclerosis is associated with better ascertaiment of internal organ disease: A retrospective cohort study. QJM. 2010;**103**(2):109-115

[33] Joven BE, Almodovar R, Carmona L, Carreira PE. Survival, causes of death and risk factors associated with mortality in Spanish systemic sclerosis patients: Results from a single University Hospital. Seminars in Arthritis and Rheumatism. 2010;**39**(4):285-293

[34] Ruangjutipopan S, Kasitanon N, Louthrenoo W, Sukitawut W, Wichainun R. Causes of death and poor survival prognostic factors in Thai patients with systemic sclerosis. Journal of the Medical Association of Thailand. 2002;**85**(11):1204-1209

[35] Czirják L, Kumánovics G, Varjú C, Nagy Z, Pákozdi A, Szekanecz Z et al. Survival and causes of death in 366 Hungarian patients with systemic sclerosis. Annals of Rheumatic Diseases. 2008;**67**:59-63

[36] Arias-Núñez MC, Llorca J, Vázquez-Rodríguez TR, Gómez-Acebo I, Miranda-Filloy JA, Martin J et al. Systemic sclerosis in northwestern Spain. Medicine. 2008;**5**:272-280

[37] Alba MA, Velasco C, Simeón CP, Fonollosa V, Trapiella L, Egurbide MV et al. Differences in clinical presentation and outcome between early versus late onset systemic sclerosis: analysis of 1037 patients. Medicine (Baltimore). 2014;**93**(2):73-81

[38] Al-Dhaher FF, Pope JE, Ouimet JM. Determinants of morbidity and mortality of systemic sclerosis in Canada. Seminars in Arthritis and Rheumatism. 2010;**39**(4):269-277

[39] Sampaio-Barros PD, Bortoluzzo AB, Marangoni RG, Rocha LF, Del Rio APT, Samara AM et al. Survival, causes of death and prognostic factors in systemic sclerosis: Analysis of 947 Brazilian patients. The Journal of Rheumatology. 2012;**39**(10):1971-1978

[40] Hoffmann-Vold A, Molberg O, Midtvedt O, Garen T, Gran JT. Survival and causes of death in an unselected and complete cohort of Norwegian patients with systemic sclerosis. The Journal of Rheumatology. 2013;**40**(7):1127-1133

[41] Vettori S, Cuomo G, Abignano G, Iudici M, Valentini G. Survival and death causes in 251 systemic sclerosis patients from a single Italian centre. Reumatismo. 2010;**62**(3):202-209

[42] Kuo CF, See LC, Yu KH, Chou IJ, Tseng WY, Chang HC et al. Epidemiology and mortality of systemic sclerosis: A nationwide population study in Taiwan. Scandinavian Journal of Rheumatology. 2011;**40**(5):373-378

[43] Rubio-Rivas M, Royo C, Simeón CP, Corbella X, Fonollosa V. Mortality and survival in systemic sclerosis: Systematic review and meta-analysis. Seminars in Arthritis and Rheumatism. 2014;**44**:208-219

[44] Ioannidis J, Vlachoyiannopoulos P, Haidich AB, Medsger TA, Lucas M, Michet CJ et al. Mortality in systemic sclerosis: An international meta-analysis of individual patient data. American Journal of Medicine. 2005;**118**:2-10

[45] Elhai M, Meune C, Avouac J, Kahan A, Allanore Y. Trends in mortality in patients with systemic sclerosis over 40 years: A systematic review and meta-analysis of cohort studies. Rheumatology. 2012;**51**:1017-1026

[46] Toledano E, Candelas G, Rosales Z, Martínez Prada C, León L, Abásolo L et al. A meta-analysis of mortality in rheumatic diseases. Reumatologia Clinica. 2012;**8**(6):334-341

[47] Komócsi A, Vorobcsuk A, Faludi R, Pintér T, Lenkey Z, Költo G, et al. The impact of cardiopulmonary manifestations on the mortality of SSc: A systematic review and meta-analysis of observational studies. Rheumatology. 2012;**51**:1027-1036

[48] Abu-Shakra M, Lee P. Mortality in systemic sclerosis. A comparison with the general population. Journal of Rheumatology. 1995;**22**(11):2100-2102

[49] Walsh SJ, Fenster JR. Geographical clustering of mortality from systemic sclerosis in the southeastern United States 1981-1990. The Journal of Rheumatology. 1997;**24**(12):2348-2352

[50] Scussel-Lonzetti L, Joyal F, Raynauld JP, Roussin A, Rich E, Goulet JR, et al. Predicting mortality in systemic sclerosis. Analysis of a cohort of 309 french Canadian patients with emphasis on features at diagnosis as predictive factors for survival. Medicine. 2002;**81**:154-167

[51] Hissaria P, Lester S, Hakendorf P, Woodman R, Patterson K, Hill C, et al. Survival in scleroderma: Results from the population-based South Australian Register. Internal Medicine Journal. 2011;**41**:381-390

[52] Mok CC, Kwok CL, Ho LY, Chan PT, Yip SF. Life expectancy, standardized mortality ratios, and causes of death in six rheumatic diseases in Hong Kong, China. Arthritis & Rheumatology. 2011;**63**:1182-1189

[53] Strickland G, Pauling J, Cavill C, Shaddick G, McHugh N. Mortality in systemic sclerosis-a single centre study from the UK. Clinical Rheumatology. 2013;**32**:1533-1539

[54] Rubio-Rivas M. Changes in the pattern of death from the Spanish Scleroderma Network [doctoral thesis]. Barcelona Autonomous University UAB; 2014

[55] Rubio-Rivas M et al. Changes in the pattern of death of 987 patients with Systemic Sclerosis from 1990 to 2009 (from the nationwide Spanish Scleroderma Registry). Clin Exp Rheumatol. 2017 Feb 6. [Epub ahead of print]

[56] Steen VD, Medsger TA. Changes in causes of death in systemic sclerosis, 1972-2002. Annals of the Rheumatic Diseases. 2007;**66**:940-944

[57] Geirsson AJ, Wollheim FA, Akesson A. Disease severity of 100 patients with systemic sclerosis over a period of 14 years: Using a modified Medsger scale. Annals of the Rheumatic Diseases. 2001;**60**:1117-1122

[58] Bond C, Pile KD, McNeil JD, Ahern MJ, Smith MD, Cleland LG et al. South Australian scleroderma register: Analysis of deceased patients. Pathology. 1998;**30**(4):386-390

[59] Vlachoyiannopoulos PG, Dafni UG, Pakas I, Spyropoulou-Vlachou M, Stavropoulos-Giokas C, Moutsopoulos HM. Systemic scleroderma in Greece: Low mortality and strong linkage with HLA-DRB1*1104 allele. Annals of the Rheumatic Diseases. 2000;**59**: 359-367

[60] Derk CT, Huaman G, Littlejohn J, Otieno F, Jiménez S. Predictors of early mortality in Systemic Sclerosis: A case-control study comparing early versus late mortality in Systemic Sclerosis. Rheumatology International. 2012;**32**:3841-3844

[61] Assassi S, Junco D, Sutter K, McNearney T, Reveille JD, Karnavas A et al. Clinical and genetic factors predictive of mortality in early systemic sclerosis. Arthritis Rheumatology. 2009;**61**(10):1403-1411

[62] Hachulla E, Carpentier P, Gressin V, Diot E, Allanore Y, Sibilia J, et al. Risk factors for death and the 3-year survival of patients with systemic sclerosis: The French ItinérAIR-Sclérodermie study. Rheumatology. 2009;**48**:304-308

[63] Sobanski V, Launay D, Hachulla E, Humbert M. Current approaches to the treatment of systemic-sclerosis-associated pulmonary arterial hypertension (SSc-PAH). Current Rheumatology Reports. 2016;**18**:10

[64] Giacomelli R, Liakouli V, Berardicurti O, Ruscitti P, Di Benedetto P, Carubbi F, Guggino G, Di Bartolomeo S, Ciccia F, Triolo G, Cipriani P. Interstitial lung disease in systemic sclerosis: current and future treatment. Rheumatology International. 2017. DOI: 10.1007/s00296-016-3636-7. Epub ahead of print

[65] Woodworth TG, Suliman YA, Furst DE, Clements P. Scleroderma renal crisis and renal involvement in systemic sclerosis. Nature Reviews Nephrology. 2016;**12**:678-691

[66] Fernández-Codina A, Simeón-Aznar CP, Pinal-Fernandez I, Rodríguez-Palomares J, Pizzi MN, Hidalgo CE, Del Castillo AG, Prado-Galbarro FJ, Sarria-Santamera A, Fonollosa-Plà V, Vilardell-Tarrés M. Cardiac involvement in systemic sclerosis: Differences between clinical subsets and influence on survival. Rheumatology International. 2017;**37**:75-84

[67] Savarino E, Furnari M, De Bortoli N, Martinucci I, Bodini G, Ghio M, Savarino V. Gastrointestinal involvement in systemic sclerosis. La Presse Medicale. 2014;**43**(10 Pt 2): e279-291

[68] Onishi A, Sugiyama D, Kumagai S. Cancer incidence in systemic sclerosis: meta-analysis of population-based cohort studies. Arthritis & Rheumatology. 2013;**65**(7):1913-1921

[69] Moinzadeh P, Fonseca C, Hellmich M, Shah AA, Chighizola C, Denton CP, Ong VH. Association of anti-RNA polymerase III autoantibodies and cancer in scleroderma. Arthritis Research and Therapy. 2014;**16**:R53

[70] Juárez M, Misischia R, Alarcón GS. Infections in systemic connective tissue diseases: Systemic lupus erythematosus, scleroderma, and polymyositis/dermatomyositis. Rheumatic Disease Clinics of North America. 2003;**29**:163-184

[71] Nandi S, Santra A, Ghoshal L, Kundu S. Interstitial lung disease in systemic scleroderma, complicated with bilateral pulmonary aspergilloma: An unusual association. Journal of Clinical and Diagnostic Research. 2015;**9**:OD11-3. DOI: 10.7860/JCDR/2015/15340.6926

[72] Au K, Singh MK, Bodukam V, Bae S, Maranian P, Ogawa R, Spiegel B, McMahon M, Hahn B, Khanna D. Atherosclerosis in systemic sclerosis: A systematic review and meta-analysis. Arthritis & Rheumatology. 2011;**63**:2078-2090

Chapter 4

Nonpharmacological Treatment in Systemic Sclerosis

Maja Špiritović and Michal Tomčík

Additional information is available at the end of the chapter

http://dx.doi.org/10.5772/intechopen.68537

Abstract

Systemic sclerosis (SSc) is a rare, severe connective tissue disease without available universal treatment. Organ involvement increases the mortality of this disease; nevertheless, skin involvement and the involvement of muscles and joints lead to loss of function, disability, and reduced quality of life.

Our experience and data from the literature suggest that physical activity interventions are an essential and integral part of treatment of patients with SSc. The limitation on most of the small number of existing studies aimed at nonpharmacological treatment for patients with SSc includes suboptimal methodological quality, low number of patients, lack of a control group or monitoring (follow-up), and short-term intervention.

The purpose of this chapter was to introduce the few studies that have examined this issue and to show that nonpharmacological therapy for diseases such as systemic sclerosis has been the focus of some research teams in recent years—the studies of which have demonstrated safety and benefits of these approaches.

Keywords: systemic sclerosis, function, disability, rehabilitation, physiotherapy, nonpharmacological interventions

1. Introduction

In the last few years, increased attention has been focused on nonpharmacological interventions in rare rheumatic diseases such as systemic sclerosis (SSc). However, there is still an unmet need to ensure medical awareness of the importance of physical therapy among patients, health professionals, rheumatologists, and other specialists to implement these nonpharmacological interventions into the daily care of patients with SSc.

Currently, physical therapy is considered a process by which patients try to restore and maintain their optimal physical, mental, social, occupational, and emotional state. It is therefore a comprehensive approach to the patient, which includes physical activity, as well as the principles of secondary prevention and healthy lifestyles, which are based on the patient's collaboration, activity, and compliance. It is beyond doubt that physical inactivity is a major risk factor for both cardiovascular and respiratory systems, but also for functional limitations and reduced quality of life.

To acknowledge the importance of prevention and adherence to healthy lifestyle even before the onset of the disease, we can draw inspiration from the results of a recently published study on another, less rare, rheumatic disease, rheumatoid arthritis (RA): about the influence of environmental factors (e.g., the intensity and frequency of physical activity, of smoking, and different exposures) showing that patients with regular physical activity before the onset of RA suffer from a milder form of the disease and that obesity reduces the chance of achieving a good response to standard pharmacological approaches in RA [1, 2].

2. Nonpharmacological interventions in patients with systemic sclerosis

Tissue fibrosis is the dominant feature of SSc and affects both the skin and internal organs—especially the lungs, heart, and gastrointestinal tract [3]. While visceral involvement is responsible for increased mortality, musculoskeletal involvement (e.g., arthralgia/arthritis, flection contractures, and muscle weakness) and skin involvement (skin thickening and tethering) pose a significant burden for the patient in terms of reduction of functionality, quality of life, and ability to work or perform activities of daily living [4].

Current recommendations for the treatment of SSc include symptomatic therapy of individual organ manifestations and complications of SSc. However, to date, we have no effective treatment of tissue fibrosis, for example, skin, lung, heart, and gastrointestinal tract. Nonpharmacological management of patients with SSc with the main focus on the musculoskeletal system and the affected skin may be useful to reduce disability and improve quality of life and contribute to reducing the burden of disease on the organism. Nevertheless, the major limitations of most of the small number of existing publications focused on physical interventions in patients with SSc include the diversity of interventions, small cohorts of patients, the absence of a control group, randomization and/or a follow-up, and a short duration of intervention [3].

The most frequently investigated nonpharmacological interventions include commonly used methods such as paraffin, manual lymphatic drainage, soft tissue techniques, stretching exercises for hands and face, massage, exercises to maintain range of motion in joints, mobilization, aerobic exercise, and strength training. Other studies focus on occupational therapy, physical therapy, sleep disturbances, sexual function, and depression.

The following paragraphs will provide an overview of the results of the available publications, which are divided according to the nature of the intervention.

2.1. Interventions using paraffin

One of the methods frequently used in physiotherapy of rheumatic diseases is paraffin treatment. Paraffin solidifies at a temperature of 52–62°C and yet gives latent heat. In order to utilize this heat, paraffin must be applied to the body in a fluid state and allowed to solidify in the course of application. There are a few studies of paraffin in SSc patients: two randomized controlled studies (RCTs), one nonrandomized controlled trial and a series of three individual case studies.

The RCT by Sandqvist et al. evaluated the difference in intervention outcomes in 17 patients with SSc who underwent therapy with paraffin in combination with exercise on one hand chosen by random, and on the other hand received only exercise. Interventions continued daily for 1 month. Hand function was assessed at the beginning of the intervention and after the first month according to hand mobility and strength, the perception of pain, stiffness and elasticity of the skin. The authors demonstrated a significant improvement in flexion and extension of the fingers, thumb abduction, plantar flexion, perceived stiffness, and elasticity of the skin in patients who underwent paraffin intervention in combination with exercise compared to baseline levels. Furthermore, significant improvement in hand function (specifically in extension deficit, perception of stiffness, and elasticity of skin) was significantly greater in the hand that was treated with paraffin in combination with exercise than in the hand treated with exercise only [5].

In another RCT study [6], 16 patients with SSc underwent 12 times paraffin wrap therapy and then were randomly assigned to the intervention and control groups. The intervention group continued with paraffin therapy for 3 months, and the control group did not. Skin thickness decreased in all patients after 12 sessions of paraffin treatment. However, at the end of 3 months therapy in the intervention group, there was no significant difference between the intervention and control group [6].

One of the first studies, a nonrandomized controlled trial by Askew et al., recruited 10 patients with SSc and examined the effectiveness of once performed interventions including paraffin, friction massage, and exercise maintaining range of motion in the joints of the wrist and hand. Compared with seven patients with SSc, who did not attend any sessions, the interventions lead to significant improvements in the articular range of motion, skin elasticity, and overall function of the hand [7].

In a series of three individual case studies [8], respondents conducted active exercises with their hands after paraffin wrap 5 times per week for 8 weeks. The authors detected clinically significant improvements in both body function/structure measurements of hand function and in their ability to participate in activities in all participants [8].

2.2. Orofacial exercises

Orofacial region has many functions. Primarily, it ensures food intake and contributes to breathing. Coordinated interplay of activity of facial muscles allows for expression of verbal, articulate speech. In the orofacial region, we find more than fifty facial muscles that enable people to communicate nonverbally, to express their feelings. No other part of the human body possesses such a social function as the orofacial region. Through this region we communicate, we speak to others, express our feelings, and create new relationships. In patients with SSc, tightening of the skin and muscle atrophy in orofacial region lead to loss of facial expressions and an appearance of a mask-like face. The affected orofacial region with skin thickening often contribute to inability of mechanical mouth opening, microstomia, which along with other symptoms, such as dry mouth, can lead to dental and mouth hygiene issues, and hampered alimentation.

In the RCT by Yuen Hon et al., the authors studied the effect of orofacial home exercise program to increase the orifice in adults with SSc. The study included 48 adult patients with SSc who were randomly divided into two groups and examined for oral aperture at baseline, 3-month, and 6-month intervals. The intervention group underwent a multifaceted oral health intervention including adaptive oral hygiene devices, instruction and demonstration on the use of the devices, brushing teeth for 2 min and flossing twice a day for 6 months. The control group received the usual dental care. Participants with orifices <40 mm in the intervention group underwent orofacial exercise program, which included manual mouth-stretching and oral augmentation exercises with a wooden stick, twice a day with a total of 6 minutes for 6 months. The results showed a significant increase in oral orifice in patients of the intervention group at 3 months, but not after 6 months evaluation. However, compliance with the program was low (48.9%), which could distort the results of this study [9].

An RCT by Maddali-Bongi et al. evaluated the effectiveness of an intervention program based on a combination of the Kabat's technique (proprioceptive neuromuscular facilitation, PNF), connective tissue massage, and kinesiotherapy specially developed for the face of SSc patients. Out of the 40 recruited SSc patients, 20 patients were randomly selected into the intervention group and underwent the intervention program for 9 weeks, 2 times a week for 1 h with a home exercise program. Twenty patients were randomly assigned into the control group, which underwent home exercise program only. Patients of both groups were evaluated at baseline, after 9 weeks and after 9 weeks of follow-up in terms of quality of life and health, stiffness of the facial area, opening of the mouth, and oral handicap. At the end of treatment, both groups showed improved orifice. However, in the follow-up period, improvement persisted only in the intervention group. The facial score in the intervention group improved both at the end of therapy and follow-up period, whereas in the control group, there were no changes. According to the results of quality of life and health status, no effect of therapy was detected in any group. A significant improvement was also found in oral handicap at the end of therapy in the intervention group, whereas in the control group, no changes were observed [10].

In an observational study by Poole et al., the authors investigated the improvement in oral hygiene in SSc patients who underwent a program involving structured oral hygiene and exercises for the face and hands. The authors recruited 17 patients with SSc who previously underwent basic dental checkup, including examination for decayed or missing teeth, calculus, sites that bleed upon probing, measures of oral aperture, and the patient hygiene performance index. The study also evaluated upper limb function involving strength, joint range and maneuverability. Participants underwent a structured exercise program including education on brushing and flossing techniques used, hand exercise of three series with five repetitions, once daily stretching, once daily facial exercise of five times stretching 3–5 seconds, individually adjusted dental equipment, and a 6-month supply of dental products. This program was performed one or two times a day for 6 months. At the end of the 6-month intervention, there were a significant improvement in oral hygiene and a significant decline in the number of teeth with calculus and a reduction in bleeding gums. There were no differences in any of the upper extremity measures or oral aperture [11].

Another observational study by Pizzo et al. examined the effects of nonsurgical exercise program in 10 patients with severe SSc-associated microstomia (maximal mouth opening ≤ 30 mm). Patients were instructed to perform an exercise program, which included mouth stretching exercises for at least 15 minutes, twice a day, and oral augmentation exercise with a stick of soft wood daily during 18 weeks. After 18 weeks, the effect of exercise was evaluated measuring the maximal mouth opening. The exercise program improved mouth opening of all subjects. At the end of the period of 18 weeks, all patients noted that eating, speaking, and oral hygiene were easier [12].

In 2009, Maddali-Bongi et al. performed two other RCTs that examined the effect of specialized intervention programs and pointed out their safety and improvements in the hands and mouth (facial). These studies will be discussed in the following sections of this chapter.

At this point, it is worth to mention a study that can be useful for dentists treating this area in such a rare disease as SSc. Alantar et al. reviewed the literature and collected expert opinion for the design of preventive and curative treatment of oral and dental disability in patients with SSc. The authors point out that prevention of oral and dental complications is a major issue in patients with SSc. Dental treatment should be tailored to limitations in mouth opening, disease severity, and on-going treatments [13].

2.3. Comprehensive physical therapy for physical and/or psychological functioning

Physiotherapy is a vital part of nonpharmacological approaches, which deals with the prevention and treatment of disorders of the musculoskeletal system. Based on a comprehensive approach, physiotherapy pays special attention to the life situations, in which the person is. The aim of comprehensive physiotherapy is to find the best way to mitigate or eliminate health problems and to maintain the current effect in a long term. There are several studies available in this area of research.

In 2009, Maddali-Bongi et al. performed two RCTs that examined the effect of a specialized intervention program in the area of hands and mouth (face). The first study aimed to evaluate the effectiveness of the intervention program based on a combination of connective tissue massage and joint manipulation according to Mc Mennell specially designed for the hands of SSc patients. Of the 40 recruited SSc patients, 20 patients were randomly assigned to intervention and underwent the exercise program for 9 weeks, twice a week for one hour, and a home exercise program. Twenty patients were randomly assigned to the control group which underwent only the home exercise program. Patients of both groups were evaluated at baseline, after 9 weeks and after 9 weeks of follow-up in terms of quality of life, hand involvement, hand functional disability, and the measurements of range of motion. The intervention group demonstrated a significant improvement in all measured parameters, whereas the home exercise program in the control group improved just closing the hand into a fist at the end of therapy [14].

The aim of the second study was to evaluate the efficacy of a specific and comprehensive rehabilitation program tailored for patients with SSc. Hand involvement was treated with a combination of connective tissue massage and Mc Mennell joint manipulation. Manual lymph drainage was applied if patients had edematous hands. Face involvement was treated with a combination of Kabat's method, connective tissue massage, and kinesiotherapy. Other techniques used in the study included hydrokinesiotherapy (for patients without ulcers), land-based rehabilitation (for patients with ulcers), and respiratory rehabilitation exercises. The authors recruited twenty patients with SSc, who were randomly divided into two groups and evaluated at baseline and after 9 weeks in terms of quality of life, health, hand function, range of motion, water volumetric test, orifice, Duruoz scale, and purpose-built-questionnaire for hand and face Involvement. The intervention group was evaluated also after 9 weeks of follow-up. The intervention group 10 patients underwent a specific rehabilitation program, one or two times per week for 9 weeks. The control group underwent only educational advice and medical information for patients with SSc. At the end of treatment, patients in the intervention group improved in all measured parameters. In follow-up, orofacial function and mobility as well as general health condition were partially lost, whereas only the mobility and function of the hand were preserved. No changes in the examined parameters were observed in the control group [15].

In a controlled clinical study by Antonioli et al., the authors evaluated the effect of a specialized individual rehabilitation program that consisted of warm-up and cool-down exercises, training of motor functions, diaphragmatic breathing, controlled coughing exercises, treadmill, freewalking, finger stretching, and occupational therapy for 2 weeks of daily 30-minute sessions (10 sessions in total). Physical therapy was also prescribed to 13 patients with joint-related problems. At-home exercise program was prescribed on days when the intervention program was terminated. Patients were reevaluated after 2 and 4 months. The control group consisted of 17 patients who did not receive any form of rehabilitation. The authors evaluated aerobic capacity, hand function, limitations in activities of daily living, quality of life, and skin-related problems. At the end of the 4-month period, the examiners observed an improvement in the perception of quality of life, better exercise tolerance, and better mobility of hand in a significant number of patients with SSc [16].

Since patients with SSc reported great need to receive support and education regarding their disease, Kwakkenbos et al. developed a short, group-based psychoeducational program, and evaluated it in an observational study using pre- and posttest design. Participants filled out a questionnaire assessing their physical and mental condition. Subsequently, patients were asked to evaluate the program content using a questionnaire. Completely filled questionnaires were available for data analysis from 41 patients. The authors detected a high satisfaction of patients with the program, smaller helplessness after the intervention, and a higher acceptance of patients' limitations. However, no differences were observed in depressed mood or in physical function. Thus, this psychoeducational program contributed to meeting the reported needs of patients and to improving the care of patients with SSc [17].

In an RCT by Schouffoer et al., the authors compared the effectiveness of a 12-week multidisciplinary nursing program with usual outpatient care for SSc patients. The multidisciplinary nursing program included individual treatment goals once a week for 12 weeks, general exercises, hand/mouth exercises, educational sessions under supervision of a local physical therapist, and a home-based exercise program at least 6 days a week for 12 weeks. Twenty-eight patients with SSc were randomly selected into the intervention group (twenty-five of them completed the treatment), and twenty-five patients were randomly assigned to the control group. The examiners evaluated the hand function, grip strength, maximal mouth opening, aerobic capacity, gait, quality of life, and health status at baseline, at the end of treatment (12 weeks), and at the end of follow up (after 24 weeks). Results showed that the 12-week daily multidisciplinary care program was more effective than regular outpatient care with regard to significant improvement in grip strength, mouth opening, gait, and quality of life after 12 weeks, whereas the results in other followed parameters showed no difference between the intervention and control group. At the end of the follow-up period, after 24 weeks, only improvement in grip strength was maintained [18].

Our own preliminary results (unpublished data) from an ongoing single-center controlled study further support the role of intensive physiotherapy in patients with SSc. Our project aimed to address some limitations of existing studies and to assess the efficacy of a long-term (24-week intervention, 24-week follow-up), intensive (1 h physiotherapy + 0.5 h occupational therapy twice weekly, and home-exercise for 0.5 h five times a week), tailored physiotherapy program on function and impairment of the hands and face, and quality of life and disability in patients with SSc. We recruited 27 SSc patients into the intervention group, which underwent the 24-week intervention, and 29 SSc patients into the control group, which received an education and textbook on home exercise at baseline only. The intervention program unit comprised several physiotherapy/occupational therapy techniques, such as warm-up with infrared lamp, manual lymphatic drainage, skin wrinkling, fascial techniques, postisometric muscle relaxation, joint mobilization, passive/active muscle stretching and exaggerated facial mimicry training, soft ball facilitation techniques, senosoric stimulation with terabeans and therapeutic plasticine. Our program not only prevented the natural course of progressive deterioration of function of hands/mouth (observed in the control group) but also led to a significant improvement in monitored parameters (e.g., delta finger to palm, hand/finger grip strength, HAMIS-Hand Mobility in Scleroderma, interincisor/lip distance), which was clinically meaningful in a substantial proportion of patients.

2.4. Stretching interventions

Stretching includes special exercises leading to increased mobility of the body that can address a variety of health-related issues. It is a method, which can gently prepare your muscles to increased physical stress, but also to very ordinary functioning of our body during daily life activities. Stretching increases performance, maintains the elasticity of muscles and tendons, prevents muscle imbalance, improves joint mobility, and helps to maintain correct posture, proper breathing, and efficient and economical movement. Furthermore, stretching reduces muscle tone and brings overall relaxation, provides prevention from muscle- and joint-related injuries, improves response and readiness, and increases resistance to fatigue. To sum up the benefits of stretching, this technique maintains overall good physical and mental condition. For patients, most of all, it is a method/technique that maintains the elasticity of tendons, muscles, and improves joint mobility. Therefore, not only in healthy individuals but also in patients with SSc, it is the only way to recover, or aim to restore physiologic length of shortened muscles.

Mugii et al., in their observational study, compared the effect of autostretching of individual fingers in patients with SSc. Forty-five patients with SSc were instructed how to autostretch their fingers. The individual fingers were held with the other hand in the stretched position for 10 s, and this was repeated 3–10 times a day. To evaluate the effect of autostretching intervention, passive range of motion of the fingers was evaluated using a goniometer during the first visit, after 1 month and 1 year of the autostretching program. Quality of life was also assessed at the first visit and after a year using the Health Assessment Questionnaire (HAQ). The authors demonstrated a significant improvement in the overall range of passive joint motion of each finger after 1 month of autostretching, which was further improved or maintained even after 1 year. Although the range of motion of the fingers was lower in patients with diffuse cutaneous (dc) SSc than in patients with limited cutaneous (lc) SSc during the first visit, the examiners detected a significant improvement regardless of the disease duration or severity of skin sclerosis. The study team noted that stretching your fingers can improve the function of fingers, because HAQ score assessing the hand function activities, such as eating and grasping, decreased significantly [19].

An RCT by Vannajak et al. recruited 28 patients with SSc who were divided into two groups of 14 patients. Both groups received the same daily home treatment with one difference: one group with gloves and the other group without gloves. The 2-week daily home intervention included a Thai massage, stretching exercises and heating. The authors assessed the function of the hand using Hand Mobility in Scleroderma (HAMIS). Both groups showed a significant improvement in the function of the hand. Wearing gloves, however, lead to greater thumb mobility [20].

2.5. Aerobic training and combined endurance/resistance training

The rehabilitation of patients with impaired cardiovascular system is based on endurance, aerobic training, that is, a prolonged dynamic loading at or below the anaerobic threshold. Regular aerobic exercise improves the efficiency of the cardiovascular system (lungs, heart, and circulatory system), and regular endurance and strength training induce characteristic changes that lead to improved physical condition. These changes represent the training effect and help to achieve greater physical load with lower heart-rate responses.

Pinto et al. in their observational study focused on the effects of 12 weeks of combined resistance and aerobic training program (concurrent training) in 11 SSc patients. Supervised concurrent training session consisted of treadmill warm-up (5 min) followed by resistance training (30 min), treadmill aerobic training (20 min), and stretching exercises (5 min). Resistance training included five exercises for the main muscle groups: bench press, leg press, latissimus pull down, leg extension, and seated row. The concurrent training program was performed in one hour sessions, twice per week for 12 weeks. The study showed that concurrent 12-week training program was safe and significantly improved muscle strength, function and aerobic capacity in SSc patients [21].

The aim of a pilot study by Alexanderson et al. was to determine the effect of 8-week intense aerobic and endurance training program in four patients (three women and one man) with SSc with 50–100% of forced vital capacity (FVC). The authors detected significantly improved muscular endurance in three participants and significantly or clinically significantly improved aerobic capacity in two participants [22].

Oliveira et al., in their prospective nonrandomized controlled trial, examined whether patients with SSc have reduced exercise capacity compared to healthy individuals, and whether aerobic exercise is safe for patients with SSc and improves their aerobic capacity. In this study, 7 patients with SSc (without interstitial lung disease) and 7 healthy controls underwent an 8-week aerobic exercise program of moderate intensity. Participants were evaluated by cardiopulmonary stress test before and after 8 weeks of training, and examined for blood lactate concentration and oxygen saturation at each visit and at rest, and quality of life. Patients with SSc and healthy controls underwent 40-min training twice weekly. The first five minutes of the exercise program were reserved for the warm-up, when the speed was gradually increased until a target heart rate. The last five minutes of exercise were represented by the cool-down with slowing down the speed to a standstill. In the first session of the program, the participants underwent 15 min of aerobic exercise at their respective target heart rate. In the second session, aerobic training was increased to 20 min, in the third session to 25 min, and in all subsequent sessions to 30 min. Both groups showed a significant improvement in peak VO2 but with no significant difference between the study groups. Furthermore, both groups improved in exercise intensity which was documented by significantly increased peak lactate concentration in blood. No significant changes in SSc skin score or quality of life were detected [23].

2.6. Interventions on lower extremities

In SSc commonly affected area of the body is the lower limbs, especially their muscular strength and function, the loss of which has an impact on quality of life of patients with SSc. Therefore, Lima et al. in their cross-sectional study assessed peripheral and respiratory muscle strength in patients with SSc and examined their correlation with the 6-minute walk test and quality of life. Secondary aim of this study was to characterize the nutritional status, lung function, functional ability and quality of life of SSc patients compared with healthy controls. The study included 20 patients with SSc and 20 healthy control subjects. Results showed that patients with SSc have significantly reduced respiratory muscle strength, decreased strength in m. quadriceps femoris, and increased fatigability compared to healthy controls [24].

2.7. Self-management programs

Poole et al., in 2013 and 2014, assessed their two self-management programs and their impact on self-management for patients with SSc. The first program (2013) consisted of a workbook and a DVD (sent by postmail) that provided information on medical aspects of the disease, dysphagia, fatigue management, advocacy, activities of daily living, oral hygiene, skin and wound care, psychosocial changes, exercises, and other features of the condition. Forty-nine participants evaluated the effect of the program providing feedback through series of questions, filling out the protocol on health condition, and through their participation in the evaluation interview. The results of the study showed a decrease in depression, fatigue and pain, and an improvement in the hand function, self-efficacy for controlling pain, and self-efficacy "other." However, the only statistically significant change was in self-sufficient pain control. Moreover, the study showed that the program was easy to use and should help individuals with SSc in self-sufficiency [25].

In another pilot study (2014), Poole et al. assessed the effectiveness of internet-based self-management program for patients with SSc. Participants logged on to a password-protected web site and completed the program, which consisted of 10 modules (e.g., coping and body image/appearance, fatigue and energy conservation, self-advocacy), an exercise video, learning activities, worksheets, and resources. Participants proceeded through the modules at their own pace over 10 weeks. Participants were encouraged to log on to the discussion board, participate in an interactive component of the web site, and respond to questions posted for each module. Participants completed pre- and postintervention questionnaires on perceived self-efficacy, health efficacy, ability to manage care, functional disability, depression, pain, and fatigue. They also completed an eight-question evaluation form regarding satisfaction with the web site, program content, discussion boards, and learning activities. Sixteen participants completed the study and postintervention measures. The authors demonstrated significant improvements in mean scores for ability to manage health care and efficacy, and significant decreases in fatigue and depression. Self-efficacy was improved as well, but not significantly [26].

2.8. Splinting interventions

Functional impairment of the hand in SSc patients is one of the major problems encountered in rehabilitation practice. Research in this area also includes splinting interventions of the hand and wrist, which aim to facilitate restoration of the lost function. In a 2-month study by Seeger et al., the authors investigated splinting effect on the secondary contractures in 19 patients with SSc. Specifically, whether dynamic splinting can improve flexion contractures in the proximal interphalangeal joints (PIP). Of the eight patients who completed the study, only one had significant improvement in range of motion as a result of PIP joint splinting, which shows that the study failed to demonstrate the use of splints as a suitable method to maintain PIP extension compared with the control hand [27].

2.9. Physical therapy

In addition to the abovementioned list of interventions, there are few studies that evaluate the effectiveness of some other nonpharmacological approaches in SSc including the use of physical therapy, which is the practical application of physical treatments procedures and methods on living organism.

Manual lymphatic drainage (MLD) stimulates the lymphatic system and reduces swelling. It is one of the main components of a combined physical therapy, which is used for the treatment of lymphedema [28]. It is a technique that applies a force to the interstitial fluid and proteins within the initial lymphatics, thereby shifting toward collaterals and/or normally functioning lymphatics [29]. This technique not only directly softens the tissues, but perhaps also removes excessive local fluid. Therefore, it is speculated that the MLD technique should modify the mechanical properties, such as strain, of the skin and subcutaneous tissue. Strain is defined as deformation of a solid due to stress and is considered to be one of the measures representing tissue hardness [30].

The effect of manual lymphatic drainage to reduce swelling, improve the functionality of the hand and the perceived quality of life (QoL) in patients with SSc in edematous stage of disease was assessed in an RCT by Bongi et al. The study recruited 35 patients with SSc who were in the edematous disease stage (swelling of the hands), 20 of which were randomly assigned to the intervention group, and underwent MLD 1h once a week for 5 weeks according to the Vodder procedures, and 15 of which served as a control group. The study demonstrated a reduction in the hand volume, improved hand function, and perceived swelling and pain. Reduction in the volume and improvement in hand function were also maintained at follow-up. Furthermore, the authors detected an improvement in overall disability and quality of life in patients who received therapy. In the control group, no improvement was observed. The authors concluded that the application of MLD is effective in the treatment of the hand in edematous SSc by reducing hand volume, edema, and pain, and improving hand function and perceived quality of life. A study on a larger cohort of patients and with a longer follow-up is needed to assess the effect of MLD on different disease subsets as well, and to verify whether the technique could be of help in preventing the transition from hand edema to fibrosis [31].

Beyond examining the effects of MLD, researchers also investigated the effects of other types of physical therapy in the rehabilitation of patients with SSc.

Sallam et al. evaluated the impact of 14-day transcutaneous electrical nerve stimulation (TENS) of gastrointestinal (GI) acupoints on GI symptoms and quality of life in 17 SSc patients. This treatment significantly increased sympathetic and vagal activity in comparison with the basal value, lead to normalization of sympathovagal balance, and increased physical function score, which is closely related to the change in the sympathovagal balance. This provides the potential to treat the upper GI tract symptoms; however, further studies are needed to support these results [32].

In a pilot study by Tinazzi et al., the authors investigated the effect of extracorporeal shock wave therapy on the skin of 30 patients with SSc. This study was based on a hypothesis that the treatment effect of extracorporeal shock wave may decrease damage to the endothelial cells and skin fibrosis in patients with SSc. The authors demonstrated rapid and sustained reduction in Rodnan skin scores and a reduction in visual analog scale. Furthermore, an improvement in skin structure and vascularization was recorded 90 days after treatment. The number of endothelial progenitor cells and circulating endothelial cells increased 60 and 90 days after treatment, whereas serological biomarkers showed no differences before and after treatment [33].

Results of a prospective RCT by Sporbeck et al. point out the beneficial impact of biofeedback and deep oscillation (three times a week for 4 weeks) on Raynaud's phenomenon in patients with SSc [34].

In an observational study by Uhlemann et al., the authors evaluated the effect of ultrasound applied to the hands with an intensity of 0.6 W/cm^2, for 6 minutes, 3 times a day for 6 days on the hand function and strength. Pain decreased in 18 of 24 patients. At the end of therapy, no increase in pain was observed, and the hand strength significantly improved in all patients [35].

Milačić et al. examined the change in volume of orifice before and after combined hyperbaric oxygen (HBO) therapy with facial physical therapy. Patients received HBO therapy ten times (2.0 ATA) and infrared phototherapy using Solux lamp 15 min before kinesiotherapy in front of mirrors daily for 10 days. This treatment targeted facial muscles. The results showed a statistically highly significant difference in improvement before and after treatment, and that use of HBO in the treatment of these patients has a significant role [36].

3. Conclusion

Chronic rheumatic diseases have a significant impact on the function, quality of life, and ability to work and represent a significant clinical and economic burden on healthcare systems. It is generally known that adequate physical activity is considered one of the adequate means to maintain or improve the quality of life, both physically and mentally. Nonpharmacological therapy plays a key role in the treatment of most rheumatic diseases. However, its effect for some of them has not been adequately studied or been little researched. A limitation of most of the small number of existing works aimed at nonpharmacological treatment for patients with SSc is low methodological quality, low number of patients, lack of a control group or monitoring (follow-up), and short-term intervention. The purpose of this chapter was to introduce the few studies that have examined this issue (**Table 1**) and to show that nonpharmacological therapies for diseases such as systemic sclerosis have been the focus of some research teams in recent years, the studies of which have demonstrated safety and benefits of these approaches.

Nonpharmacological therapy in patients with SSc includes, in particular, methods commonly used, for example, paraffin, manual lymphatic drainage, massage, stretching exercises to maintain range of motion in joints, mobilization, aerobic exercises, specially developed programs for the face and hands, self-management programs, splinting, and physical therapy. Other studies also investigated occupational therapy, sexual dysfunction, education, psychosocial status, and nutrition in patients with SSc.

Quality of treatment depends on the cooperation of a multidisciplinary team. A physician should properly choose the right medical treatment. A physiotherapist must select an adequate therapy to be individually tailored for a specific patient. An exercise program should be feasible even in the home environment, and patient's family or partner should get involved. Modifications to the home and work environments should be consulted with an occupational therapist. A psychologist or a psychosomatic medicine specialist can help not only the patient

Name of study	Author, year	Study design	Type of intervention	Description of intervention in intervention group	Description of intervention in control group	Number of individuals in intervention group	Number of individuals in control group	Duration of the intervention	Postintervention assessment	Results
Evaluation of paraffin bath treatment in patients with systemic sclerosis [5]	SANDQVIST, 2004	RCT	Paraffin	Paraffin in combination with exercise	Only exercise	17 SSc patients	17 SSc patients	1 month daily	After 1 month	The results showed that hand exercise in combination with paraffin bath seemed to be a suitable form of treatment in the effort to improve mobility and perceived hand stiffness
Paraffin hand bath for scleroderma [6]	PILS, 1991	RCT	Paraffin	12 times paraffin wrap therapy which continued for next 3 months	12 times paraffin wrap therapy	8 SSc patients	8 SSc patients	3 months	After 3 months	Skin thickness decreased in all patients after 12 sessions of paraffin treatment. However, at the end of 3 months therapy in the intervention group, there was no significant difference between the intervention and control group
Objective evaluation of hand function in scleroderma patients to assess effectiveness of physical therapy [7]	ASKEW, 1983	CCT	Paraffin	Paraffin, friction massage and exercise maintaining ROM in the joints of the wrist and hand	–	10 SSc patients	7 SSc patients	Once performed interventions	After 2 hours	Significant improvement in the articular ROM, skin elasticity and overall function of the hand
The effect of paraffin and exercise on hand function in persons with scleroderma: a	MANCUSO and POOLE, 2009	3x single case study	Paraffin	Active exercises with hands after paraffin wrap	-	3 SSc patients	-	5 times per week for 8 weeks	1 month and at 2 months after intervention	The results of this study suggest clinical efficacy of paraffin and exercises to

Name of study	Author, year	Study design	Type of intervention	Description of intervention in intervention group	Description of intervention in control group	Number of individuals in intervention group	Number of individuals in control group	Duration of the intervention	Postintervention assessment	Results
series of single case studies [8]										improve activity/ participation involving the use of the hands
Effect of orofacial exercises on oral aperture in adults with systemic sclerosis [9]	YUEN, 2012	RCT	Orofacial treatment	Multifaceted oral health intervention	Usual dental care	26 SSc patients	22 SSc patients	Twice a day with a total of 6 minutes for 6 months	After 3 months, and 6 months	A significantly larger increase in oral aperture for participants receiving the orofacial exercise program was found when compared to those in the usual care at 3 months, but not at 6 months evaluation. Participants' adherence rate to the exercise program was low (48.9%)
The rehabilitation of facial involvement in systemic sclerosis: efficacy of the combination of connective tissue massage, Kabat's technique and kinesitherapy [10]	MADDALI-BONGI, 2011	RCT	Orofacial treatment	Combination of the Kabat's technique, connective tissue massage, and kinesiotherapy specially developed for the face of SSc patients with a home exercise program	Only home exercise program	20 SSc patients	20 SSc patients	9 weeks, 2 times a week for 1 hour	After 9 weeks and after 9 weeks of follow-up	The combination of connective tissue massage, Kabat's technique, kinesiotherapy, and home-based exercises was more effective than a home exercise program alone in the rehabilitative treatment of SSc facial involvement
Oral hygiene in scleroderma: the effectiveness of a	POOLE, 2010	OD	Orofacial treatment	Structured oral hygiene and exercises for the face and hands	–	17 SSc patients	–	6 months daily	After 6 month intervention	There was a significant improvement in

Name of study	Author, year	Study design	Type of intervention	Description of intervention in intervention group	Description of intervention in control group	Number of individuals in intervention group	Number of individuals in control group	Duration of the intervention	Postintervention assessment	Results
multidisciplinary intervention program [11]										oral hygiene and a significant decrease in the number of teeth that bled on probing and in subgingival calculus
Effects of a nonsurgical exercise program on the decreased mouth opening in patients with systemic scleroderma [12]	PIZZO, 2003	OD	Orofacial treatment	Mouth stretching exercises for at least 15 minutes, twice a day, and oral augmentation exercise with a stick of soft wood daily	–	10 SSc patients	–	18 weeks	After 18 weeks	The exercise program improved the mouth opening of all subjects. At the end of the 18 week period, all patients commented that eating, speaking and oral hygiene measures were easier
Efficacy of connective tissue massage and Mc Mennell joint manipulation in the rehabilitative treatment of the hands in systemic sclerosis [14]	BONGI, 2009	RCT	Comprehensive physical therapy for physical and/or psychological functioning	Combination of connective tissue massage and joint manipulation according to Mc Mennell specially designed for the hands, and a home exercise program	Only home exercise program	20 SSc patients	20 SSc patients	9 weeks twice a week, 1 h per session	After 9 weeks, and after 9 weeks of follow-up	The combination of connective tissue massage, Mc Mennell joint manipulation and home exercise program was effective in the rehabilitative treatment of SSc hands. This combined treatment may lead to an improvement in hand function and QoL
Efficacy of a tailored rehabilitation	BONGI, 2009	RCT	Comprehensive physical therapy for	Combination of connective tissue massage and Mc	Educational advices and	10 SSc patients	10 SSc patients	One or two times per week for 9 weeks	After 9 weeks and after 9 weeks of follow-up	The association of disease-specific and global

Name of study	Author, year	Study design	Type of intervention	Description of intervention in intervention group	Description of intervention in control group	Number of individuals in intervention group	Number of individuals in control group	Duration of the intervention	Postintervention assessment	Results
program for systemic sclerosis [15]			physical and/or psychological functioning	Mennell joint manipulation (MLD if patients had edematous hands. Face involvement was treated with a combination of Kabat's method, connective tissue massage, and kinesiotherapy. Hydrokinesiotherapy (for patients without ulcers) or land-based rehabilitation (for patients with ulcers), and respiratory rehabilitation exercises)	medical information					rehabilitative techniques designed and tailored for SSc patients improved disability, HRQoL, hand and face disability and functionality, with its effects partially maintained at the follow-up
An individualized rehabilitation program in patients with systemic sclerosis may improve quality of life and hand mobility [16]	ANTONIOLI, 2009	CCT	Comprehensive physical therapy for physical and/or psychological functioning	Rehabilitation program that consisted of warm-up and cool-down exercises, training of motor functions, diaphragmatic breathing, controlled coughing exercises, treadmill, freewalking, finger stretching, and occupational therapy (physical therapy was also prescribed to 13 patients with articular problems) and home exercise program	–	16 SSc patients	17 SSc patients	2 weeks daily 30-minute sessions (10 sessions in total)	After 2 and 4 months	This study suggests that a significant proportion of patients with SSc experience an improvement in their perception of QoL, a better exercise tolerance, and a better hand mobility after a rehabilitation program consisting of a 2-week period of daily individual 30-min sessions of outpatient care, followed by at-home exercise program

Name of study	Author, year	Study design	Type of intervention	Description of intervention in intervention group	Description of intervention in control group	Number of individuals in intervention group	Number of individuals in control group	Duration of the intervention	Postintervention assessment	Results
Addressing patient health care demands in systemic sclerosis: pre- and postassessment of a psychoeducational group programme [17]	KWAKKENBOS, 2011	OD	Comprehensive physical therapy for physical and/or psychological functioning	A short, group-based psychoeducational program	–	41 SSc patients	–	The intervention was scheduled over 3 weekends	6 weeks after the intervention and 6 months postintervention	Patients reported less helplessness after the intervention, and higher acceptance of their limitations. However, no difference in depressed mood and physical functioning was observed. Patients reported high satisfaction with the content of the program
Randomized comparison of a multidisciplinary team care program with usual care in patients with systemic sclerosis [18]	SCHOUFFOER, 2011	RCT	Comprehensive physical therapy for physical and/or psychological functioning	Multidisciplinary team care program (1 day per week; individual treatments, group exercises, and group education)	Regular outpatient care	25 SSc patients	25 SSc patients	12 weeks	0, 12, and 24 weeks	In patients with SSc, a 12-week multidisciplinary day patient treatment program was more effective than regular outpatient care
The efficacy of self-administered stretching for finger joint motion in Japanese patients with systemic sclerosis [19]	MUGII, 2006	OD	Stretching	Autostretching (individual fingers were maintained in a stretched position using the opposite hand for 10 seconds and this was repeated 3–10 times)	-	45 SSc patients	-	1 year	After 1 month and 1 year	The total passive ROM was significantly improved in each finger after 1 month of finger stretching and 1 year after the first visit. Eating and gripping was also significantly improved
The short-term effect of gloving in	VANNAJAK, 2014	RCT	Stretching	The home program combined traditional	Same program	14 SSc patients	14 SSc patients	2 weeks daily	After intervention	Both groups showed a

Name of study	Author, year	Study design	Type of intervention	Description of intervention in intervention group	Description of intervention in control group	Number of individuals in intervention group	Number of individuals in control group	Duration of the intervention	Postintervention assessment	Results
combination with traditional Thai massage, heat, and stretching exercise to improve hand mobility in scleroderma patients [20]				Thai massage with stretching exercises and heat with gloves	without gloves					significant improvement in hand mobility after 2 weeks of daily home exercise program. Wearing the glove, however, resulted in better thumb mobility
Efficacy and safety of concurrent training in systemic sclerosis [21]	PINTO, 2011	OD	Aerobic training and combined endurance/ resistance training	Combined resistance and aerobic training program (concurrent training)	–	11 SSc patients	–	12 weeks	After intervention	This study demonstrates that a 12-week concurrent training program is safe and substantially improves muscle strength, function, and aerobic capacity in SSc patients
Intensive aerobic and muscle endurance exercise in patients with systemic sclerosis: a pilot study [22]	ALEXANDERSON, 2014	Pilot study	Aerobic training and combined endurance/ resistance training	Intense aerobic and endurance training program	–	4 SSc patients	–	6 weeks (noninterventional baseline period) and 8 weeks (exercise intervention period 3× a week)	Every other week throughout the 14-week study	Three participants improved significantly in muscular endurance, and two participants improved significantly or clinically relevantly in aerobic capacity. All other variables remained unchanged, except for a trend toward reduced fatigue
Aerobic exercise is safe and effective in	OLIVEIRA, 2009	CCT	Aerobic training and combined endurance/	Aerobic exercise program of moderate intensity	Aerobic exercise program of	7 SSc patients	7 healthy volunteers	8 weeks	Pre- and posttest	Both groups showed a significant

Name of study	Author, year	Study design	Type of intervention	Description of intervention in intervention group	Description of intervention in control group	Number of individuals in intervention group	Number of individuals in control group	Duration of the intervention	Postintervention assessment	Results
systemic sclerosis [23]			resistance training		moderate intensity					improvement in peak VO2 but with no significant difference between the study groups. Furthermore, both groups improved in exercise intensity which was documented by significantly increased peak lactate concentration in blood. No significant changes in SSc skin score or QoL were detected
Lower limb muscle strength is associated with functional performance and quality of life in patients with systemic sclerosis [24]	LIMA, 2015	Cross-sectional study	Lower extremities treatment	Study assesses the peripheral and respiratory muscle strength in individuals with SSc and investigates their correlation with the 6MWD and QoL measurements		20 SSc patients	20 healthy volunteers	April 2013 and January 2014		Patients with SSc exhibited reduced respiratory muscle and quadriceps strength and an increase in its fatigability. In these individuals, there was a relationship between quadriceps strength, functional capacity, and QoL
Evaluation of a mail-delivered, print-format, self-management program for persons with systemic sclerosis [25]	POOLE, 2013	Pilot study	Self-management program	The program consisted of a workbook and exercise DVD that provided information on medical aspects of the disease, dysphagia, fatigue	–	49 SSc patients	–	4–6 weeks	–	Participants consistently reported that the program was easy to use. Depression, fatigue, and pain decreased, and hand function, self-

Name of study	Author, year	Study design	Type of intervention	Description of intervention in intervention group	Description of intervention in control group	Number of individuals in intervention group	Number of individuals in control group	Duration of the intervention	Postintervention assessment	Results
				management, advocacy, activities of daily living, oral hygiene, skin and wound care, psychosocial changes, exercises, and other features of the condition						efficacy for controlling pain, and self-efficacy "other" improved; however, the only statistically significant change was in self-efficacy for pain
Taking charge of systemic sclerosis: a pilot study to assess the effectiveness of an internet self-management program [26]	POOLE, 2014	Pilot study	Self-management program	The program consisted of 10 modules (e.g. coping and body image/ appearance, fatigue and energy conservation, self-advocacy), an exercise video, learning activities, worksheets, and resources	–	16 SSc patients	–	Over 10 weeks	–	There were significant improvements in mean scores for ability to manage care and health, and significant decreases in fatigue and depression. Self-efficacy improved, but not significantly
Effects of splinting in the treatment of hand contractures in progressive systemic sclerosis [27]	SEEGER, 1987	Pilot study	Splinting interventions	Dynamic splinting of the hand daily for 8 hours (could decrease proximal interphalangeal (PIP) flexion contractures?)	The nonsplinted hand	8 SSc patients	8 SSc patients	2 months	After 1 and 2 months	Just one of eight patients experienced a statistically significant improvement in PIP range of motion as a result of the splinting. There was no evidence that the use of the splints served to maintain PIP extension when compared with the control hand

Name of study	Author, year	Study design	Type of intervention	Description of intervention in intervention group	Description of intervention in control group	Number of individuals in intervention group	Number of individuals in control group	Duration of the intervention	Postintervention assessment	Results
Manual lymph drainage improving upper extremity edema and hand function in patients with systemic sclerosis in edematous phase [31]	BONGI, 2011	RCT	Physical therapy	MLD 1 session a week (lasting 1 hour)	–	20 SSc patients	15 SSc patients	14 weeks: 5 weeks of rehabilitation and 9 weeks of follow-up	At the end of the treatment, and after a follow-up of 9 weeks	The application of MLD is effective in the treatment of the hand in edematous SSc by reducing hand volume, edema, and pain, and improving hand function and perceived QoL
Transcutaneous electrical nerve stimulation (TENS) improves upper GI symptoms and balances the sympathovagal activity in scleroderma patients [32]	SALLAM, 2007	CCT	Physical therapy	Home use TENS application at two GI acupoints on GI symptoms and QoL		17 SSc patients	9 healthy controls	14 days	The electrocardiogram was recorded for two intervals: baseline and TENS application	Prolonged TENS application improved GI symptoms and restored the sympathovagal balance, with an impressive correlation with improved physical functioning scores
Effects of shock wave therapy in the skin of patients with progressive systemic sclerosis: a pilot study [33]	TINAZZI, 2011	CCT	Physical therapy	ESWT of the arm and the hand of one arm	Second arm was without intervention	30 SSc patients	30 SSc patients	Three sittings	Before and immediately after ESWT and at 7, 30, 60, and 90 days after the treatment	The results of this study suggest that ESWT is a novel and efficacious treatment that can be added to the pharmacological therapy in order to decrease endothelial cell damage and skin fibrosis in patients with SSc. This treatment is well tolerated and can be repeated without side effects; in the

Name of study	Author, year	Study design	Type of intervention	Description of intervention in intervention group	Description of intervention in control group	Number of individuals in intervention group	Number of individuals in control group	Duration of the intervention	Postintervention assessment	Results
										majority of cases it determines a rapid improvement in skin elasticity and skin wellness, even if the effects tend to reduce during the time
Effect of biofeedback and deep oscillation on Raynaud's phenomenon secondary to systemic sclerosis: results of a controlled prospective randomized clinical trial [34]	SPORBECK, 2012	RCT	Physical therapy	The effect of deep oscillation and biofeedback on RP secondary to SSc	No intervention or therapies with an expected effect	8 SSc patients biofeedback and 10 SSc patients—deep oscillation	10 SSc patients	3 times per week for 4 weeks	After 4 and 12 weeks	Biofeedback resulted in an improvement in RP as determined by score reduction of visual analogue scale compared with patients of the control group, whereas deep oscillation revealed a tendency for improvement. The study underlines the beneficial role of physiotherapy for the treatment of SSc-related RP
Multiple daily ultrasound treatment of patients with progressive systemic scleroderma [35]	UHLEMANN, 1990	OD	Physical therapy	Ultrasound therapy of the hands with an intensity of 0.6W/cm^2, 6 minutes per region	–	24 SSc patients	–	3 times a day during 6 days	After 6 days	Pain decreased in 18 of 24 patients. At the end of therapy, no increase in pain was observed, and the hand strength significantly improved in all patients

Name of study	Author, year	Study design	Type of intervention	Description of intervention in intervention group	Description of intervention in control group	Number of individuals in intervention group	Number of individuals in control group	Duration of the intervention	Postintervention assessment	Results
Mouth opening scope in the patients with systemic sclerosis: Simultaneous application of a hyperbaric oxygenation and physical therapy [36]	MILAČIĆ, 2014	Prospective study	Physical therapy	Combined HBO therapy with facial physical therapy	–	13 SSc patients	–	Daily 10 days	After intervention	The therapy showed a statistically significant difference and proved that the combination of HBO therapy and physical therapy has its place in treating these patients

Acronyms: SSc, systemic sclerosis; RCT, randomized controlled trial; CCT, controlled clinical trial; OD, observational design; QoL, quality of life; HRQoL, health-related quality of life; ROM, range of motion; VO2, oxygen uptake; MLD, manual lymphatic drainage; 6MWD, 6-min walk distance; TENS, transcutaneous electrical nerve stimulation; GI, gastrointestinal; ESW, extracorporeal shock wave; ESWT, extracorporeal shock wave therapy; RP, Raynaud's phenomenon; HBO, hyperbaric oxygenation.

Table 1. Overview of available studies on nonpharmacological interventions in patients with systemic sclerosis.

but also the family or a partner to solve the psychological problems that could be associated with the establishment of the diagnosis.

It is clear from the systematic literature search of available studies that nonpharmacological treatment for these patients has its positive results and has been investigated worldwide. However, since it is a rare disease, the strength of evidence of efficacy of nonpharmacological treatment is limited. The aforementioned limitations suggest that there is an unmet need for international multicentric cooperation, teamwork, and unified projects with a solid design in order to explore this area to arrive at definite conclusions and treatment recommendations. Thus, even nonpharmacological approaches could offer specific techniques that could be implemented and would effectively contribute to greater self-sufficiency, and easier self-management of patients with SSc.

It is also important to carry out further studies to assess other neglected areas such as psycho-social status, depression or sexual dysfunction in order to provide a complex therapy by a team of specialist offering a versatile assistance to patients with SSc.

Acknowledgements

This chapter was supported by grant projects AZV 16-33542A, AZV 16-33574A, SVV for FTVS UK 2017, UNCE, PRVOUK P38, GAUK 214615, and the Ministry of Health of the Czech Republic [Research Project No. 00023728].

Author details

Maja Špiritović[1,2] and Michal Tomčík[2*]

*Address all correspondence to: michaltomcik@yahoo.com

1 Faculty of Sport and Physical Education, Department of Physiotherapy, Charles University, Prague, Czech Republic

2 Institute of Rheumatology and Department of Rheumatology, First Faculty of Medicine, Charles University, Prague, Czech Republic

References

[1] Sandberg ME, Bengtsson C, Kallberg H, Wesley A, Klareskog L, Alfredsson L, et al. Overweight decreases the chance of achieving good response and low disease activity in early rheumatoid arthritis. Annals of the Rheumatic Diseases. 2014;**73**(11):2029-2033

[2] Sandberg MEC, Wedren S, Klareskog L, Lundberg IE, Opava CH, Alfredsson L, et al. Patients with regular physical activity before onset of rheumatoid arthritis present with milder disease. Annals of the Rheumatic Diseases. 2014;**73**(8):1541–1544

[3] Gabrielli A, Avvedimento EV, Krieg T. Mechanisms of disease: scleroderma. New England Journal of Medicine. 2009;**360**(19):1989–2003

[4] Mau W, Listing J, Huscher D, Zeidler H, Zink A. Employment across chronic inflammatory rheumatic diseases and comparison with the general population. Journal of Rheumatology. 2005;**32**(4):721–728.

[5] Sandqvist G, Akesson A, Eklund M. Evaluation of paraffin bath treatment in patients with systemic sclerosis. Disability and Rehabilitation. 2004;**26**(16):981–987

[6] Pils K, Graninger W, Sadil F. Paraffin hand bath for scleroderma. Physical Medicine and Rehabilitation. 1991;**1**(1):19–21

[7] Askew LJ, Beckett VL, An KN, Chao EY. Objective evaluation of hand function in scleroderma patients to assess effectiveness of physical therapy. British Journal of Rheumatology. 1983;**22**(4):224–32

[8] Mancuso T, Poole JL. The effect of paraffin and exercise on hand function in persons with scleroderma: a series of single case studies. Journal of Hand Therapy. 2009;**22**(1):71–7; quiz 8

[9] Yuen HK, Marlow NM, Reed SG, Mahoney S, Summerlin LM, Leite R, et al. Effect of orofacial exercises on oral aperture in adults with systemic sclerosis. Disability and Rehabilitation. 2012;**34**(1):84–89

[10] Maddali-Bongi S, Landi G, Galluccio F, Del Rosso A, Miniati I, Conforti ML, et al. The rehabilitation of facial involvement in systemic sclerosis: Efficacy of the combination of connective tissue massage, Kabat's technique and kinesitherapy: A randomized controlled trial. Rheumatology International. 2011; **31**(7):895–901

[11] Poole J, Conte C, Brewer C, Good CC, Perella D, Rossie KM, et al. Oral hygiene in scleroderma: The effectiveness of a multi-disciplinary intervention program. Disability and Rehabilitation. 2010;**32**(5):379–384

[12] Pizzo G, Scardina GA, Messina P. Effects of a nonsurgical exercise program on the decreased mouth opening in patients with systemic scleroderma. Clinical Oral Investigations. 2003;**7**(3):175–178

[13] Alantar A, Cabane J, Hachulla E, Princ G, Ginisty D, Hassin M, et al. Recommendations for the care of oral involvement in patients with systemic sclerosis. Arthritis Care and Research (Hoboken). 2011;**63**(8):1126–1133

[14] Bongi SM, Del Rosso A, Galluccio F, Sigismondi F, Miniati I, Conforti ML, et al. Efficacy of connective tissue massage and Mc Mennell joint manipulation in the rehabilitative treatment of the hands in systemic sclerosis. Clinical Rheumatology. 2009;**28**(10):1167–1173

[15] Bongi SM, Del Rosso A, Galluccio F, Tai G, Sigismondi F, Passalacqua M, et al. Efficacy of a tailored rehabilitation program for systemic sclerosis. Clinical and Experimental Rheumatology. 2009;**27**(3):S44–S50

[16] Antonioli CM, Bua G, Frige A, Prandini K, Radici S, Scarsi M, et al. An individualized rehabilitation program in patients with systemic sclerosis may improve quality of life and hand mobility. Clinical Rheumatology. 2009;**28**(2):159–165

[17] Kwakkenbos L, Bluyssen SJM, Vonk MC, van Helmond AF, van den Ende CHM, van den Hoogen FHJ, et al.: Addressing patient health care demands in systemic sclerosis: pre-post assessment of a psycho-educational group programme. Clinical and Experimental Rheumatology. 2011;**29**(2):S60–S65

[18] Schouffoer AA, Ninaber MK, Beaart-van de Voorde LJJ, van der Giesen FJ, de Jong Z, Stolk J, et al. Randomized comparison of a multidisciplinary team care program with usual care in patients with systemic sclerosis. Arthritis Care and Research. 2011;**63**(6):909–917

[19] Mugii N, Hasegawa M, Matsushita T, Kondo M, Orito H, Yanaba K, et al. The efficacy of self-administered stretching for finger joint motion in Japanese patients with systemic sclerosis. Journal of Rheumatology. 2006; **33**(8):1586–1592

[20] Vannajak K, Boonprakob Y, Eungpinichpong W, Ungpansattawong S, Nanagara R. The short-term effect of gloving in combination with Traditional Thai Massage, heat, and stretching exercise to improve hand mobility in scleroderma patients. Journal of Ayurveda and Integrative Medicine. 2014;**5**(1):50–55

[21] Pinto AL, Oliveira NC, Gualano B, Christmann RB, Painelli VS, Artioli GG, et al. Efficacy and safety of concurrent training in systemic sclerosis. The Journal of Strength and Conditioning Research. 2011;**25**(5):1423–1428

[22] Alexanderson H, Bergegard J, Bjornadal L, Nordin A. Intensive aerobic and muscle endurance exercise in patients with systemic sclerosis: A pilot study. BMC Research Notes. 2014;**7**:86

[23] Oliveira N, dos Santos Sabbag L, de Sa Pinto A, Borges C, Lima F. Aerobic exercise is safe and effective in systemic sclerosis. International Journal of Sports Medicine. 2009;**30**(10): 728–732

[24] Lima TR, Guimaraes FS, Carvalho MN, Sousa TL, Menezes SL, Lopes AJ. Lower limb muscle strength is associated with functional performance and quality of life in patients with systemic sclerosis. Brazilian Journal of Physical Therapy. 2015;**19**(2):129–136

[25] Poole JL, Skipper B, Mendelson C. Evaluation of a mail-delivered, print-format, self-management program for persons with systemic sclerosis. Clinical Rheumatology. 2013;**32**(9):1393–1398

[26] Poole JL, Mendelson C, Skipper B, Khanna D. Taking charge of systemic sclerosis: A pilot study to assess the effectiveness of an internet self-management program. Arthritis Care & Research (Hoboken). 2014;**66**(5):778–782

[27] Seeger MW, Furst DE. Effects of splinting in the treatment of hand contractures in progressive systemic sclerosis. The American Journal of Occupational Therapy. 1987;**41**(2): 118–121

[28] ISL I. The Diagnosis and Treatment Of Peripheral Lymphedema: 2013 Consensus Document of the International Society Of Lymphology. Lymphology. 2009;**46**(1):1–11

[29] Baulieu F, Bourgeois P, Maruani A, Belgrado JP, Tauveron V, Lorette G, et al. Contributions of SPECT/CT imaging to the lymphoscintigraphic investigations of the lower limb lymphedema. Lymphology. 2013;**46**(3):106–119

[30] Hall TJ. AAPM/RSNA physics tutorial for residents: topics in US: Beyond the basics: Elasticity imaging with US. Radiographics. 2003;**23**(6):1657–1671

[31] Bongi SM, Del Rosso A, Passalacqua M, Miccio S, Cerinic MM. Manual lymph drainage improving upper extremity edema and hand function in patients with systemic sclerosis in edematous phase. Arthritis Care & Research (Hoboken). 2011;**63**(8):1134–1141

[32] Sallam H, McNearney TA, Doshi D, Chen JD. Transcutaneous electrical nerve stimulation (TENS) improves upper GI symptoms and balances the sympathovagal activity in scleroderma patients. Digestive Diseases and Sciences. 2007;**52**(5):1329–1337

[33] Tinazzi E, Amelio E, Marangoni E, Guerra C, Puccetti A, Codella OM, et al. Effects of shock wave therapy in the skin of patients with progressive systemic sclerosis: A pilot study. Rheumatology International. 2011;**31**(5):651–656

[34] Sporbeck B, Mathiske-Schmidt K, Jahr S, Huscher D, Becker M, Riemekasten G, et al. Effect of biofeedback and deep oscillation on Raynaud's phenomenon secondary to systemic sclerosis: Results of a controlled prospective randomized clinical trial. Rheumatology International. 2012;**32**(5):1469–1473

[35] Uhlemann C, Abendroth K, Callies R, Gassel M. Multiple daily ultrasound treatment of patients with progressive systemic scleroderma. Dermatologische Monatschrift. 1990; **176**(5–6):323

[36] Milačić DM, Čobeljić KP, Isaković RU. Mouth opening scope in the patients with systemic sclerosis: Simultaneously application of a hyperbaric oxygenation and physical therapy. Homeopathic Materia Medica. 2014;**30**(3):1186–1189

Chapter 5

Videocapillaroscopy in Connective Tissue Diseases

Simone Parisi and Maria Chiara Ditto

Additional information is available at the end of the chapter

http://dx.doi.org/10.5772/intechopen.69520

Abstract

Videocapillaroscopy is a noninvasive, quick, and easy examination method to indicate if there is clinical suspicion of microangiopathy. It provides the rheumatologist indispensable information on the microcirculation state. Recently with the development of the new classification criteria of systemic sclerosis (ACR 2013), capillaroscopy has become even more important. It is currently the only instrumental test whose result is pathognomonic for diagnosis of systemic sclerosis. During videocapillaroscopy, the following parameters are evaluated: density, structure, hemosiderin deposition, bloodstream, presence of megacapillaries, presence of subpapillary venous plexus, and edema. It can distinguish several patterns, especially scleroderma pattern, as follows: (1) "Early" pattern: few enlarged/giant capillaries, few capillary hemorrhages, relatively well-preserved capillary distribution, no evident loss of capillaries; (2) "Active" pattern: frequent giant capillaries, frequent capillary hemorrhages, moderate loss of capillaries, mild disorganization of the capillary architecture, absent or mild ramified capillaries; (3) "Late" pattern: irregular enlargement of the capillaries, few or absent giant capillaries and hemorrhages, severe loss of capillaries with extensive avascular areas, disorganization of the normal capillary array, ramified/bushy capillaries. Although capillaroscopic examination is easy to perform, it is essential that the operator has been properly trained on the instrument's function and on correct method of image acquisition to avoid misinterpretation.

Keywords: nailfold capillaroscopy, Raynaud's phenomenon, scleroderma pattern, prognostic score

1. Introduction

Capillaroscopy is a noninvasive, fast, and easy imaging technique to evaluate the assessment of the microcirculation. It is indicated in patients with suspect of microangiopatia [1].

It gives precise information about capillaries' conditions and related diseases to rheumatologist.

Recently, after the development of new systemic sclerosis classifications criteria [2], the role of capillaroscopy became more important. In fact a score of two out of nine is assigned in the case of significant capillaroscopic abnormalities to diagnose this disease (**Table 1**).

In the past, the study of capillaries was performed by instruments that could zoom, take pictures, or film the blood microcirculation, such as the ophthalmoscope and the dermatoscope, the stereo microscope, and tools for macrophotography.

The modern capillaroscopy, equipped with optical probes, is today commonly used in rheumatological and dermatological practice, and it is able to zoom (magnificat) capillaries in order of 200×, obtaining much qualitative measurements that could be reproducible.

The instrument consists of an optical probe fitted with an adjustable magnification and illumination ring for focusing and a personal computer (with high resolution color screen) with software for data processing. Several new models interface with iOS or Android system, and they are more portable (**Figure 1**).

Although capillaroscopic examination is easy to perform, it is essential that the operator has been properly trained about the instrument's functioning and correct method of image acquisition to avoid misinterpretation [3].

2013 ACR / EULAR Criteria For The Classification Of Systemic Sclerosis (Scleroderma)*

Item	Sub-items(s)	Weight/score †
Skin thickening of the fingers of both hands extending proximal to the metacarpophalangeal joints *(sufficient criterion)*	-	9
Skin thickening of the fingers *(only count the higher score)*	Puffy fingers	2
	Sclerodactyly of the fingers (distal to the metacarpophalangeal joints but proximal to the proximal interphalangeal joints)	4
Fingertip lesions *(only count the higher score)*	Digital tip ulcers	2
	Fingertip pitting scars	3
Telangiectasia	-	2
Abnormal nailfold capillaries	-	2
Pulmonary arterial hypertension and/or interstitial lung disease *(maximum score is 2)*	Pulmonary arterial hypertension	2
	Interstitial lung disease	2
Raynaud's phenomenon	-	3
SSc-related autoantibodies (anticentromere, anti–topoisomerase I [anti-Scl-70], anti–RNA polymerase III) *(maximum score is 3)*	Anticentromere 3 Anti–topoisomerase I Anti–RNA polymerase III	3

* The criteria are not applicable to patients with skin thickening sparing the fingers or to patients who have a scleroderma-like disorder that better explains their manifestations (e.g., nephrogenic sclerosing fibrosis, generalized morphea, eosinophilic fasciitis, scleredema diabeticorum, scleromyxedema, erythromyalgia, porphyria, lichen sclerosis, graft-versus-host disease, diabetic cheiroarthropathy).

† The total score is determined by adding the maximum weight (score) in each category.
Patients with a total score of ≥ 9 are classified as having definite scleroderma.

Sensitivity 91% Specificity 92%

Van den Hoogen et al. 2013 Classification Criteria for Systemic Sclerosis. Arthritis and Rheumatism. Vol. 65, No. 11, November 2013, pp 2737–2747

Table 1. Systemic sclerosis classification criteria 2013.

http://dx.doi.org/10.5772/intechopen.69520

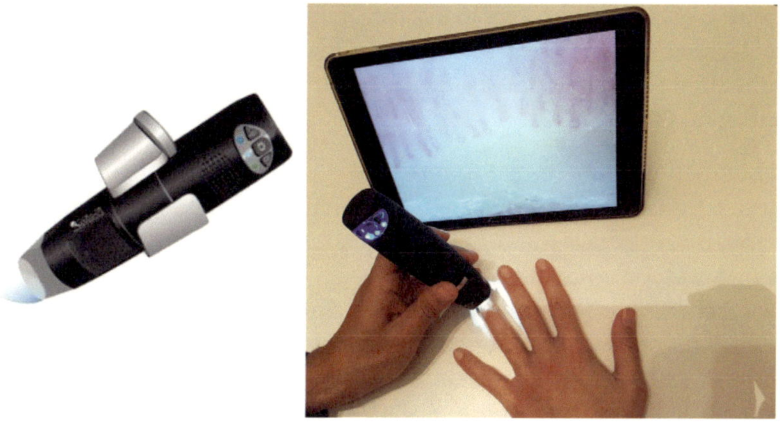

Figure 1. Example of Wi-fi capillaroscope.

2. The capillaroscopic technique

Capillaroscopy should be always performed in conditions of constant temperature. By convention, it is considered that the patient needs an acclimatization of at least 15 min at the temperature of 21–24°C before performing the examination.

When booking the videocapillaroscopy, it is necessary to give to the patient a few suggestions, especially to avoid the manicure in 7–10 days prior to the examination and application of nail polish.

At the time of the examination, the patient should be sat with his hands gently resting on the table on the palm with the fingers slightly apart.

Before starting the exam, it is necessary to apply a drop of oil (usually cedar oil) on the nail fold of each district that should be examined. At this level, the capillaries shall run parallel to the skin plane and, therefore, in normal subjects, are visible an afferent branch, a loop and an efferent branch (capillary hairpin).

Usually, they are investigated four districts in each hand leaving the first finger that usually has a bad view of the vascular widespread and nonspecific alterations. Furthermore, several studies have shown that, even in the presence of Raynaud phenomenon exclusively localized at the foot, capillaroscopy of the hands provides the same information that would be obtained by investigating the lower limbs and, therefore, for convenience, the examination, even in these cases, is usually performed exclusively in the hand level.

Modern software let you select on the monitor the investigation from time to time in the district, so you can compare any changes in respect of each finger. Also, they include measuring systems for dimensional analysis [4].

Although there are some parameters to indicate a normal/healthy capillaroscopic, it is important to consider that there is great variability in the capillary structure both interindividual and intraindividual. This variability depends on many factors such as employment, racial, and environmental.

In particular, in patients underwent to repeated microtrauma for professional reasons, such as typists, jackhammer users, pianists, etc., it is not uncommon to observe widespread phenomena of microhemorrhages and neoangiogenesis. As well as, patients who smoke have often shortened and tortuous capillaries. Moreover, in patients with dark or very dark skin color (e.g., for racial factors), it is often difficult to correctly visualize the capillaries and almost impossible to see the subpapillary venous plexus. Modern capillaroscopies with editable light intensity solve this problem in part. It is also important that the capillaroscopic be set from time to time for each patient calibrating on the "contrast", "range," and "saturation" functions to obtain an image that is as clear as possible [5].

3. The capillaroscopic parameters in normal/healthy conditions

A good capillaroscopic examination is achieved by positioning the probe plumb to the district under consideration and to obtain the correct visualize of the dermal papilla roughly between the middle and the upper third of the monitor (photo 2—correct assessment of the image). The area of interest is in fact just the dermal papilla and the capillaries residing there, or should reside within it, although the outside alterations are also important [6–8].

During capillaroscopy, the following parameters are evaluated:

- Density
- Structure
- Microhemorrhages
- Bloodstream
- Edema (soft focus effect)
- Subpapillary venous plexus

Density: In a healthy subject, the number of capillaries per millimeter is equal to 11 ± 2 while the number of capillaries for dermal papilla is equal to 2 ± 1 (picture 3: number of capillaries normal, equal to 12 per mm). The conditions under which this number is reduced may be described simply as "density reduction capillary" up to extreme situations of complete absence capillary describable as "areas avascular" or, in the case of a specific papilla, "vacuous papilla" (**Figure 2**: normal density; **Figure 3**: (a) and (b) area avascular papillary or "papillae vacuous.")

Structure: The capillaries of the healthy subject, in most cases, have an aspect so-called "hairpin shape" or "U-shaped" and are well aligned, in an orderly manner, the one beside the other with a "comb arrangement" (**Figure 4**: distribution capillary ordered to comb with

http://dx.doi.org/10.5772/intechopen.69520

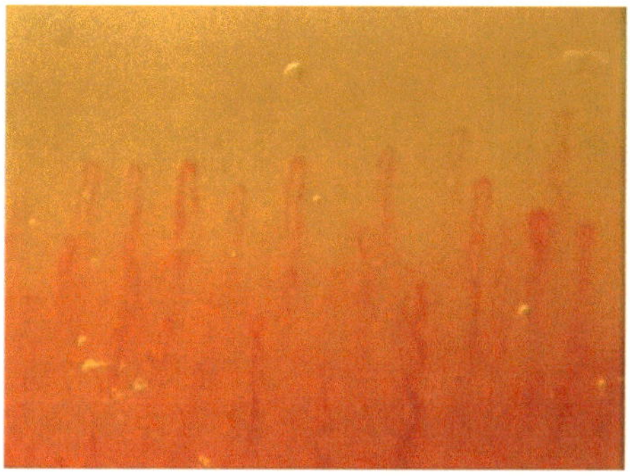

Figure 2. Example of normal pattern.

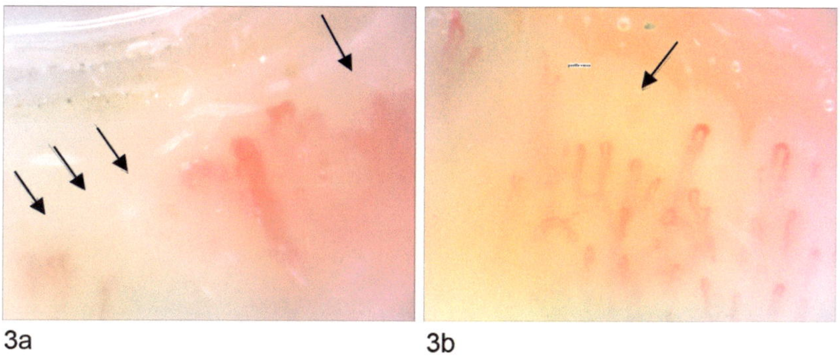

Figure 3. (a) and (b) Black arrows indicate papillae vacuous.

aspect hairpin), all similar in form and with some dimensional variability (length approximately between 200 and 500 μm).

You can observe the modest structural disorganization even in healthy individuals. Instead, the complete subversion of it is attributable to pathological conditions.

They should not be present ramifications that often indicate a poor vascularization with angiogenesis to provide the blood supply of avascular areas.

Tortuosities are often found, for the most in apical zone, and the capillary has a distorted aspect. It manifested as single or multiple cross/overs and/or patterns described as "trefoil," "antler," "glomerular loop," and "treble clef." These anomalies can be isolated or diffuse (**Figure 5**: tortuosities).

The apical tortuosities, by themselves, are not a pathologic finding. They are frequently found in heavy smokers, in patients underwent to repeated microtrauma, in patients with psoriasis and in various other conditions.

Otherwise, the tortuosity can be contextualized within a framework frankly altered or a real scleroderma pattern.

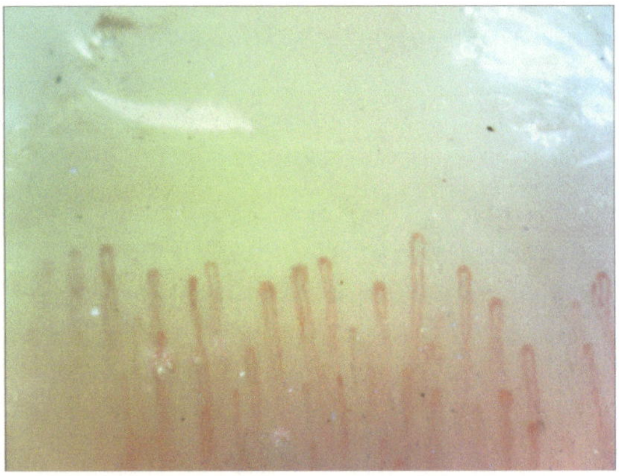

Figure 4. Normal structure: hairpin shape.

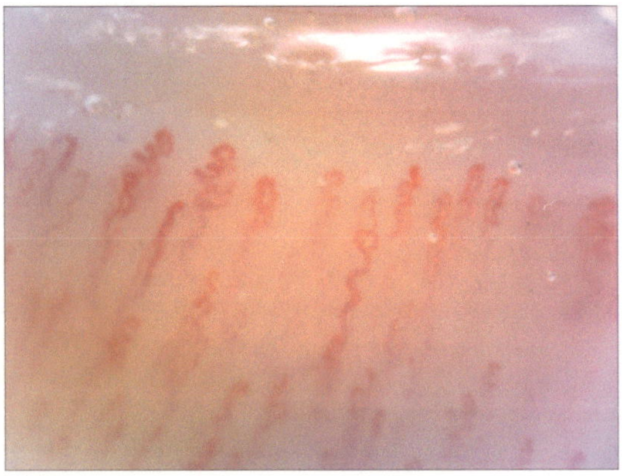

Figure 5. Tortuosity in apical zone.

The capillary branches (afferent and efferent loop) of the healthy subject normally have a diameter between 8 and 20 μm depending on the capillary portion considered. In fact, usually, the loop efferent, due to venous stasis, is slightly larger than that afferent.

They are defined "enlarged" capillaries with a diameter between 30 and 50 μm measured at the level of the two branches and the loop, "mega" capillaries with diameter >50 μm at the level of the two branches and the loop, and "giant" capillaries with diameters >100 μm wide and the two branches of the loop (**Figure 6**: megacapillaries and giant capillaries).

Morphostructural minor anomalies (e.g., tortuosity) are found in approximately 10–20% of healthy subjects.

Among irregularly enlarged capillaries, loop size can vary considerably in different segments, with normal portions alternating with extremely enlarged areas, sometimes giving a "micro-aneurysmatic" or "rosary-like" appearance (**Figure 7**).

Microhemorrhages: Although the microhemorrhages are frequent elements in the pathological or scleroderma pattern, it is not uncommon to observe them in healthy individuals as a

http://dx.doi.org/10.5772/intechopen.69520

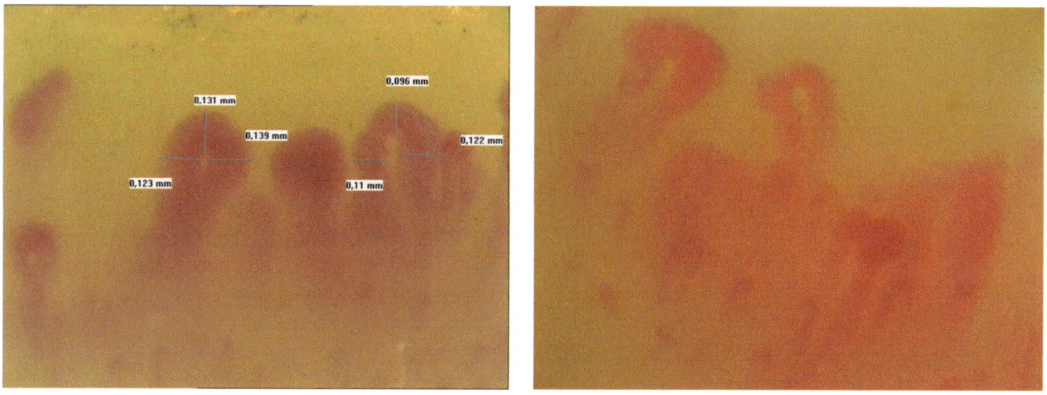

Figure 6. (a) and (b) Megacapillaries and giant capillaries.

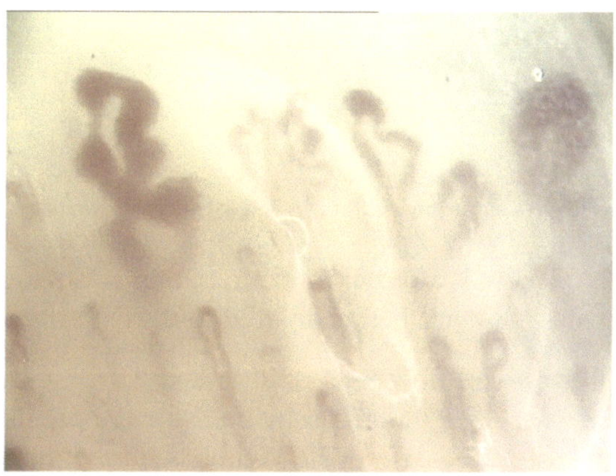

Figure 7. Capillaries with "rosary-like" aspect.

result of trauma. In these cases, bleeding is well-defined, unique, and usually transient, not necessarily directly related to the underlying capillaries. It is also not uncommon to observe very distant from the papilla or much below it.

The extravasation blood of pathological capillaries assumes a characteristic aspect in the supply chain "a strung pearls" (**Figure 8a** and **b**: microhemorrhages to "strung pearls"), or mold on the capillary (**Figure 8c** and **d**: "Napoleonic hat").

It can get an idea more or less realistic age of bleeding based on the analysis of the same color that tends to move from dark red to light yellow before disappearing altogether.

In the case of disease patterns may be encountered persistent deposits hemosiderin standing.

Nailfold microbleeds may also be related to capillary thrombosis which can occur in some pathological conditions and is often misinterpreted as hemorrhages. A key distinguishing feature of capillary thrombosis is the configuration of the dark area, which mirrors that of the capillary loops.

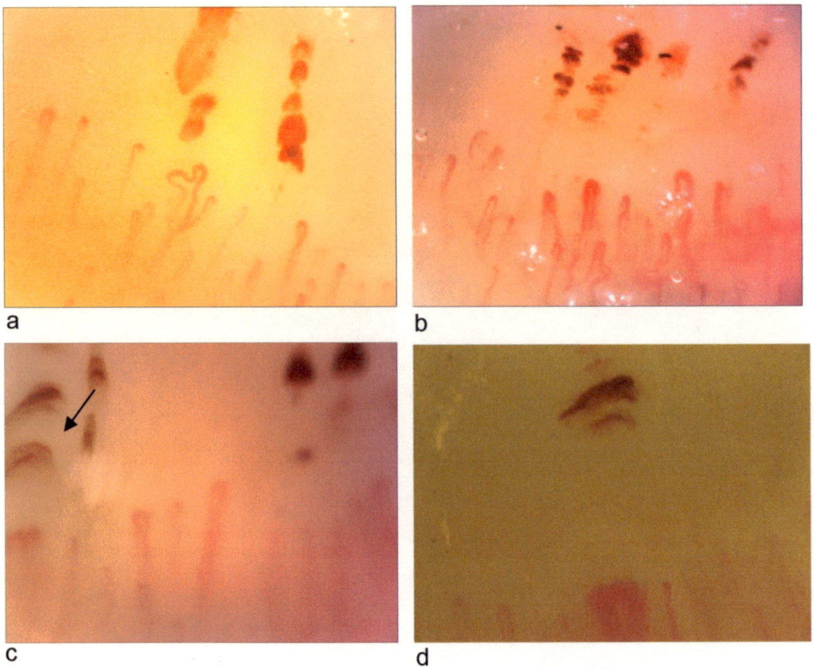

Figure 8. (a) and (b) Microhemorrhages to "strung pearls"; (c) and (d) microhemorrhages to "Napoleonic hat."

Bloodstream: The capillaroscopy is a dynamic examination and allows to study blood flow, although in an approximate manner when compared to the Doppler technique.

A capillary with continuous blood flow is normal index. It will appear constantly full, and in the case when pressure is exerted by the probe on the same papilla, these will quickly fill the cessation of the stimulus. In the case of slowed blood flow, this will assume a granular appearance in particular in correspondence of the capillary walls and, in the case a pressure is exerted with the capillaroscopic probe the capillary will fill up slowly to cease the stimulus.

In the case where there is capillary thrombosis, typical of giant capillaries or megacapillari, the flow will appear static, and neither the pressure exerted by the probe nor the subsequent stop of the stimulus will show variations in the capillary which will appear always full.

Edema (soft focus effect): The flou effect in photography is a special effect that is achieved by reducing the contrast of the image without really being blurred. In capillaroscopy, it is talking about flou effect when, at the subpapillary, capillaries appear poorly visible in an edematous context of vascular congestion.

Occasionally, it is seen in healthy subjects. Alone it does not constitute a significant fault (**Figure 9**: flou effect).

Subpapillary venous plexus: The plexus is visible in the case of good skin transparency and is best viewed in the extreme ages of life (**Figure 10(a)** and **(b)**).

The venous plexus vessels have a perpendicular progress to the capillaries and are larger.

Figure 9. Black arrow → indicates flou effect.

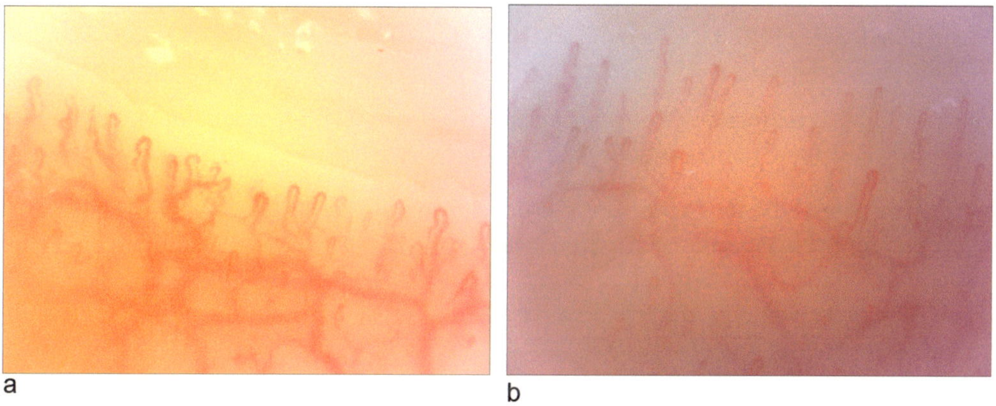

Figure 10. (a) and (b) Good visibility of the subpapillary venous plexus.

In cases of serious and widespread destruction capillaries, such as in the advanced stages of systemic sclerosis, the subpapillary venous plexus may constitute the only identifiable vascular element.

In healthy individuals, it is not always detectable.

4. Capillaroscopy in pathologic subjects

4.1. Introduction

Secondary Raynaud's phenomenon refers to the clinical manifestation in the presence of an underlying systemic disease.

Among the diseases of rheumatologic interest, the more strongly and inseparably linked to Raynaud's phenomenon is the systemic sclerosis, even if this appears also in the presence of other autoimmune diseases such as systemic lupus erythematosus, dermatomyositis, undifferentiated connective, and mixed connective, in a small percentage of cases, in the presence of rheumatoid, psoriatic, or juvenile idiopathic arthritis.

Capillaroscopy does not constitute, in itself, a diagnostic test. Especially not usefull to diagnostic Raynaud's phenomenon, whose diagnosis is exclusively linked to the clinic. The examination provides a specific view on the state of the microcirculation and in particular on its integrity and is always related to the clinical and laboratory data. Then we can determine whether the Raynaud's phenomenon is referable to a damage of the microcirculation [8, 9].

However, capillaroscopy plays a key role in the diagnosis of connective tissue diseases and especially of the scleroderma spectrum disorders, which include, in addition to systemic sclerosis, the dermatomyositis, the undifferentiated, and mixed connective tissue disease [10, 11].

In fact, historically, the typical capillaroscopic alterations for scleroderma spectrum disorders have always played a fundamental role in the diagnosis of systemic sclerosis, being included in all the diagnostic criteria formulated over the years for this condition, including the latest ACR criteria of 2013.

In contrast to what happens in the case of primitive Raynaud's phenomenon, in the presence of secondary Raynaud's phenomenon, the capillaroscopy is able to reveal specific anomalies.

Over the years, we have been implemented many efforts in an attempt to identify specific capillaroscopic paintings for a specific pathology. These efforts have hesitated in identifying a capillaroscopic pattern defined as "scleroderma pattern." More than 95% of patients with overt systemic sclerosis have morphological markers of microvascular disorganization, including giant capillaries, microhemorrhages, loss of capillaries, avascular areas, and angiogenesis [12–14].

4.2. Systemic sclerosis

Specific capillaroscopic alterations are found in the majority of cases of systemic sclerosis and often several years before diagnosis. The key element that distinguishes the scleroderma pattern is megacapillare. Another common finding is typical microhemorrhage called "pearls strung" or "Napoleon hat" usually overlying dilated capillaries or megacapillaries. Third distinctive element is represented by avascular areas. In 2000, the group of Genoa, headed by professor Cutolo, has identified three types of scleroderma pattern, referred to as "early," "active," and "late" [15–17].

We analyze below a capillaroscopic examination as a "scleroderma pattern."

Density: As is known in a healthy subject, the number of capillaries per millimeter is equal to 11 ± 2 while the number of capillaries for dermal papilla is equal to 2 ± 1. In the case of scleroderma, pattern is common to find a reduction in the number of capillaries. In particular, the reduction of the density can range from focused frameworks (e.g., to a single papilla "vacuous papilla") to framework of rarefied widespread, until the total disappearance of capillaries with large subpapillary vascular areas. The most dramatic paintings are typical of late stages or framework identified by Cutolo et al. as "late," even if similar findings can be found in patients with recent symptoms onset, especially in progressive cases.

Structure: The most significant finding of scleroderma pattern, as said, is the megacapillare or a capillary which measures a greater diameter than 50 μm in correspondence with the two branches of the ascending and descending loops. In the case of diameters greater than 100 μm, it is called the capillary giant. The presence of only one megacapillare within a normal framework is not sufficient to define scleroderma pattern although suggests the need a follow up. The presence of two or more megacapillaries leads to a scleroderma pattern even in the absence of microhemorrhages or avascular areas.

Generally, the presence of megacapillari in the context of apparently normal capillaries, with few or absent microhemorrhages, characterizes the earliest stages of the disease and it is identified by Cutolo et al. as "early." Instead, in the presence of numerous or ubiquitous megacapillari in the context of rare normal capillaries or ectatic capillaries, in the presence of numerous microhemorrhages in more districts, we will be faced to a capillary framework called "active."

In the late stages of systemic sclerosis are sometimes pathognomonic capillary ramifications, with elongated and bizarre capillaries, or overgrowth of the subpapillary venous plexus, last attempt to make up for the total or almost total disappearance of the subpapillary capillaries. This framework configures the "late" scleroderma pattern.

Other detectable morphostructural abnormalities in scleroderma pattern are ectasia (capillaries in the range from 30 to 50 μm), the tortuosities, identifying, based on the forms as "staghorn," "a clef,""a glomerulus,""ball," etc. and microaneurysms. These alterations are not specific and can also be found in healthy subjects.

Microhemorrhages: They constitute an extremely common finding in the scleroderma pattern and, especially in the one called "active". The typical hemorrhages of the scleroderma pattern may look as a mold, overlooking a megacapillare, or a giant capillary, or an aspect to "strung pearls" that are stacked in succession in the subpapillary and extrapapillary, never in deep seat. The microhemorrhages indicated breaking of capillary wall and are a sign of microvascular damage. There may be bleeding in the absence of megacapillari. The lonely bleeding are not considered sufficient for the identification of scleroderma pattern although, the presence of diffuse bleeding, even in the absence of further alterations, suggests necessarily the follow up.

The microhemorrhages should not be confused with traumatic hemorrhages that have a very heterogeneous presentation, generally overlying or adjacent to completely normal capillaries. Usually, they have a greater extension and can be found in the subpapillary-, deep-or extrapapillary segment.

Flow: The typical flow scleroderma patterns abnormalities are linked to the structural damage, in particular to megacapillaries. In these cases, the blood flow can appear slow or granular or even static. In the case of slow or static flow, a stimulus as the modest pressure exercised by the capillaroscopy probe is sufficient to make empty capillaries, and the capillaries will become fills when pressure is stopped. However, megacapillaries, giant capillaries, and the microaneurismatic capillaries remain completely filled both in the presence and in the absence of pressure stimulus, indicating a wall thickening causing static flow.

Edema (soft focus effect): Subpapillary edema is a constant finding in the case of capillaries vasodilatation in particular in the presence of megacapillaries and giant capillaries, so it is a typical finding in the scleroderma pattern. Edema could be mild, moderate, or severe and in these cases, subpapillary nous plexus is hardly visible.

Subpapillary venous plexus: It is clearly visible in healthy subjects and the extreme ages of life, can be seen in the case of early scleroderma pattern, is usually barely visible or not visible in the "active" phase, and is the only detectable findings in the late stage, where papillary capillaries are absent. Bizarre capillary ramifications are frequent findings in the late stage, as a last attempt to overcome the vascular deficit.

Scleroderma pattern:

- Early scleroderma pattern (**Figure 11(a–c)**): framework characterized by the presence of dilated capillaries and some megacapillaries. Microhemorrhages are poorly represented or absent. No reduction in capillary density.
- Active scleroderma pattern (**Figure 12(a)** and **(b)**: framework characterized by the widespread presence of megacapillaries and/or giant capillaries. A large number of microhemorrhages. No reduction in capillary density or occasional finding of "papilla vacua" in the presence of angiogenesis phenomena.
- Late scleroderma pattern (**Figure 13(a)** and **(b)**: framework characterized by the presence of rare lasts megacapillaries, abundant ramifications. Rare or absent microhemorrhages. Large avascular areas. Exuberance of the subpapillary venous plexus.

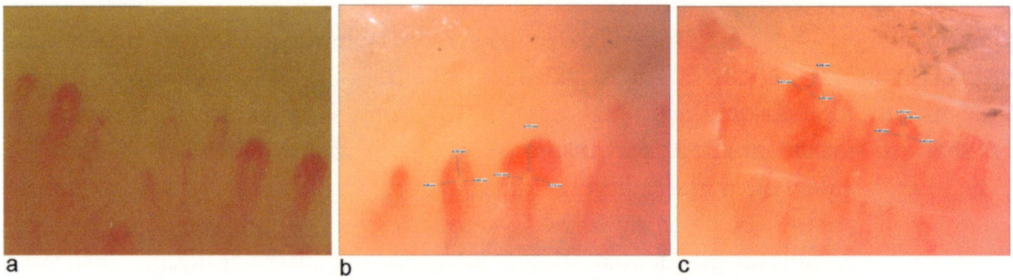

a b c

Figure 11. (a–c) Few megacapillaries without microhemorrhages.

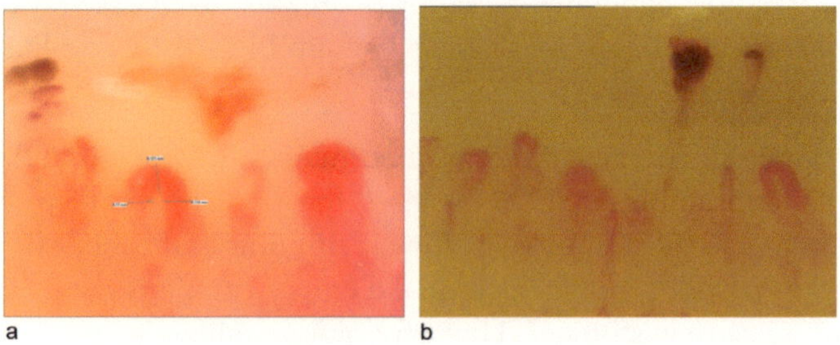

a b

Figure 12. (a) and (b) Diffuse megacapillaries with microhemorrhages.

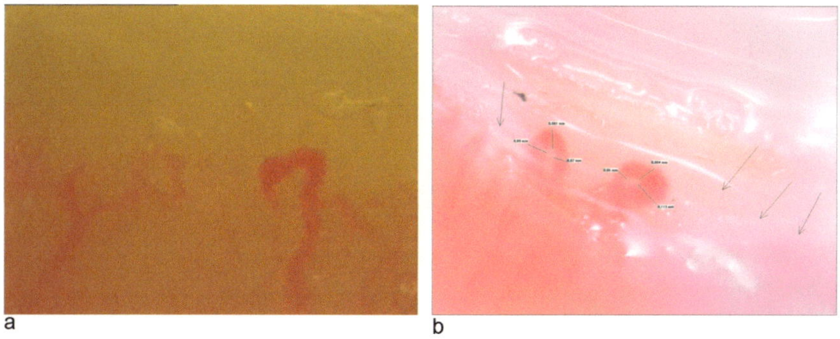

Figure 13. (a) and (b) "Papilla vacua," diffuse or localized loss of capillaries.

5. Capillaroscopy in other rheumatic diseases

As mentioned, all of rheumatic diseases included in the scleroderma spectrum disorders may present a capillaroscopic framework suggesting for scleroderma pattern. However, in some diseases, there are typical capillary feature presentations. For example, in rheumatoid arthritis, extremely elongated capillaries are the principal findings (**Figure 14**) [18, 19].

In dermatomyositis, the most frequent findings are dilated and giant capillaries with tree-like appearance (**Figure 15(a)** and **(b)**).

Even in the case of psoriatic arthritis, capillaries appear rather short and stubby (**Figure 16**).

However, these features are not enough specific to identify a defined framework.

5.1. Scoring method

In present-day clinical practice, capillaroscopic surveys are usually analyzed qualitatively in order to show patterns of disease (as previously stated). However, some authors share the idea that a normalization of the capillaroscopic pattern may be positive.

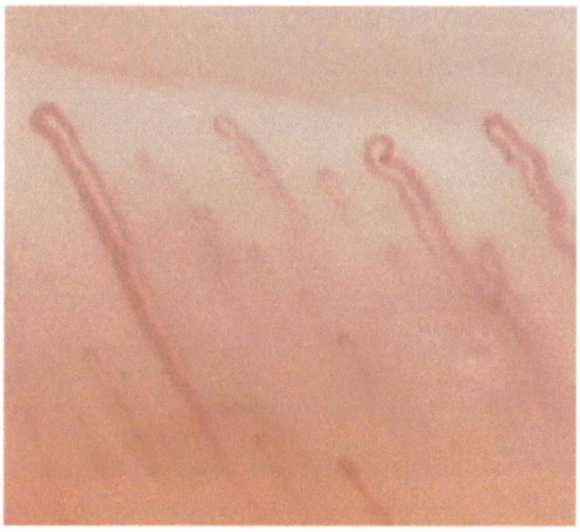

Figure 14. Capillaroscopy in rheumatoid arthritis.

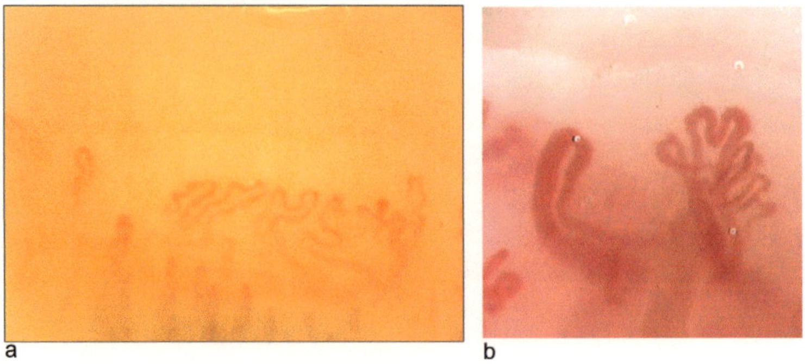

Figure 15. (a) and (b) Tree pattern in dermatomyositis.

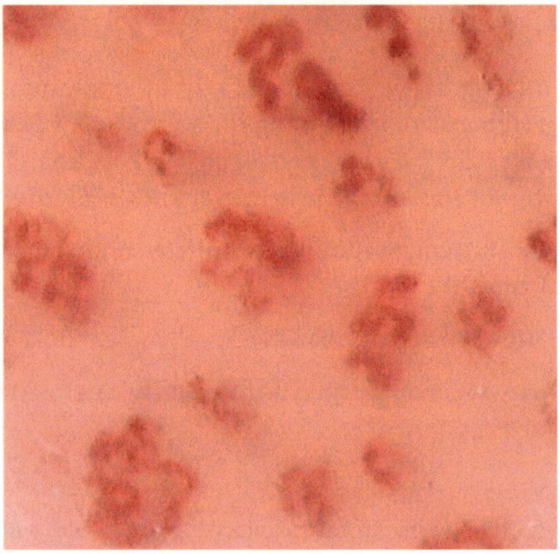

Figure 16. Capillaroscopy pattern in psoriatic arthritis.

Different scoring methods have been proposed to prospectively evaluate both the trend and the gravity of the scleroderma microangiopathy.

5.2. Semiquantitative method

One of these methods is the semiquantitative assessment which contemplates the analysis of the following capillaroscopic parameters:

1. Loss of capillaries: reduction of the number of capillaries to less than 9 per mm
2. Disorganization of the capillary architecture: irregular loops distribution, orientation, and morphology
3. Tree-like capillary network: capillaries with skein-like or shrub-like branched loops.

Each parameter is given a score based on the given impairment:

- 0: no alteration
- 1: capillary impairment up to 33%
- 2: capillary impairment higher than 33% and up to 66%
- 3: capillary impairment higher than 66%

The average score for each parameter comes from the analysis of four conterminous capillaroscopic areas (each area consisting of a 1 mm^2 surface) in the central part of the II, III, IV, and V finger of each hand.

The final score of each parameter is given by adding up the average scores of each finger; then the result is divided by 8. Lastly, the sum of the three scores constitutes the *microangiopathy evolution score* whose value may vary from 0 to 9.

On the basis of the capillaries loss only, such score is easier to determine and has been proposed as a predictor of digital ulcers. An average score of the capillaries number decrease is obtained by using capillary density as only parameter if a 1 mm^2 surface on eight fingers is analyzed. Scores that appear to be higher than 1.67 are shown to be a predictive factor of digital ulcers (Se 70%, Sp 69.77%, with a positive likelihood ratio of 2.32 and a negative likelihood ratio of 0.43) since such ulcers occur within 6–12 months after the capillaroscopic evaluation [20] (**Figure 17**).

5.3. Quantitative method

This method needs a strict standardization to be reproducible and comparable through time. As of today, the only quantitative score to be validated for both replicabilities and the predictive value is the *Capillaroscopy Skin Ulcer Risk Index* (CSURI), which is predictive for the incoming appearance of digital ulcers (which are already present within 3 months of the capillaroscopy) and for the nonfulfillment of their recovery (Se 92.3%, Sp 81.4 %, NPV 97.2%, TPV 84.3% with a PPV higher than 81% in the subgroup of patients with a history of ulcers appeared within a year).

The calculation is carried out by analyzing the whole nailfold area (from the II to the V finger of each hand, saving at least an image for each finger). Of all selected images, the one with the highest number of capillaries and the one with the lowest number of megacapillaries are to be considered; then the following formula has to be used: M×DN2 (with M: numbers of capillaries, D: maximum diameter, N: numbers of megacapillaries). Having at least a visible capillary is a prerequisite (otherwise the formula would be equal to 0; in fact, it is not possible to use it in 5% of patients. In this case, the formula is considered positive in principle). The analyzed area must be 1.57 mm wide. CSURI calculation is based on one image chosen between the saved one (the image with the lowest number of capillaries should be preferred) (**Figures 18** and **19**).

Capillaroscopic parameters are defined in a strict way so that reproducibility and replicability are optimized:

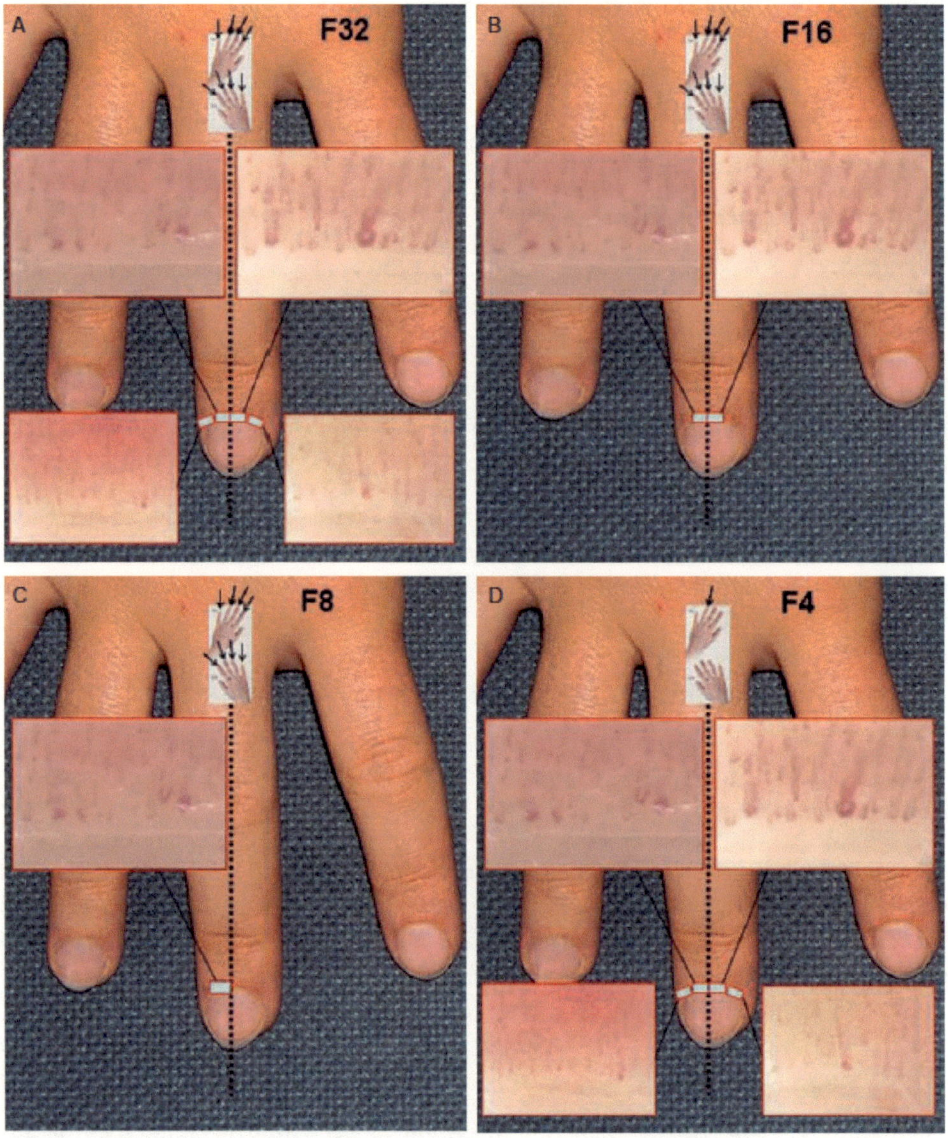

Figure 17. Number of fields studied: gold standard (F32) and successive simplifications (F16-F8-F4). (A) F32: eight fingers (arrows), four fields of 1 mm per finger, giving a total of 32 fields. (B) F16: eight fingers (arrows), two fields of 1 mm per finger, giving a total of 16 fields. (C) F8: eight fingers (arrows), one filed of 1 mm per finger, giving a total of eight fields. (D) F4: one finger (arrows), four fields of 1 mm in that finger, giving a total of four fields [20].

- Number of capillaries: all the capillaries in the first row (the ones closest to the papilla) must be counted even if they are all different depths.
- Megacapillary: maximum measurable diameter in the first row (microaneurysms should not be included).
- Tree-like morphology: a tree-like capillary is equivalent to the number of taken papillae or to the number of observable loops.

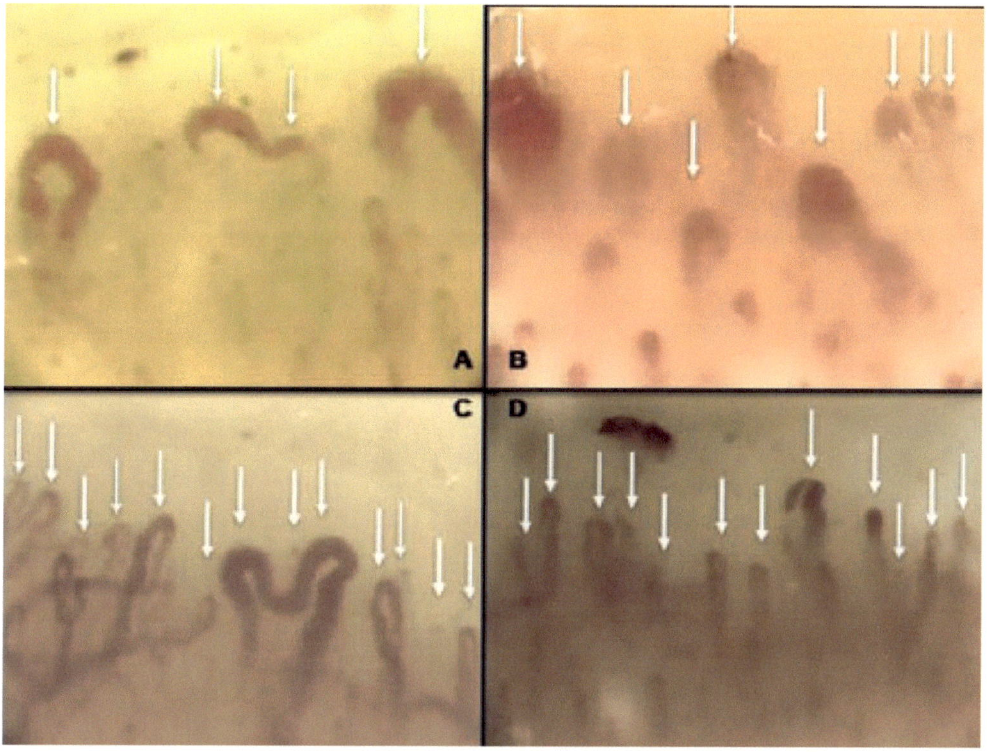

Figure 18. Examples of capillaroscopic finding measurements. (A) 4 capillaries, 3 giant capillaries (1 ramified giant capillaries occupying both dermal papillae). (B) 8 capillaries, 5 giant capillaries (every capillary was counted in the distal row even if it was not on the same level). (C) 13 capillaries, 1 giant capillary (1 ramified giant capillary computed as 2 in the total number count). (D) 12 capillaries, 1 giant capillaries (every capillary was counted in the distal row even if it was not on the same level) [14].

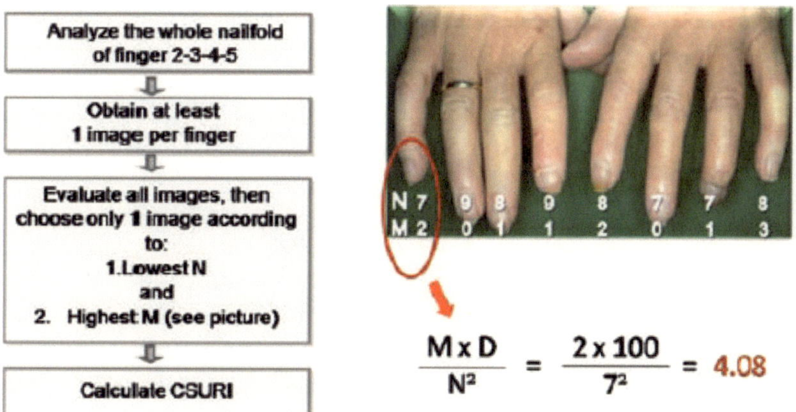

Figure 19. Algorithm for capillaroscopic skin ulcer risk index (CSURI) evaluation. D, Maximum diameter of mega capillary; M, number of megacapillaries (diameter ≥ 50 μm); N, number of capillaries [14].

The CSURI value per patient is the maximum computable if the whole nailfold area is analyzed so that the highest score of microangiopathy is defined. PROs: number of false negatives <3%. CONs: a higher risk of increasing the false positives.[21].

5.4. Prognostic index

The *Prognostic Index for Nailfold Capillaroscopic Examination* (PRINCE: **Table 2**) allows to stratify the risk of development of a scleroderma spectrum disorder over a period of 5 years in

Parameters	Value	Log HR		Score
A. Megacapillaries	Absent=0 Present=1	0.46	A	N x 0.46
B. Microemorragies	Absent=0 Present=1	0.57	B	N x 0.57
C. Number of Capillaries	linear	0.41	C	N x 0.41 + (t1+t2+t3)
	Non linear (t1+t2+t3)			
	No. ≤3.8	t1 0 t2 0 t3 0		
	No. 3.9 to 7.2	t1 -0.41x[(N3.8)/3.45]^3 t2 0 t3 0		
	No. 7.3 to 10.2	t1 -0.41x[(N3.8)/3.45]^3 t2 6.4x[(N-7.25)/3.45]^3/2.95 t3 0		
	No ≥ 10.3	t1 -0.41x[(N3.8)/3.45]^3 t2 6.4x[(N-7.25)/3.45]^3/2.95 t3 3.45x[(N-10.2)/3.45]^3		
Total Score	A + B + C			

N.: mean number of capillaries/mm

Table 2. Prognostic parameters of PRINCE index.

patients with Raynaud syndrome by analyzing the three main capillaroscopic anomalies (with the survey of a 1 mm area per finger):

- Presence of megacapillaries
- Presence of microhemorrhages
- Numbers of capillaries per mm

The inclusion of antinuclear antibodies allowed to develop an additional predictive model with the following risk categories: high (50+ %), medium (10–50%) and low risk (<10%) (**Figure 20**) [22].

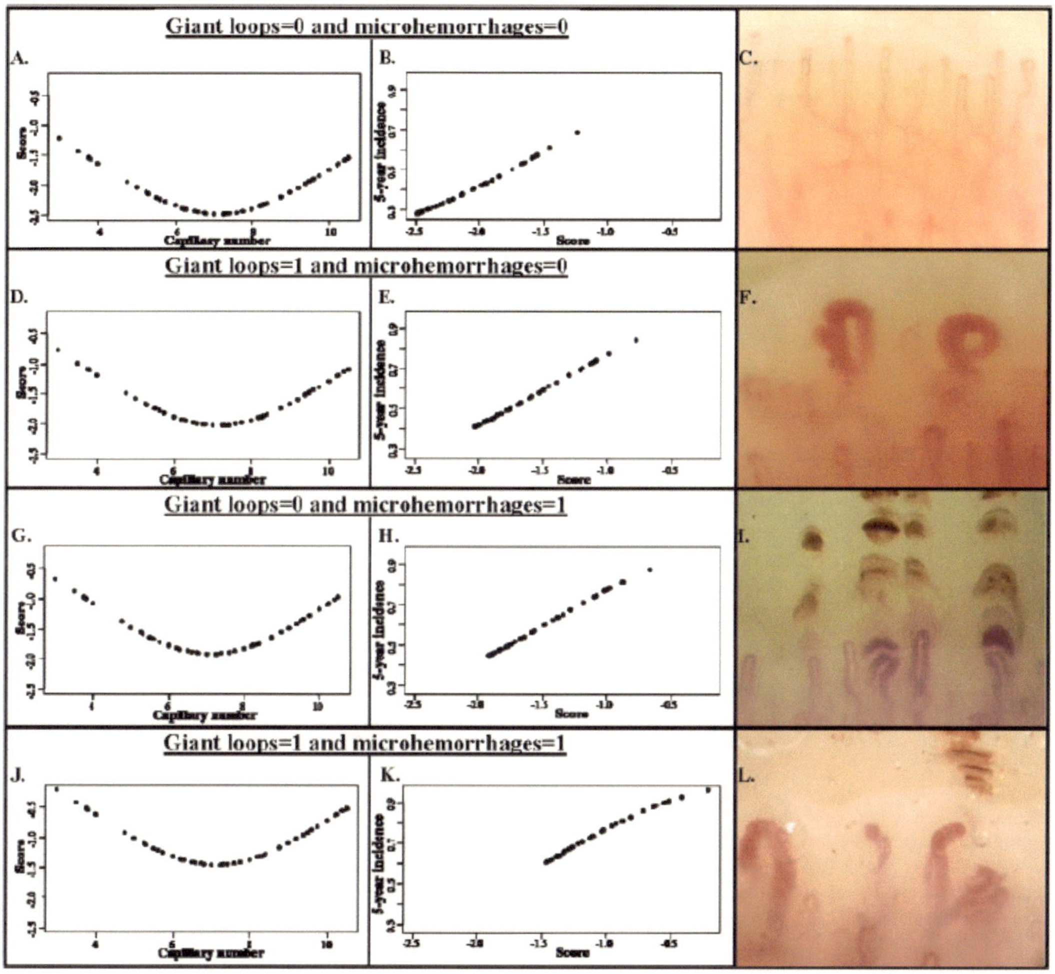

Figure 20. Prognostic Index for Nailfold Capillaroscopic Examination (PRINCE). A, D, G, and J: possible combination of giant loops and microhemorrhages (0 = absent, 1 = present). The score (on the y-axis) is obtained as a function of the number of capillaries (represented on the x-axis). B, E, H, and K: data used with the corresponding scores in A, D, G, and J to obtain the incidence and thus deduce the risk of developing Raynaud's phenomenon secondary to a scleroderma spectrum disorder. C, F, I, and L: examples of capillaroscopic patterns [22].

6. The role of capillaroscopy in the early diagnosis of systemic sclerosis

The role of capillaroscopy has been considered over the years more and more attention, especially in the early diagnosis of systemic sclerosis. Then, to detect valid predictors of early systemic sclerosis, the European Scleroderma Trials and Research group (EUSTAR) identified three red flags, thanks to the VEDOSS program (very early diagnosis of systemic sclerosis): Raynaud's phenomenon (RP), antinuclear antibodies (ANA) positivity, and puffy fingers are the main elements to suspect systemic sclerosis. In the case of these three flags performing, further tests to confirm the diagnosis, in particular nailfold video-capillaroscopy and evaluation of specific disease antibodies (anticentromere and antitopoisomerase I), are mandatory. The challenge of VEDOSS program is to identify patients who will develop an established systemic sclerosis.

Very recently, the first results of the VEDOSS project were processed and new EULAR/ACR (American College of Rheumatology) classification criteria have been validated and published (2013), in which the capillaroscopic characteristic changes have been included (requiring at least two, or better, all four items to be present) (**Figure 21**) [23, 24].

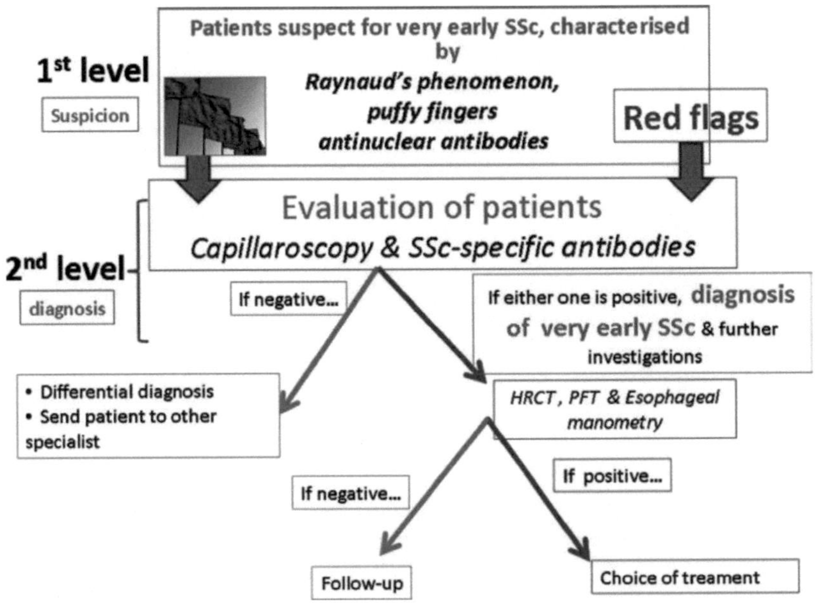

Figure 21. A behavioral flow chart for patients in whom the very early diagnosis of systemic sclerosis (SSc) should be considered is proposed. Red flags should trigger the differential diagnosis of SSc and guide the general practitioner to send the patient to the referral center where capillaroscopy and specific autoantibodies are ordered and the diagnosis of very early SSc is made. HRCT, high resolution CT; PFT, pulmonary function tests [23].

7. Conclusions

Capillaroscopy is an easily tolerable, noninvasive, important angiologic examination method. In the case of Raynaud's phenomenon, associated or not with signs or symptoms suggestive for connective tissue disorders or in the presence of autoantibodies (in particular, antinuclear antibodies (ANA) and extractable nuclear antigens (ENA)), capillaroscopy is a crucial examination that adds irreplaceable information to formulate a diagnosis. In the meantime, capillaroscopy has achieved a firm status in the early diagnosis of systemic sclerosis (SSc).

7.1. Capillaroscopic template

The report should include capillaroscopic terms understandable to nonexperts and should be as standardized as possible, using both qualitative and quantitative parameters that reliable and establishing normal limits (**Figure 22**). In the presence of capillaroscopic, more alterations (megacapillaries, microhemorrhages, neoangiogenesis, density decrease,) a greater degree of detail is required, indicating although these alterations are present on only one or a few fingers.

CAPILLAROSCOPIC TEMPLATE

Patient personal data: ___________

Medical History: Duration of Raynaud's Phenomenon, Concomitant Medication, Digital Ulcers, ecc..

Side: right ☐ – left ☐

- Structure: homogeneous/normal ☐ – inhomogeneous/abnormal ☐
- Microhaemorrhages: present ☐ – absent ☐ – number _ _
- Edema (soft focus effect): present ☐ – absent ☐
- Sub-papillary venous plexus: visible ☐ – not visible ☐
- Decreased Density: absent ☐ – localized ☐ or diffuse ☐, <30% ☐ 30-70% ☐ >70% ☐
- Tortusity: present ☐ – absent ☐
- Megacapillaries: present ☐ – absent ☐ – number _ _
- Neoangiogenesis: present ☐ – absent ☐

Conclusion/Pattern: Aspecific ☐ Scleroderma Early ☐ Scleroderma Active ☐ Scleroderma Late ☐

Prognostic Index: MES ☐ – PRINCE ☐ – CSURI ☐ Score _ _

Comments: ______________________________

Figure 22. Example of Capillaroscopic Template.

Author details

Simone Parisi* and Maria Chiara Ditto

*Address all correspondence to: simone.parisi@hotmail.it

Rheumatology Unit, Azienda Ospedaliera Universitaria Città della Salute e della Scienza di Torino, Turin, Italy

References

[1] De Angelis R, Ferri C, Sebastiani M, Manfredi A, Grassi W. La capillaroscopia in reumatologia. Lesioni elementari e metodi di scoring 2012 Mattioli 1885 Editore. ISBN: 9788862613194

[2] Van den Hoogen F, et al. Classification criteria for systemic sclerosis: An American College of Rheumatology/European League against Rheumatism collaborative initiative. Arthritis & Rheumatology. 2013 Nov;**65**(11):2737-2747

[3] Anderson ME, et al. Computerized nailfold video capillaroscopy—A new tool for assessment of Raynaud's phenomenon. Journal of Rheumatology. 2005 May;**32**(5):841-848

[4] Cutolo M. Atlas of Capillaroscopy in Rheumatic Disease. Elsevier 2010 ISBN: 9788821433917

[5] Fahrig C, et al. Capillary microscopy of the nailfold in healthy subjects. International Journal of Microcirculation. 1995 Nov-Dec;**15**(6):287-292

[6] Batticciotto A, et al. Feet nailfold capillaroscopy is not useful to detect the typical scleroderma pattern. Clinical and Experimental Rheumatology. 2012 Mar-Apr;**30**(2 Suppl 71): S116-S117

[7] Cutolo M, Sulli A, Pizzorni C, Accardo S. Nailfold videocapillaroscopy assessment of microvascular damage in systemic sclerosis. J Rheumatol. 2000 Jan;**27**(1):155-60

[8] Hoerth C, et al. Qualitative and quantitative assessment of nailfold capillaries by capillaroscopy in healthy volunteers. Vasa. 2012 Jan;**41**(1):19-26

[9] Kabasakal Y, et al. Quantitative nailfold capillaroscopy findings in a population with connective tissue disease and in normal healthy controls. Annals of the Rheumatic Diseases. 1996 Aug;**55**(8):507-512

[10] De Angelis R, et al. A growing need for capillaroscopy in rheumatology. Arthritis & Rheumatology. 2009 Mar 15;**61**(3):405-410

[11] LeRoy EC, Medsger TA Jr. Criteria for the classification of early systemic sclerosis. Journal of Rheumatology. 2001 Jul;**28**(7):1573-1576

[12] Anderson ME, Allen PD, Moore T, Jayson MI, Herrick AL. Computerized nailfold videocapillaroscopy—A new tool for assessment of Raynaud's phenomenon. Journal of Rheumatology. 2005;**32**:841-848

[13] Sulli A, Secchi ME, Pizzorni C, Cutolo M. Scoring the nailfold microvascular changes during the capillaroscopic analysis in systemic sclerosis patients. Annals of the Rheumatic Diseases 2008;**67**:885-887

[14] Sebastiani M, Manfredi A, Vukatana G, Moscatelli S, Riato L, Bocci M, Iudici M, Principato A, Mazzuca S, Del Medico P, De Angelis R, D'Amico R, Vicini R, Colaci M, Ferri C. Predictive role of capillaroscopic skin ulcer risk index in systemic sclerosis: A multicentre validation study. Annals of the Rheumatic Diseases. 2012 Jan;**71**(1):67-70

[15] Bellando-Randone S, Guiducci S, Matucci-Cerinic M. Very early diagnosis of systemic sclerosis. Polskie Archiwum Medycyny Wewnętrznej. 2012;**122**(Suppl 1):18-23

[16] Lambova S1, Hermann W, Muller-Ladner U. Nailfold capillaroscopy—Its role in diagnosis and differential diagnosis of microvascular damage in systemic sclerosis. Current Rheumatology Reviews. 2013;**9**(4):254-260

[17] Valentini G, Marcoccia A, Cuomo G, Iudici M, Vettori S. The concept of early systemic sclerosis following 2013 ACR\EULAR criteria for the classification of systemic sclerosis. Current Rheumatology Reviews. 2014;**10**(1):38-44

[18] Selva O'Callaghan A, Fonollosa-Pla V, Trallero-Araguas E, Martinez-Gomez X, Simeon Aznar CP, Labrador-Hornillo M, Vilardell-Tarres M. Nailfold capillary microscopy in adults with inflammatory myopathy. Seminars in Arthritis and Rheumatism. 2010;**39**:398-404

[19] De Angelis R, Cutolo M, Gutierrez M, Bertolazzi C, Salffi F, Grassi W. Different microvascular involvement in dermatomyositis and systemic sclerosis. A preliminary study by a tight videocapillaroscopic assessment. Clinical and Experimental Rheumatology. 2012;**30**(2 Suppl 71):S67-S70

[20] Smith V, De Keyser F, Pizzorni C, Van Praet JT, Decuman S, Sulli A, Deschepper E, Cutolo M. Nailfold capillaroscopy for day-to-day clinical use: Construction of a simple scoring modality as a clinical prognostic index for digital trophic lesions. Clinical and Experimental Rheumatology. 2011 Jan;**70**(1):180-183

[21] Sebastiani M, Manfredi A, Colaci M, D'amico R, Malagoli V, Giuggioli D, Ferri C. Capillaroscopic skin ulcer risk index: A new prognostic tool for digital skin ulcer development in systemic sclerosis patients. Arthritis & Rheumatology. 2009 May 15;**61**(5):688-694

[22] Ingegnoli F, Boracchi P, Gualtierotti R, Lubatti C, Meani L, Zahalkova L, Zeni, S, Fantini F. Prognostic model based on nailfold capillaroscopy for identifying Raynaud's phenomenon patients at high risk for the development of a scleroderma spectrum disorder: PRINCE (prognostic index for nailfold capillaroscopic examination). Arthritis & Rheumatology. 2008 Jul;**58**(7):2174-282

[23] Avouac J, Fransen J, Walker UA, Riccieri V, Smith V, Muller C, Miniati I, Tarner IH, Randone SB, Cutolo M, Allanore Y, Distler O, Valentini G, Czirjak L, Müller-Ladner U, Furst DE, Tyndall A, Matucci-Cerinic M; EUSTAR Group. Preliminary criteria for the very early diagnosis of systemic sclerosis: Results of a Delphi Consensus Study from EULAR Scleroderma Trials and Research Group. Annals of the Rheumatic Diseases. 2011 Mar;**70**(3):476-481

[24] Guiducci S, Bellando-Randone S, Matucci-Cerinic M. A new way of thinking about systemic sclerosis: The opportunity for a very early diagnosis. The Israel Medicine Association Journal. 2016 Mar-Apr;**18**(3-4):141-143

Chapter 6

Ophthalmological Manifestations and Tear Investigations in Systemic Sclerosis

Aniko Rentka, Krisztina Koroskenyi, Jolan Harsfalvi, Zoltan Szekanecz, Gabriella Szucs, Peter Szodoray and Adam Kemeny-Beke

Additional information is available at the end of the chapter

http://dx.doi.org/10.5772/intechopen.69909

Abstract

Systemic sclerosis (SSc) is a chronic autoimmune disorder characterized by widespread small vessel vasculopathy, immune dysregulation with production of autoantibodies, and progressive fibrosis. There are only few reports available concerning ophthalmological complications in the course of SSc, although ocular manifestations, e.g., dry eye syndrome (DES), occurs frequently and decreases the quality of life of these patients. Vascular endothelial growth factor (VEGF), the major pro-angiogenic factor, plays a key role in the pathomechanism of SSc. Although elevated levels of VEGF in sera have already been demonstrated, VEGF analysis in tears of patients with SSc has not been performed in previous studies. VEGF in the tears of patients with SSc was found to be decreased by 20%, compared to healthy controls. The reason why the VEGF levels are not elevated in the tears of patients with SSc needs further investigations, as does the sera of the same patients. The cytokine array results revealed a shift in the cytokine profile characterized by the predominance of inflammatory mediators. Our current data depict a group of cytokines and chemokines, which play a significant role in ocular pathology of SSc; furthermore, they might function as excellent candidates for future therapeutic targets in SSc with ocular manifestations.

Keywords: systemic sclerosis, dry eye syndrome, tear, vascular endothelial growth factor, cytokine, tear sampling, total protein, enzyme-linked immunosorbent assay, cytokine array, multiplex bead assay

1. Introduction

There are few reports, mainly case reports, available concerning ophthalmological complications in the course of systemic sclerosis (SSc). Overall studies are even fewer involving only a small number of patients, since SSc is a rare disease [1, 2]. Changes in the organ of vision are thought to be the consequences of systemic complications of scleroderma or adverse effects of the immunosuppressive treatment applied. Ocular symptoms may occur at any stage of the disease and may involve numerous ocular tissues. Their course can be clinically latent or very intensive. The most prevalent clinical manifestations of soft tissue fibrosis and inflammation in patients with SSc include increased tonus and telangiectasia of the eyelid skin. The most common lesions reported include periorbital edema, palpebral ectropion, and madarosis [3].

The most frequent ocular manifestation of SSc in our studies was dry eye syndrome (DES).

DES is a major healthcare problem because it affects the patient's quality of life. DES in SSc is believed to be caused by fibrosis-related impairment of lacrimal gland secretion, namely, the reduction of the water portion of the tear film. Furthermore, lipid layer disorder is caused by chronic blepharitis and meibomian gland dysfunction (MGD), while increased evaporation of tears from the ocular surface is the consequence of restricted eyelid mobility and the consecutive reduced blinking [2]. DES was recently redefined as a multifactorial disease of the tears and ocular surface that results in symptoms of discomfort, visual disturbance, tear film instability, and last but not least damage to the ocular surface [4]. Increased osmolality of the tear film [5] and inflammation of the ocular surface [6] are the two major characteristic features of this ocular surface disease. The most important laboratory findings [6] are increased levels of several inflammatory cytokines. Accordingly, tear cytokine levels are regarded as potential markers of inflammation in DES.

The ophthalmological manifestations in patients with SSc are frequently underestimated and not or not correctly treated. In order to better understand the ocular features and use this body fluid as a potential tool for monitoring these important biomarkers, we have turned our attention to tear investigations.

Precorneal tears as a biological fluid are very easily accessible with non- or very low-invasive methods at a relatively low cost. Tears not only lubricate the ocular surface carrying secreted molecules from corneal epithelial cells and tissues producing tear components but also represent the whole physiological status of the body. Due to the very limited amount of samples and the relative instability of the components, sample collection is a critical step in tear research and diagnostics.

Although tear analysis is of increasing interest in ophthalmology, no studies have investigated tears of patients with SSc as yet, possibly because of the technical challenge posed by the extremely small sample volumes available [7].

Quantitative determination of tear proteins is of increasing interest in ophthalmology, but a technical problem still remains due to small tear sample volumes available on the one hand and the complexity of their composition on the other [7, 8]. Tear sampling performed either directly or indirectly is definitely a major challenge or has a most significant influence on the precision and reproducibility of the analytical results as seen in the summary below.

1.1. Direct sampling methods

Direct sampling methods use microcapillary tubes [9] or micropipettes for sampling. This requires previous stimulation or instillation of different volumes of saline (100–200 μl) into the cul-de-sac and collecting after appropriate mixing. The procedure causes dilution and may not permit collection of samples from specific sites of the ocular surface [10].

Kalsow et al. investigated the tear cytokine response to multipurpose solutions in contact lens [11] wearing. Before tear collection, contact lens was removed, and then NST tears were collected from both eyes from the inferior lateral conjunctival cul-de-sac using a 10-μl flame-polished glass micropipette. The collection, a 5.5-μl tear volume, was immediately transported to a sterile 0.2-ml tube containing 49.5 μl of storage solution to produce a 1:10 tear dilution for immediate storage at −80°C [11].

Guyette et al. compared low-abundance biomarker levels in capillary-collected NST tears and washout (WO) tears of aqueous-deficient and normal patients. 10-microliter polished micropipettes were used to collect tears from the inferior marginal strip, taking special care to minimize ocular surface contact. Tear collection rate was continuously monitored. Individual NST tear samples were collected in 10-min aliquots and immediately transferred to a sterile polymerase chain reaction (PCR) tube. An equal volume of assay buffer was added, and the sample was stored at −86°C. A total of at least 6.5-μl NST tears were collected from each study participant, and each 10-min aliquot was transferred into a separate PCR tube and put in the freezer without delay. Prior to WO tear sample collection, 10-μl sterile physiologic saline solution was added to the lower conjunctiva by a digital pipette. The patient was instructed to gently close the eyes and avoid any eye movements for one minute. Tears were then collected using the same method as for NST samples, but a shorter collection time of 5 min per aliquot was used to make up the 6.5-μl minimum volume required. Tear collection volume and time were continuously monitored to measure tear collection rate [12].

There have been several research projects focusing on dry eye syndrome, and nowadays the emphasis has shifted toward the role of inflammation in the anterior surface of the eye [13]. Since inflammatory mediators originating from various ocular surface sources and the main lacrimal gland do not constitute a totally homogenous mix, the way the tears are collected will influence the resulting biomarker profile. NST tear samples from the inferior marginal strip cover a broader spectrum of the sources, whereas ST samples contain a higher proportion of the lacrimal gland secretion [14]. Explicit protein profile differences between NST and ST tears demonstrate that these two sample types are not equivalent [15, 16]. Although NST tears represent specifically the inflammatory status of the ocular surface, the volume of NST tears is limited, especially in aqueous-deficient dry eye. Even though tear sampling frequently makes use of capillaries as they are less irritating and the resulting sample is an exact representative concentration of molecules, the main limitation of the method is the volume of sample (2–3 μl) to be gained [17].

One way to increase the available tear sample volume is to add fluid (e.g., sterile saline) to the eye prior to sample collection, effectively "washing out" ocular surface molecules [18, 19].

In an experimental dry eye study, Luo et al. collected tears from mice with tear fluid washing [20]. Tear fluid washings were collected by a method previously reported by Song et al. [21]. Briefly, 1.5 μl of phosphate buffered saline (PBS) containing 0.1% bovine serum albumin (BSA) was instilled into the conjunctival sac. The tear fluid and buffer were collected with a 10-μl volume glass capillary tube by capillary action from the tear meniscus in the lateral canthus. The 2-μl sample of tear washings was pooled from both eyes of each mouse and was stored at −80°C until zymography and enzyme-linked immunosorbent assay (ELISA) were performed.

Validity of the WO method depends on the extent to which it changes the NST tear biomarker profile. By determining tear sIgA, inducement of reflex tearing is easily detected because tear sIgA levels decrease with reflex tear flow rate [16]. Markoulli et al. found equal tear sIgA-total tear ratios in WO and NST tears, which suggests that WO tear samples do not significantly induce reflex tearing [19]. Guyette's study evaluated WO tear collection as a replacement for microcapillary NST tear collection and applied this to compare biomarker levels between aqueous-deficient (AD) dry eye and non-AD patients [12, 15, 22].

1.2. Indirect methods

An indirect method means that collection of precorneal tear film (PTF) is carried out using absorbing supports such as Schirmer test strips (STS), filter paper disks, cellulose sponges, and polyester rods. STS collection is the most commonly used method among them [23].

Acera et al. analyzed the inflammatory markers in the PTF of patients with ocular surface disease. 10 μl of tear samples was collected by a Weck-Cel sponge [24]. The concentrations of IL-1β, IL-6, and pro-MMP-9 were measured by ELISA, and the MMP-9 activity was evaluated by gelatin zymography.

Inic-Kanada et al. compared ophthalmic sponges and extraction buffers for quantifying cytokine profiles in tears using Luminex technology. They found that Luminex detection of cytokine/chemokine profiles of tears collected with Merocel sponges may be useful in clinical studies, for instance, to assess cytokine profile evaluation in ocular surface diseases [25].

Samples obtained from the Schirmer test procedure have been found to have a higher mucus, lipid, and cellular content than microcapillary (MC) samples [26]. STS also suffers from incomplete, nonuniform elution of proteins from the filter matrix [23]. Although micropipette and STS collection provide different biomarker profiles for a given donor, the correctly applied micropipette method has proved to be more consistent [27]. STS is widely applied as the volume of sample collected with this method is larger than other methods, but it can cause reflexive tearing due to irritation, which increases the volume of the samples, thus aggravating the detection of the investigated tear component(s), e.g., drug levels [9].

In comparative studies, the tears of the same patient are collected using several collection methods to determine the same biomarkers from the different tear samples.

Green-Church et al. collected tears using small volume (1–5 μl) Drummond glass MC tubes with 1.6× slit-lamp magnification. Non-reflex tears were collected from the inferior tear prism without contact with the lower lid until a total of 5 μl had been collected. During a separate visit, tear collection was performed by placing an STS over the lower lid. The lid was canthus. The subject was instructed to close his/her eyes for the 5-min test duration; the wet length was not recorded but was observed to be within normal ranges in all cases. The STS was then placed in 1.6-ml amber Eppendorf tube and stored at 4°C until analysis [27].

Lee et al. used two collection techniques for the comparative analysis of polymerase chain reaction assay for herpes simplex virus 1 detection [28]. Tear samples were collected from the lower fornix using STS for 5 min, a method adopted in a previous study of Satpathy et al. [29]. The other collection method they used was micropipetting tears, after irrigating 100-μl saline in the lower fornix, a method that was described in a previous study of Markoulli et al. [19], who validated the "flush" tear collection technique as a viable alternative to basal and reflex tear collection.

2. "Main body of the paper"

The aims of our studies were the following:

1. To select an appropriate sampling method to investigate vascular endothelial growth factor (VEGF) and cytokines in tears of SSc patients.
2. To detect VEGF in tears of SSc patients.
3. To compare VEGF levels in tears of patients with SSc to those in healthy controls.
4. To determine a wider panel of cytokines and chemokines that have a role in immunopathogenesis and inflammatory processes in tears of patients with SSc.
5. To compare the levels of identified mediators in tears of these patients and controls and to select the most significantly differing ones for further investigations.
6. To determine the selected mediators with the help of a more sensitive and specific laboratory method in tears of both patients and controls.

2.1. Patients and healthy controls

In the first study, 43 patients with SSc (40 female and 3 men) and 27 healthy controls were included. In the second study, we enrolled 9 patients and 12 controls. Mean (SD) age of the patients was 61.85 (48–74) years. SSc was diagnosed based on the corresponding international criteria. Patients were enrolled from the outpatient clinic at the Department of Rheumatology. They went through ophthalmological examination and basal tear sample collection at the Department of Ophthalmology. None of the patients had secondary Sjögren's syndrome. The healthy control groups were composed of age- and gender-matched volunteers with no history of any autoimmune or ocular disorder. Patients did not take immunosuppressive medications at the time of the tear sampling.

Written informed consent was obtained from all patients and controls. Study protocol was approved by the local bioethics committee and followed the tenets of the declaration of Helsinki.

2.2. Tear sample collection

Unstimulated, open-eye tear samples were gently collected from the inferior temporal meniscus of both eyes, using glass capillary tubes (Haematokritkapillare, 75 μL, L 75 mm, Hirschmann Laborgerate, Germany), minimizing irritation of the ocular surface or lid margin as much as possible.

In the course of the first study, samples were collected between 11 a.m. and 16 p.m. by the same physician. Tear-secretion velocity was counted by dividing the volume of collected sample with time of secretion. Volume was calculated from the lengths of the fluid column in the capillary tube, measured with a vernier caliper, and from the known diameter of the tube. Time of tear collection was measured with a stopwatch.

In the course of the second study, tear collection was performed between 9 and 11 a.m.

Tears were transferred into low-binding-capacity Eppendorf tubes by the help of a sterile syringe and a needle, carried on dry ice to the laboratory and stored at −80°C until assessment. The samples were obtained from both eyes of each individual and were pooled due to the small volume available.

2.3. Quantification of total protein and VEGF levels in tear samples of patients with SSc

First, as a point of reference for VEGF, total tear protein concentrations were determined using the microplate method of the bicinchoninic acid (BCA) Protein Assay Kit (Pierce Biotechnology, Rockford, USA) adapted to a 384-well microplate due to the small sample amounts. The kit is a two-component, high-precision, detergent-compatible assay. Total protein concentration determination was based on color intensity measurement proportional to the peptide bound and the protein provided with the reagent set. The reaction absorbs visible light, namely, the wavelength 562 nm.

We used a human VEGF immunoassay kit by Quantikine (R&D Systems, Minneapolis, MN, USA) for the quantitative determination of VEGF in tear fluid. This assay employs the quantitative sandwich enzyme immunoassay technique.

2.4. Membrane array and multiplex bead analysis of tear cytokines in SSc

To remove cells, cellular debris, and contaminant particles, tear samples were centrifuged (10 min, 15,000 rpm, 4°C) prior to use.

Tear samples of controls and patients were used for cytokine profiling. The relative levels of 102 different cytokines were determined by Proteome Profiler Human XL Cytokine Array Kit (R&D Systems) using 50-μl samples according to the manufacturer's instructions. The pixel density in each spot of the array was determined by ImageJ software.

Alternatively, the absolute levels of MCP-1, complement factor D (CFD), IP-10, and C-reactive protein (CRP) were determined from diluted tear samples (CFD, MCP-1, and CRP, 1:10; IP-10, 1:40) by Human Luminex Performance Assays (R&D Systems) according to the manufacturer's instructions. The measurement was run on Bio-Plex 200 Systems (Bio-Rad) workstation.

2.5. Results

2.5.1. Vascular endothelial growth factor in tear samples of patients with systemic sclerosis

The average tear secretion velocity in patients was 4.53 μl/min with a median of 3.8 μl/min (1.5–25.6).

Duration of tear sample collection from patients varied between 20 and 313 s, until 5 μl, the minimally required volume was reached.

The average collected tear fluid volume was 10.4 μl (1.6–31.2) in patients and 15.63 μl (3.68–34.5) in controls.

In tear samples of patients with SSc, the average total protein level was 6.9 μg/μl (1.8–12.3), and the average concentration of VEGF was 4.9 pg/μl (3.5–8.1) in the case of basal tear secretion.

Control tears contained on average 4.132 μg/μl (0.1–14.1) protein and 6.15 pg/μl (3.84–12.3) VEGF.

2.5.2. Membrane array and multiplex bead analysis of tear cytokines in systemic sclerosis

2.5.2.1. Cytokine array results

Nonstimulated tear cytokine profiles of the control groups and patients with SSc were analyzed by cytokine array detecting 102 different cytokines. Array results revealed a shift in cytokine profile characterized by the predominance of inflammatory mediators. The following 9 out of the 102 analyzed molecules were significantly increased in tears of patients with SSc: complement factor D (CFD), chitinase-3-like protein 1 (CHI3L1), C-reactive protein (CRP), epidermal growth factor (EGF), interferon-γ-inducible protein 10 (IP-10, also called CXCL-10), monocyte chemoattractant protein-1 (MCP-1), monokine induced by gamma interferon (MIG), matrix metallopeptidase 9 (MMP-9), and vitamin D binding protein (VDBP) (**Table 1**).

Integrated density values were normalized to positive control spots and total protein content of the samples. Cytokine array data are representative of four control and four SSc samples.

Name of the cytokines and chemokines	Normalized density—patients with SSc	Normalized density—healthy controls	Significance of the difference (p)
CFD	50.35 (23.17–53.76)	22.33 (18.39–24.75)	0.002072
CHI3L1	94.41 (31.9–95.98)	31.06 (20.37–45.85)	0.000000
CRP	25.98 (15.28–53.16)	4.55 (4.35–4.66)	0.018250
EGF	53.42 (34.86–70.23)	34.04 (20.42–47.61)	0.032818
IP-10	123.42 (93.81–152.35)	21.99 (12.12–29.01)	0.000000
MCP-1	19.93 (5.38–42.44)	1.72 (1.44–2.27)	0.044726
MIG	22.85 (5.6–64.14)	3.58 (3.29–3.88)	0.033787
MMP-9	49.10 (4.24–129.04)	12.74 (10.29–17.56)	0.000068
VDBP	31.35 (11.87–64.68)	10.18 (8.3–13.84)	0.019733

Mean total protein values did not differ significantly in tears of patients and controls. Mean total protein value was 40.9239 μg/ml in tears of patients with SSc and 42.536 μg/ml in tears of healthy controls (p = 0.863604).

Table 1. Normalized densities of cytokines and chemokines in patients with SSc and healthy controls.

2.5.2.2. Multiplex cytokine bead assay results

By using the more sensitive and more specific Luminex bead assay, 4 selected molecules were determined in tears of 9 healthy controls and 12 patients with SSc.

Based on the Luminex bead results, mean CRP levels were 103.44 (3.57–359.02) μg/mg protein in tears of patients with SSc and 7.41 (0.87–18.03) μg/mg protein in tears of healthy controls.

Mean IP-10 levels were 564.78 (252.62–1107.2) μg/mg protein in tears of patients with SSc and 196.118 (101.66–514.37) μg/mg protein in tears of healthy controls.

Mean MCP-1 levels were 2626.83 (457.84–5619.4) μg/mg protein in tears of patients with SSc and 661.27 (397.87–1171.4) μg/mg protein in tears of healthy controls.

Mean CFD levels were 15.27 (5.00–35.28) μg/mg protein in tears of patients with SSc and 23.31 (5.18–106.63) μg/mg protein in tears of healthy controls.

Except for CFD all results were significant at p = 0.01 for CRP, p = 0.001 for IP-10, and p = 0.01 for MCP-1, respectively.

Values represent the mean (±SD) of the 9 control and 12 patient samples, which are the fold change of normalized cytokine levels.

The difference between total protein values of control and SSc tear samples was not significant (p = 0.37263). Mean total protein was 818.46 (779.94–1162.4) μg/ml in tears of patients and 872.46 (771.78–1359.5) μg/ml in tears of controls.

Based on both the cytokine array and the multiplex bead assay results, concentrations of IP-10 showed the most significant difference in tears of patients and controls.

http://dx.doi.org/10.5772/intechopen.69909

2.6. Discussion

Although ocular manifestations in systemic autoimmune diseases have significant debilitating effects, tear analysis has been missing from the repertoire of investigations. Since tears represent the local homeostasis of the ocular surface better than serum, this makes tears ideal for assessing ocular pathology in the disease. There are two possible ways for cytokines to appear in the precorneal tear film. Some are locally produced and diffuse into the tear film from the corneal and conjunctival epithelia; others leak into the tear film from the conjunctival blood vessels [30]. Tear investigation is a challenging research field; though sample collection is noninvasive, it has an almost insurmountable limitation, the quantity of the sample obtainable [31].

Tear investigation studies have been performed in different ocular and systemic disorders [30, 32, 33]. Leonardi et al. assessed multiple mediators, such as cytokines, matrix metalloproteases, and angiogenic and growth factors in tears of patients with vernal keratoconjunctivitis. These analyses identified previously unreported factors in tears of patients, including MMP-3 and MMP-10 and multiple proteases, growth factors and cytokines, which may all be instrumental in the pathogenesis of conjunctival inflammation. Different molecules were identified in human tear samples that were involved in the development and maintenance of corneal neovascularization. Concentrations of the pro-angiogenic cytokines such as IL-6, IL-8, VEGF, MCP-1, and Fas ligand were determined in blood and tear samples using flow cytometry-based multiplex assay. These investigations resulted in significantly higher concentrations of pro-angiogenic cytokines in human tears compared to their concentrations in serum; furthermore highest levels were revealed in basal tear samples [30]. These findings lend further support to the importance of our current studies.

After reviewing the literature on direct and indirect tear sampling methods in various ocular and systemic disorders, we have chosen the microcapillary method for tear sampling in patients with SSc, since it is safely applicable for the collection of nonstimulated tears. In order to transfer the tear fluid from the microcapillary tube to the collection tube, we applied a sterile syringe and a needle. This tear sampling method proved to be suitable for our experiments on tear cytokines.

2.6.1. VEGF in tear samples of patients with SSc

VEGF is one of the components of normal tear fluid [34]. Vesaluoma et al. determined VEGF concentrations in healthy tears. The median VEGF concentration was 5 pg/μl (4–11) consistent with our results, as control tears contained an average of 6.15 pg/μl (3.84–12.3) VEGF [35].

They calculated the average tear fluid secretion in healthy controls, which was 8.1 μl/min (0.7–20.8), using the same tear collecting method as we did in our study. Results show that patients with SSc have significantly decreased tear secretion that could be explained by DES, which is a probable sequel of the disease or to the side effects of the therapeutic drugs [36].

Tear-secretion velocity was lower by 67% in patients with SSc than in healthy controls. The difference was significant ($p < 0.01$). The reason for this sign could be explained by the pathophysiology of the disease, namely, fibrotic processes of the lacrimal gland.

Total protein values in patients with SSc were higher by 42% than in healthy controls. This may indicate that total protein production—or simply protein concentration, since patients with SSc have a decreased tear secretion velocity—is only increased because of the smaller tear volume. VEGF in the tears of patients with SSc decreased by 20%, which can be explained also by the decreased tear secretion of patients [36].

The question why contrary to our expectations VEGF levels are not higher in patients with SSc than in the healthy group needs further investigation.

2.6.2. Membrane array and multiplex bead analysis of tear cytokines in SSc

Based on our cytokine array results, nine cytokines and chemokines had significantly higher levels in tears of patients with SSc. This screening method was performed for the assortment of 102 cytokines, selecting the most relevant ones in the pathogenesis of SSc for further experiments. All molecules which appeared to be significantly higher in tears of patients are molecular players of the immune responses and inflammatory processes, which confirms the presence of ocular surface inflammation in patients with SSc possibly as a consequence of DES [36].

CHI3L1, a protein which takes part in the processes of inflammation and tissue remodeling, has not been previously described in relation to the pathomechanism of SSc. We have found elevated levels of CHI3L1 in patients with SSc. This result correlates well with the fact that inflammation and tissue injury caused by hypoxia and oxidative stress are always present in the course of SSc.

In fact, different pathways may lead to vascular dysfunction processes in SSc, such as direct vascular damage or pro-inflammatory responses. Studies in different diseases have shown functional links between activated complement molecules and these pathways. CFD, a serine protease, also known as adipsin, plays a key role in these processes [37, 38]. CFD is the rate-limiting enzyme in the activation cascade of the alternative pathway, and its level in the blood is quite low. Our cytokine array results showed increased CFD levels, which confirm the role of the complement system in the ocular pathology of SSc.

Levels of EGF were also elevated in tear samples of patients with SSc. EGF is a growth factor that stimulates cell growth, proliferation, and differentiation [39]. Elevation of EGF may be explained by the above processes of vasculopathy. The next molecule, which appeared to be higher in patients' tears, is matrix metallopeptidase-9 (MMP-9). As a protease of the MMP family, it is involved in the breakdown of extracellular matrix in normal physiological processes, such as embryonic development, reproduction, angiogenesis, bone development, wound healing, cell migration, as well as in pathological processes, such as intracerebral hemorrhage, arthritis, and metastasis [40–42]. In a study of Kim et al., serum MMP-9 concentrations were found to be elevated in patients with SSc correlating well with skin scores [43]. Their results suggest that increased MMP-9 concentrations may be due to their overproduction by dermal fibroblasts and also that the enhanced production of MMP-9 may contribute to fibrogenic remodeling during the progression of skin sclerosis in SSc. Our results of tear cytokine array are parallel with the finding that MMP-9 is increased in the course of SSc.

In a previous study, expression of antiangiogenic chemokines and their receptors were determined in the sera and skin of patients with SSc [44]. Based on their results, MIG and its receptor are elevated in serum and highly expressed in the skin of patients with SSc. We have also found increased levels of MIG in tear samples of patients, which confirm the fact that dysregulated angiogenesis is an important feature in the pathomechanism of SSc. The next protein that appeared to be higher is VDBP, a member of the albumin gene family. VDBP is a multifunctional protein found in plasma, ascitic and cerebrospinal fluid and on the surface of many cell types. It binds to vitamin D and its plasma metabolites and transports them to target tissues [45]. Others have measured significant quantities of VDBP-actin complexes in the plasma following injury [46]. The presence of tissue injury is likely to be the explanation of our results, namely, the elevated levels of VDBP in the tears of patients with SSc.

Based on our results of multiplex bead assay, the three molecules that showed significant differences in tears of patients and controls were IP-10, MCP-1, and CRP. Previous studies have already demonstrated elevated levels of these markers in the sera of patients with SSc.

General markers of inflammation, such as CRP, are expected to be higher in a disease like SSc. In earlier trials, CRP appeared to be elevated in the sera of patients with SSc and was associated with poor survival. Therefore, it may be a useful indicator of disease activity and severity in SSc [47, 48].

Another inflammatory chemokine, IP-10, also called CXCL-10, has often been investigated in SSc studies [44, 49, 50]. IP-10 has an angiostatic function as it suppresses neovascularization; furthermore, it is involved in immune regulation [51].

Recent reports have shown that the serum and/or the tissue expressions of IP-10 are increased in various bacterial, viral, fungal, and protozoal infections [52] and also in autoimmune diseases like rheumatoid arthritis, systemic lupus erythematosus, multiple sclerosis, autoimmune thyroid diseases, type 1 diabetes mellitus, Addison's disease, and SSc [50, 53–55]. CXCL10 is secreted by CD4+, CD8+, natural killer and natural killer T cells and is dependent on interferon-γ. CXCL10 can also be secreted by several other cell types, including endothelial cells, fibroblasts, keratinocytes, thyrocytes, preadipocytes, etc. Detecting a high level of CXCL10 in peripheral fluids is therefore a marker of host immune response [48], which correlates well with our results of cytokine bead assay measurements.

Finally, MCP-1, which is a key participant of the fibrotic processes in SSc, also appeared to be higher in patients' tears. MCP-1, which recruits monocytes, memory T cells, and dendritic cells to the sites of inflammation, is produced by either tissue injury or infection [56]. It is known as one of the most pathogenic chemokines during the development of inflammation and fibrosis in SSc [57]. MCP-1 is not only a chemoattractant molecule for monocytes and T cells, but it also induces Th2 cell polarization and stimulates collagen production by fibroblasts [58]. Hasegawa et al. have previously shown that serum MCP-1 levels are elevated when the skin and lung are affected in patients with SSc [59]. It has also been reported that cultured dermal fibroblasts from patients with SSc show augmented expressions of MCP-1 mRNA and protein [60].

Of the last three molecules, IP-10 and MCP-1 are the ones whose molecular characteristics single them out as potential candidates for therapies against the pathological consequences of diseases such as SSc.

2.7. Novel findings

1. After reviewing the literature of tear sampling techniques, we labored the adequate tear sampling methods and collected tears with capillary system from SSc patients in order to investigate VEGF molecule and cytokines.
2. We were the first to demonstrate the presence and concentration of VEGF, an element that plays an important vascular role in the pathogenesis of SSc, with the help of a method that is based on a quantitative sandwich immunoassay technique.
3. By the help of our survey, which is based on a quantitative sandwich immunoassay technique, we were able to verify a 20% reduction in the VEGF concentration in tears of SSc patients compared to healthy controls.
4. We were the first to establish a wide cytokine profile in tears of SSc patients using an array that monitors 102 cytokines simultaneously.
5. Based on our cytokine array results, we revealed that 9 out of the 102 cytokines and chemokines had significantly higher levels in tears of patients with SSc. All of them are molecular players of the immune responses and the inflammatory processes. These findings legitimate the existence of ocular surface inflammations which are quite frequent in patients with SSc. In addition, they are in accordance with former study results regarding the pathomechanism of SSc.
6. By using a highly sensitive and specific multiplex bead assay, we were the first to demonstrate increased levels of IP-10, MCP-1, and CRP in tear samples of patients with SSc. Previous studies have already demonstrated elevated levels of these biomarkers in the sera of these patients; therefore tear analysis is to be raised as a potential means in dealing with diagnostic, prognostic, and maybe even therapeutic challenges of SSc.

2.8. Future plans

Angiogenesis impairment in SSc has been proved by several researchers. A number of serum investigations have been carried out regarding this phenomenon, but there are only scant data concerning tears of SSc patients.

The issue why the VEGF levels are not higher in SSc patients than in the healthy group needs further investigation. Other biochemical methods, like PCR, would be feasible to confirm array results. Furthermore, a longer-term prospective study in a larger population with extension of the ophthalmological examinations is needed to confirm clinical utility.

Our current data depict a group of inflammatory mediators, which may play a significant role in ocular pathology of SSc. Monitoring these factors in the tears of patients with SSc can be a noninvasive alternative to serum investigation. Additionally, in patients with ocular manifestations, such as DES, tear analysis is far more informative; it provides information of the ocular surface; hence it could help us choose the appropriate treatment, in particular artificial tears or anti-inflammatory eye drops [36]. Further studies are needed to understand the signaling pathways regulating pro-inflammatory cytokines, with the aim of developing new interventions against autoimmune diseases mediated by cytokines and chemokines, as well as inventing novel therapeutic possibilities for the ocular manifestations of SSc. New inflammatory mediators are to be searched that might function as excellent candidates for future therapeutic targets in SSc with ocular manifestations.

Acknowledgements

Parts of this chapter are reproduced from authors' recent work mentioned in the "Reference" section and properly cited in the body of the chapter (Refs. [34, 36]). Permission from authors/publishers for the usage of the content of their articles has been obtained.

Nomenclatures

AD	Aqueous deficient
BCA	Bicinchoninic acid
CD	Cluster of differentiation
CFD	Complement factor D
CHI3L1	Chitinase-3-like protein 1
CRP	C-reactive protein
CXCL	Chemokine (C-X-C motif) ligand
DES	Dry eye syndrome
EGF	Epidermal growth factor
ELISA	Enzyme-linked immunosorbent assay
IFN	Interferon
IL	Interleukin
ILD	Interstitial lung disease
IP-10	Interferon gamma-induced protein-10
MC	Microcapillary tubes
MCP	Monocyte chemoattractant protein
MGD	Meibomian gland dysfunction
MIG	Monokine induced by gamma interferon
MMP	Matrix metalloproteinase
mRNA	Messenger ribonucleic acid
NST	Nonstimulated tear

PCR	Polymerase chain reaction
PTF	Precorneal tear filmRNARibonucleic acid
RNP	Ribonucleoprotein
sIgA	Secretory immunoglobulin A
SSc	Systemic sclerosis
ST	Stimulated tear
STS	Schirmer test strip
TGF-β	Transforming growth factor-beta
TNF-α	Tumor necrosis factor-alpha
TRIM	Tripartite motif
VDBP	Vitamin D binding protein
VEGF	Vascular endothelial growth factor
WO	Washout

Author details

Aniko Rentka[1], Krisztina Koroskenyi[2], Jolan Harsfalvi[3], Zoltan Szekanecz[4], Gabriella Szucs[4], Peter Szodoray[5] and Adam Kemeny-Beke[1]*

*Address all correspondence to: kemenyba@med.unideb.hu

1 Department of Ophthalmology, Faculty of Medicine, University of Debrecen, Debrecen, Hungary

2 Department of Biochemistry and Molecular Biology, Signaling and Apoptosis Research Group, Hungarian Academy of Sciences, Research Center of Molecular Medicine, University of Debrecen, Debrecen, Hungary

3 Department of Biophysics and Radiation Biology, Semmelweis University, Budapest, Hungary

4 Department of Rheumatology, Institute of Medicine, Faculty of Medicine, University of Debrecen, Debrecen, Hungary

5 Institute of Immunology, Rikshospitalet, Oslo University Hospital, Oslo, Norway

References

[1] Gomes Bde A, Santhiago MR, Magalhaes P, Kara-Junior N, Azevedo MN, Moraes HV, Jr. Ocular findings in patients with systemic sclerosis. Clinics (São Paulo, Brazil). 2011;**66**(3):379-385

[2] Waszczykowska A, Gos R, Waszczykowska E, Dziankowska-Bartkowiak B, Jurowski P. Prevalence of ocular manifestations in systemic sclerosis patients. Archives of Medical Science. 2013;**9**(6):1107-1113

[3] Albert D, Jakobiec, FA. Principles and Practice of Ophthalmology. 5th ed. Philadelphia: W.B.Saunders Company; 2000

[4] Plastiras S. The definition and classification of dry eye disease: Report of the definition and classification subcommittee of the international dry eye workshop (2007). The Ocular Surface. 2007;**5**(2):75-92

[5] Farris RL, Stuchell RN, Mandel ID. Tear osmolarity variation in the dry eye. Transactions of the American Ophthalmological Society. 1986;**84**:250-268

[6] Pflugfelder SC, Jones D, Ji Z, Afonso A, Monroy D. Altered cytokine balance in the tear fluid and conjunctiva of patients with Sjogren's syndrome keratoconjunctivitis sicca. Current Eye Research. 1999;**19**(3):201-211

[7] Li K, Chen Z, Duan F, Liang J, Wu K. Quantification of tear proteins by SDS-PAGE with an internal standard protein: A new method with special reference to small volume tears. Graefes Archive for Clinical and Experimental Ophthalmology. 2010;**248**(6):853-862

[8] Geerling G, Maclennan S, Hartwig D. Autologous serum eye drops for ocular surface disorders. Br J Ophthalmol. 2004;**88**(11):1467-74

[9] Pistillo MP, Ferrara GB, Reed E, Brensilver J, McCabe R, Benvensity A, et al. Detection of anti-idiotypic antibodies to HLA (anti-anti-HLA antibodies) by use of human monoclonal antibodies. Transplantation Proceedings. 1989;**21**(1 Pt 1):760-761

[10] Small D, Hevy J, Tang-Liu D. Comparison of tear sampling techniques for pharmacokinetics analysis: Ofloxacin concentrations in rabbit tears after sampling with schirmer tear strips, capillary tubes, or surgical sponges. Journal of Ocular Pharmacology and Therapeutics. 2000;**16**(5):439-446

[11] Kalsow CM, Reindel WT, Merchea MM, Bateman KM, Barr JT. Tear cytokine response to multipurpose solutions for contact lenses. Clinical Ophthalmology. 2013;**7**:1291-1302

[12] Guyette N, Williams L, Tran MT, Than T, Bradley J, Kehinde L, et al. Comparison of low-abundance biomarker levels in capillary-collected nonstimulated tears and washout tears of aqueous-deficient and normal patients. Investigative Ophthalmology & Visual Science. 2013;**54**(5):3729-3737

[13] Research in dry eye: Report of the Research Subcommittee of the International Dry Eye WorkShop (2007). The Ocular Surface. 2007;**5**(2):179-193

[14] Tiffany JM. The normal tear film. Developments in Ophthalmology. 2008;**41**:1-20

[15] Fullard RJ, Snyder C. Protein levels in nonstimulated and stimulated tears of normal human subjects. Investigative Ophthalmology & Visual Science. 1990;**31**(6):1119-1126

[16] Fullard RJ, Tucker D. Tear protein composition and the effects of stimulus. Advances in Experimental Medicine and Biology. 1994;**350**:309-314

[17] Mishima S, Gasset A, Klyce SD, Jr., Baum JL. Determination of tear volume and tear flow. Investigative Ophthalmology. 1966;**5**(3):264-276

[18] Bjerrum KB, Prause JU. Collection and concentration of tear proteins studied by SDS gel electrophoresis. Presentation of a new method with special reference to dry eye patients. Graefes Archive for Clinical and Experimental Ophthalmology. 1994;**232**(7):402-405

[19] Markoulli M, Papas E, Petznick A, Holden B. Validation of the flush method as an alternative to basal or reflex tear collection. Current Eye Research. 2011;**36**(3):198-207

[20] Luo L, Li DQ, Doshi A, Farley W, Corrales RM, Pflugfelder SC. Experimental dry eye stimulates production of inflammatory cytokines and MMP-9 and activates MAPK signaling pathways on the ocular surface. Investigative Ophthalmology & Visual Science. 2004;**45**(12):4293-4301

[21] Song XJ, Li DQ, Farley W, Luo LH, Heuckeroth RO, Milbrandt J, et al. Neurturin-deficient mice develop dry eye and keratoconjunctivitis sicca. Investigative Ophthalmology & Visual Science. 2003;**44**(10):4223-4229

[22] Senchyna M, Wax MB. Quantitative assessment of tear production: A review of methods and utility in dry eye drug discovery. Journal of Ocular Biology, Diseases, and Informatics. 2008;**1**(1):1-6

[23] VanDerMeid KR, Su SP, Krenzer KL, Ward KW, Zhang JZ. A method to extract cytokines and matrix metalloproteinases from Schirmer strips and analyze using Luminex. Molecular Vision. 2011;**17**:1056-1063

[24] Acera A, Rocha G, Vecino E, Lema I, Duran JA. Inflammatory markers in the tears of patients with ocular surface disease. Ophthalmic Research. 2008;**40**(6):315-321

[25] Inic-Kanada A, Nussbaumer A, Montanaro J, Belij S, Schlacher S, Stein E, et al. Comparison of ophthalmic sponges and extraction buffers for quantifying cytokine profiles in tears using Luminex technology. Molecular Vision. 2012;**18**:2717-2725

[26] Choy CK, Cho P, Chung WY, Benzie IF. Water-soluble antioxidants in human tears: Effect of the collection method. Investigative Ophthalmology & Visual Science. 2001;**42**(13):3130-3134

[27] Green-Church KB, Nichols KK, Kleinholz NM, Zhang L, Nichols JJ. Investigation of the human tear film proteome using multiple proteomic approaches. Molecular Vision. 2008;**14**:456-470

[28] Lee SY, Kim MJ, Kim MK, Wee WR. Comparative analysis of polymerase chain reaction assay for herpes simplex virus 1 detection in tear. Korean Journal of Ophthalmology. 2013;**27**(5):316-321

[29] Satpathy G, Mishra AK, Tandon R, Sharma MK, Sharma A, Nayak N, et al. Evaluation of tear samples for Herpes Simplex Virus 1 (HSV) detection in suspected cases of viral keratitis using PCR assay and conventional laboratory diagnostic tools. The British Journal of Ophthalmology. 2011;**95**(3):415-418

[30] Zakaria N, Van Grasdorff S, Wouters K, Rozema J, Koppen C, Lion E, et al. Human tears reveal insights into corneal neovascularization. PLoS One. 2012;**7**(5):e36451

[31] Leonardi A, Sathe S, Bortolotti M, Beaton A, Sack R. Cytokines, matrix metalloproteases, angiogenic and growth factors in tears of normal subjects and vernal keratoconjunctivitis patients. Allergy. 2009;**64**(5):710-717

[32] Leonardi A, Tavolato M, Curnow SJ, Fregona IA, Violato D, Alio JL. Cytokine and chemokine levels in tears and in corneal fibroblast cultures before and after excimer laser treatment. Journal of Cataract and Refractive Surgery. 2009;**35**(2):240-247

[33] Liu J, Shi B, He S, Yao X, Willcox MD, Zhao Z. Changes to tear cytokines of type 2 diabetic patients with or without retinopathy. Molecular Vision. 2010;**16**:2931-2938

[34] Rentka A, Harsfalvi J, Berta A, Koroskenyi K, Szekanecz Z, Szucs G, et al. Vascular endothelial growth factor in tear samples of patients with systemic sclerosis. Mediators of Inflammation. 2015;**2015**:573681

[35] Vesaluoma M, Teppo AM, Gronhagen-Riska C, Tervo T. Release of TGF-beta 1 and VEGF in tears following photorefractive keratectomy. Current Eye Research. 1997;**16**(1):19-25

[36] Rentka A, Harsfalvi J, Szucs G, Szekanecz Z, Szodoray P, Koroskenyi K, et al. Membrane array and multiplex bead analysis of tear cytokines in systemic sclerosis. Immunologic Research. 2016;**64**(2):619-626

[37] Ricklin D, Hajishengallis G, Yang K, Lambris JD. Complement: A key system for immune surveillance and homeostasis. Nature Immunology. 2010;**11**(9):785-797

[38] Zipfel PF, Skerka C. Complement regulators and inhibitory proteins. Nature Reviews Immunology. 2009;**9**(10):729-740

[39] Hackel PO, Zwick E, Prenzel N, Ullrich A. Epidermal growth factor receptors: Critical mediators of multiple receptor pathways. Current Opinion in Cell Biology. 1999;**11**(2):184-189

[40] John A, Tuszynski G. The role of matrix metalloproteinases in tumor angiogenesis and tumor metastasis. Pathology and Oncology Research. 2001;**7**(1):14-23

[41] Johnson C, Sung HJ, Lessner SM, Fini ME, Galis ZS. Matrix metalloproteinase-9 is required for adequate angiogenic revascularization of ischemic tissues: Potential role in capillary branching. Circulation Research. 2004;**94**(2):262-268

[42] Kotani T, Takeuchi T, Takai S, Yoshida S, Hata K, Nagai K, et al. Serum levels of matrix metalloproteinase (MMP) 9, a risk factor for acute coronary syndrome, are reduced independently of serum MMP-3 by anti-TNF-alpha antibody (infliximab) therapy in patients with rheumatoid arthritis. Journal of Pharmacological Sciences. 2012;**120**(1):50-53

[43] Kim WU, Min SY, Cho ML, Hong KH, Shin YJ, Park SH, et al. Elevated matrix metalloproteinase-9 in patients with systemic sclerosis. Arthritis Research & Therapy. 2005;**7**(1):R71-R79

[44] Rabquer BJ, Tsou PS, Hou Y, Thirunavukkarasu E, Haines GK, 3rd, Impens AJ, et al. Dysregulated expression of MIG/CXCL9, IP-10/CXCL10 and CXCL16 and their receptors in systemic sclerosis. Arthritis Research & Therapy. 2011;**13**(1):R18

[45] Chun RF. New perspectives on the vitamin D binding protein. Cell Biochemistry and Function. 2012;**30**(6):445-456

[46] Ge L, Trujillo G, Miller EJ, Kew RR. Circulating complexes of the vitamin D binding protein with G-actin induce lung inflammation by targeting endothelial cells. Immunobiology. 2014;**219**(3):198-207

[47] Muangchan C, Harding S, Khimdas S, Bonner A, Baron M, Pope J. Association of C-reactive protein with high disease activity in systemic sclerosis: results from the Canadian Scleroderma Research Group. Arthritis Care and Research (Hoboken). 2012;**64**(9):1405-1414

[48] Liu X, Mayes MD, Pedroza C, Draeger HT, Gonzalez EB, Harper BE, et al. Does C-reactive protein predict the long-term progression of interstitial lung disease and survival in patients with early systemic sclerosis? Arthritis Care and Research (Hoboken). 2013;**65**(8):1375-1380

[49] Hasegawa M, Fujimoto M, Matsushita T, Hamaguchi Y, Takehara K, Sato S. Serum chemokine and cytokine levels as indicators of disease activity in patients with systemic sclerosis. Clinical Rheumatology. 2011;**30**(2):231-237

[50] Lee EY, Lee ZH, Song YW. CXCL10 and autoimmune diseases. Autoimmunity Reviews. 2009;**8**(5):379-383

[51] Neville LF, Mathiak G, Bagasra O. The immunobiology of interferon-gamma inducible protein 10 kD (IP-10): A novel, pleiotropic member of the C-X-C chemokine superfamily. Cytokine & Growth Factor Reviews. 1997;**8**(3):207-219

[52] Liu M, Guo S, Hibbert JM, Jain V, Singh N, Wilson NO, et al. CXCL10/IP-10 in infectious diseases pathogenesis and potential therapeutic implications. Cytokine & Growth Factor Reviews. 2011;**22**(3):121-130

[53] Narumi S, Takeuchi T, Kobayashi Y, Konishi K. Serum levels of ifn-inducible PROTEIN-10 relating to the activity of systemic lupus erythematosus. Cytokine. 2000;**12**(10):1561-1565

[54] Hanaoka R, Kasama T, Muramatsu M, Yajima N, Shiozawa F, Miwa Y, et al. A novel mechanism for the regulation of IFN-gamma inducible protein-10 expression in rheumatoid arthritis. Arthritis Research & Therapy. 2003;**5**(2):R74-R81

[55] Fujii H, Shimada Y, Hasegawa M, Takehara K, Sato S. Serum levels of a Th1 chemoattractant IP-10 and Th2 chemoattractants, TARC and MDC, are elevated in patients with systemic sclerosis. Journal of Dermatological Science. 2004;**35**(1):43-51

[56] Yoshimura T, Yuhki N, Moore SK, Appella E, Lerman MI, Leonard EJ. Human monocyte chemoattractant protein-1 (MCP-1). Full-length cDNA cloning, expression in mitogen-stimulated blood mononuclear leukocytes, and sequence similarity to mouse competence gene JE. FEBS Letters. 1989;**244**(2):487-493

[57] Distler JH, Akhmetshina A, Schett G, Distler O. Monocyte chemoattractant proteins in the pathogenesis of systemic sclerosis. Rheumatology (Oxford). 2009;**48**(2):98-103

[58] Gu L, Tseng S, Horner RM, Tam C, Loda M, Rollins BJ. Control of TH2 polarization by the chemokine monocyte chemoattractant protein-1. Nature. 2000;**404**(6776):407-411

[59] Hasegawa M, Sato S, Takehara K. Augmented production of chemokines (monocyte chemotactic protein-1 (MCP-1), macrophage inflammatory protein-1alpha (MIP-1alpha) and MIP-1beta) in patients with systemic sclerosis: MCP-1 and MIP-1alpha may be involved in the development of pulmonary fibrosis. Clinical and Experimental Immunology. 1999;**117**(1):159-165

[60] Matsunaga K, Klein TW, Newton C, Friedman H, Yamamoto Y. Legionella pneumophila suppresses interleukin-12 production by macrophages. Infection and Immunity. 2001;**69**(3):1929-1933

Chapter 7

Biological Therapy in Systemic Sclerosis

Joana Caetano, Susana Oliveira and
José Delgado Alves

Additional information is available at the end of the chapter

http://dx.doi.org/10.5772/intechopen.69326

Abstract

Systemic sclerosis is the autoimmune connective tissue disease with the highest morbidity and mortality, through the combination of inflammation, vasculopathy and fibrosis leading to severe internal organ involvement. Currently, there are no approved disease-modifying therapies, and treatment is based on organ-specific treatment and broad immunosuppression, with disappointing long-term results in most cases. Recent research has helped to improve knowledge of the pathogenesis of systemic sclerosis and to optimize treatment based on specific physiopathological targets, and a new era of biological agents in systemic sclerosis has now begun. Promising results are emerging from targeting specific cytokine signalling, especially IL-6, and cellular subpopulations such as B cells, with anti-CD20 therapy, and T-cells, with inhibition of T-cell co-stimulation. Other approaches under evaluation are based on the modulation of profibrotic pathways by anti-TGF-β agents. In this chapter, we discuss the available evidence to support the use of each biological agent in systemic sclerosis based on data from basic and translational research and on results from clinical studies.

Keywords: systemic sclerosis, biological therapy, cytokines, immune dysfunction, targeted treatment

1. Introduction

Systemic sclerosis (SSc) is a rare multisystem connective tissue disease in which inflammation, fibrosis, vasculopathy and autoimmunity are the principal features leading to diverse organ-based injuries [1]. The complex physiopathology, the substantial clinical heterogeneity, the unknown determinants of organ involvement and severity and the different individual outcomes that are frequently independent of therapeutic interventions make SSc one of the most challenging autoimmune diseases to treat [2–4].

With increasing understanding of the mechanisms and the targets underlying the immune dysregulation in many autoimmune connective tissue diseases, substantial therapeutic advances have been achieved in the past few years, including the development of biological therapies [5]. Biological agents have indeed significantly changed the prognosis of different conditions not only in rheumatology [rheumatoid arthritis (RA), seronegative spondyloarthropathies and systemic lupus erythematous (SLE)] but also in neurological, dermatological and gastrointestinal diseases [6–8].

The available treatment approved for SSc is still directed towards organ-associated manifestations, with cyclophosphamide and mycophenolate mofetil being the main therapeutic options. While these treatments may reduce the progression of organ damage, especially cardiac and lung disease, their effects are often not sustained [3, 4]. Therefore, the use of targeted therapy such as biological agents, acting on the central pathways of the disease, could be considered as a true disease-modify treatment for SSc, halting fibrosis and preventing disease progression [5].

In this chapter, we provide an update of the biological agents available for clinical treatment of SSc. First, we briefly review the pathogenic pathways that help clarify the targets for such therapeutic agents, followed by an overview of the available evidence for the use of each biological agent in SSc.

2. Main physiopathological mechanisms with specific treatment potential in systemic sclerosis

Vasculopathy, inflammation, autoimmunity and fibrosis are the basis of SSc pathophysiology. However, the relative contribution of each of these processes varies, leading to protean manifestations and clinical phenotypes. Hence, the use of specific targeted therapies in SSc is complicated by the heterogeneous nature of the disease across patients [2, 3]. Recently, a more integrated model based on the interplay between all these processes has been suggested, with sequential immune activation and vasculopathy leading to fibrosis, although the primary triggering event is still unknown (**Figure 1**) [4, 9].

Immune activation is thought to be an early event, with circulating and tissue activated CD4+ T-cells, production of T helper 2 (Th2) cell-derived cytokines (interleukins 4, 10 and 13) and subsequent skin infiltration by macrophages. Differentiation of T helper 17 (Th17) lymphocytes may also be an important process in SSc, promoting fibrosis [9, 10]. Gourh et al. analysed the levels of 13 cytokines in 444 SSc patients and compared with 216 healthy donors. They found that SSc patients had higher plasma levels of tumour necrosis factor-α (TNF-α) ($p < 0.0001$) and interleukin-6 (IL-6) ($p < 0.001$), and lower levels of interleukin-23 (IL-23) ($p = 0.014$). Additionally, cytokine profiles differed in SSc patients based on the presence of specific autoantibodies, with IL-6 being elevated in patients with positive anti-topoisomerase I and anti-RNA polymerase antibodies, but not in anti-centromere-positive patients. Moreover, disease duration also influenced cytokines levels: IL-6 and TNF-α were significantly elevated in SSc patients with disease duration between 0 and 10 years, with no difference compared with healthy controls for disease duration of more than 10 years. In contrast, levels of interleukin-10

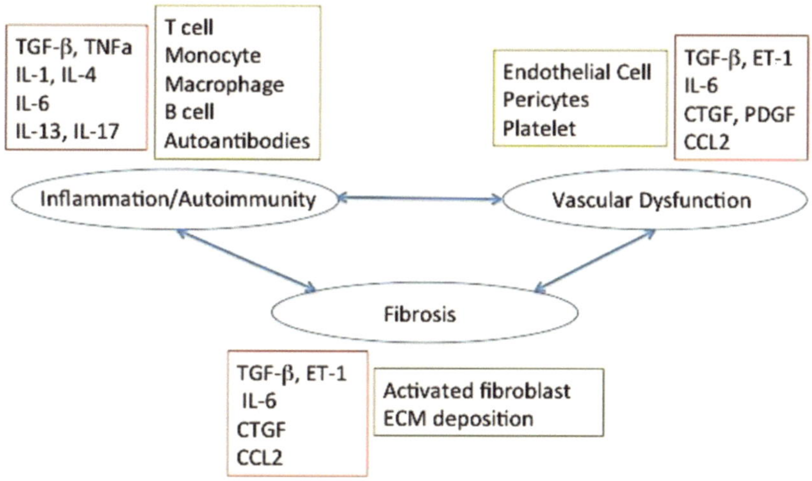

Figure 1. Integrated pathogenesis and target molecules in systemic sclerosis. Abbreviations: CCL2, chemokine ligand 2; CTGF, connective tissue growth factor; ECM, extracellular matrix; ET-1, endothelin-1; IL-1, interleukin-1; IL-4, interleukin-4; IL-6, interleukin-6; IL-13, interleukin-13; IL-17, interleukin-17; PDGF, platelet-derived growth factor; TGF-β, transforming growth factor β and TNF-α, tumour necrosis factor α.

(IL-10), interleukin-5 (IL-5) and interferon-γ (IFN-γ) were significantly increased in later stages of the disease (>10 years), compared with healthy controls [10].

Although immune activation is more common in the early disease phases, it persists in later stages, with B-cells promoting not only the production of antibodies but also interfering with antigen presentation, T-cell response and cytokine secretion, mostly through the secretion of IL-6 and transforming growth factor (TGF-β). In the tight skin mouse (tsk) model of SSc, B-cell depletion leads to suppression of skin fibrosis and downregulation of Th2 cytokines, suggesting a key role of B-cells in SSc pathogenesis and providing a link between autoimmunity and fibrosis [11].

Vascular dysfunction and remodelling can also occur early in SSc, resulting from disrupted and inappropriate repair processes following endothelial injury, with upregulation of angiogenic factors including platelet-derived growth factor (PDGF), vascular endothelial growth factor (VEGF), endothelin-1 (ET-1), TGF-β and chemokine ligand 2/chemoattractant protein 1 (CCL2/MCP-1) [9]. These processes lead to a reduction in the number of capillaries and a narrowing of the vessels, impairing blood flow and resulting in tissue hypoxia. The abnormal vascular repair may initiate uncontrolled and persistent tissue remodelling, culminating in fibrosis [12].

Among all the cytokines found to be up-regulated in SSc, especially in the skin and lung, TGF-β is a potent stimulator of extracellular matrix production and has been widely studied and reviewed [13]. It plays an important role in wound healing and tissue repair, and an aberrant regulation of TBG-β is associated with inherited conditions, such as hereditary haemorrhagic telangiectasia, familial pulmonary hypertension and Marfan syndrome, and with fibrotic diseases, such as liver cirrhosis and idiopathic pulmonary fibrosis. In SSc, TBG-β plays a major role in fibroblast activation and differentiation and contributes to altered extracellular matrix deposition, creating a persistent state of activation. Additionally, TGF-β influences endothelial cells and the production of anti- and pro-angiogenic factors (increasing VEGF and ET-1 expression and downregulating inducible nitric oxide synthase), hence contributing to the complex vascular phenotype seen in SSc patients, with proliferative and obliterative vascular lesions occurring simultaneously [12, 13].

Many of these molecules are potential targets for biological therapy in SSc. Indeed, many of these cytokines are known to correlate with specific organ-based complications in SSc. In the study by Gourh et al. described previously, higher serum levels of IL-6 were associated with interstitial lung disease (ILD) and pulmonary hypertension (PH), whereas patients with increased serum levels of TNF-α were more likely to have SSc renal crisis. IL-6 was also associated with higher total skin scores and IL-17 with arthritis [10].

The main effects of the biological agents are (**Table 1**) [7, 8]:

1. Neutralization of pro-inflammatory cytokines
2. Blockage of co-stimulation between antigen-presenting cells and T-cells
3. B-cell depletion

Most of these biological agents are already approved for the treatment of many autoimmune diseases, and for some of them, there are on-going clinical trials in SSc, based on pre-clinical work showing the relevance of each of their respective targets in the pathogenesis of SSc.

In the following section, we will review the available evidence to support the use of each biological agent in SSc, based on data from basic and translational research and on results from clinical studies. At the end of this chapter, **Tables 2** and **3** summarize the reported experience from observational studies and clinical trials for each biological agent in SSc.

Biological agent	Biological target
Infliximab, etanercept, adalimumab, golimumab	TNF-α
Tocilizumab	IL-6
Rilonacept	IL-1
Ixekizumab	IL-17
Brodalumab	IL-17 receptor
Tralokinumab	IL-13
Fresolimumab	TGF-β
Abatacept	CTLA-4 (T-cell)
Rituximab	CD20 (B-cell)
Belimumab	BAAF (B-cell)

Abbreviations: BAAF, B-cell activating factor; CTLA-4, cytotoxic T-lymphocyte-associated protein-4; IL-1, interleukin-1; IL-6, interleukin-6; IL-13, interleukin-13; IL-17, interleukin-17; TGF-β, transforming growth factor β and TNF-α, tumour necrosis factor α.

Table 1. Potential targets for current biological therapies in SSc.

Biological agent	First author, Year [Ref]	Study type	Patients, *n*	Organ involvement	Treatment, dose and duration	Outcome
Tocilizumab	Shima, 2010 [18]	CS	2 dcSSc (patients A and B)	ILD (A) SRC (B)	8 mg/Kg/ monthly Duration: 6 months	mRSS reduction: 27→13 (A); 26→20 (B) Internal organ stable (A,B)
	Elhai, 2013 [19]	CHS	15 SSc	Polyarthritis ($n = 15$)	8 mg/Kg/ monthly Duration: 5 months	DAS-28 score improvement ($n = 10$): 5.2→2.8 Stopped due to inefficacy ($n = 2$)
	Fernandes das Neves, 2015 [20]	CS	2 dcSSc (patients A and B) 1 lcSSc (patient C)	ILD (A,B,C)	8 mg/Kg/ monthly Duration: 6 months	mRSS reduction: 17→11(A); 41→25(B); 7→5(C) ILD: stable (A,B); progression (C) Patient VAS score reduction: 70→40(A); 70→30(B); 60→10(C)
Anti-TNF-α	Distler, 2011 [25]	CS	65 SSc	ILD* Polyarthritis* Myositis*	INF ($n = 30$) ETA ($n = 29$) ADA ($n = 6$) Duration: not specified	Organ involvement: improvement ($n = 48$) - stable ($n = 10$) - worsened ($n = 7$) – mainly ILD
	Allanore, 2006 [27]	CR	1 lcSSc	ILD and polyarthritis	ADA (40 mg sc/every 2 weeks) Duration: 7 months	DAS-28 score improvement: 7.8→5.1 ILD progression Dead from respiratory failure
Abatacept	Elhai, 2013 [19]	CHS	12 SSc	Polyarthritis ($n = 12$) Myositis ($n = 7$)	10 mg/Kg/ monthly Duration: variable 11–18 months	DAS-28 score improvement ($n = 12$) Median score: 5.2→2.8 Myopathy stable ($n = 7$)
	Paoli, 2014 [49]	CS	4 dcSSc (patients A, B, C and D)	Extensive skin fibrosis (A, B, C, D) ILD (A,B)	500–750 mg/ dose at weeks 0,2 and 4, then every 4 week Duration: variable 12–15 months	mRSS reduction: 37→8 (A); 32→20 (B); 35→17 (C); 30→15 (D) ILD regression (B)
Rituximab	Daoussis, 2012 [63]	CHS	8 dcSSc	ILD ($n = 8$)	375 mg/m^2 at baseline, and at 6, 12 and 18 months	At 24 months: ILD improvement ($n = 8$) mRSS reduction (mean score): 13.5 ± 12.42→4.87 ± 0.83

Abbreviations: CS, case series; CHS, cohort study; CR, case report; dcSSc, diffuse cutaneous systemic sclerosis; lcSSc, limited cutaneous systemic sclerosis; ILD, interstitial lung disease, mRSS, modified Rodnan skin score; SRC, scleroderma renal crisis; TCZ, tocilizumab, RTX, rituximab; ADA, adalimumab; ETA, Etanercept; INF, infliximab; VAS, visual analogue scale and DAS-28, Disease Activity Score for 28 joints.

*Number of patients not specified.

Table 2. Observational studies and case series reporting the experience of biological therapy in SSc.

Biological agent	First author, year [Ref]	Study type	Patients, *n*	Control Y/N (n)	Treatment	Study duration	Aim/primary end-point	Outcome
Tocilizumab	Khanna, 2016 [21]	RCT	87 dcSSc	Y (n = 44)	162 mg sc weekly	48 weeks (followed by open-label weekly TCZ for 48 weeks)	Change in mRSS at week 24	Reduction in mRSS at w24: TCZ −3.92 vs placebo −1.22, (−2.70, p = 0.0915) Fewer patients on TCZ with FVC decline vs placebo (w24, p = 0.009, w48 p = 0.03)
Infliximab	Denton, 2009 [24]	OL	16 dcSSc	N	5 mg/Kg at week 0, 2,6, 14 and 22	26 weeks	Safety assessment and potential efficacy	No change in mRSS Frequent AEs (19 treatment-related)
Metelimumab (CAT-129)	Denton, 2007 [46]	RCT	45 dcSSc	Y (n = 11)	0.5, 5 or 10 mg/Kg every 6 weeks	24 weeks	Safety assessment	No change in mRSS AEs more frequent in treatment group
Fresolimumab	Rice, 2015 [47]	OL	15 dcSSc	N	2 × 1 mg/kg (4 weeks apart), or 1 × 5 mg/Kg	24 weeks	Safety assessment Effect on TGF-β responsive skin gene expression	Downregulation of all TGF-β skin gene expression Reduction in mRSS: w11 (−6, p = 0.0005); w17 (−9, p = 0.0024) Frequent bleeding events (n = 11)
Abatacept	Chakravarty, 2011 [50]	RCT	10 dcSSc	Y (n = 3)	500–750 mg/dose at week 0, 2 and 4, then every 4 weeks	24 weeks	Safety assessment and change in mRSS at week 24	Reduction in mRSS vs placebo: −8.6 vs −2.3, p = 0.059 No serious AEs
	Chakravarty, 2015 [51]	RCT	10 dcSSc	Y (n = 3)	500–750 mg/dose at week 0, 2 and 4, then every 4 weeks	24 weeks	Safety assessment and potential efficacy Effect on skin gene expression	Reduction in mRSS vs placebo: −9.8, p = 0.0014 Decreased inflammatory-related intrinsic skin gene expression

Biological agent	First author, year [Ref]	Study type	Patients, n	Control Y/N (n)	Treatment	Study duration	Aim/primary end-point	Outcome
Rituximab	Bosello, 2010 [59]	OL	9 dcSSc	N	1000 mg day 1 and 15 (with 100 mg MPDN each)	36 months	Safety assessment and change in mRSS and serum IL-6 levels	At 6 months: Reduction in mRSS: 21.1 ± 9.0 to 12.0 ± 6.1, $p = 0.001$ Decrease in serum IL-6 ($p = 0.02$) No significant change in FVC or DLCO
	Smith, 2010 [60]	OL	8 dcSSc	N	1000 mg day 1 and 15 (with 100 mg MPDN each)	24 weeks	Safety and potential efficacy assessment	At w24 Reduction in mRSS: 24.8 ± 3.4–14.3 ± 3.5, $p < 0.001$ No significant change in FVC or DLCO Decrease in myofibroblast score on skin biopsy
	Lafyatis, 2009 [61]	OL	15 dcSSc	N	1000 mg day 1 and 15	12 months	Safety and potential efficacy assessment Change in mRSS	No significant change in mRSS or in FVC or DLCO at 6 months
	Jordan, 2015 [62]	MCNCC	35 dcSSc 11 lcSSc	Y ($n = 25$)	Variable most received 1000 mg at day 1 and 15	Variable: 7 months (5–9)	Change in mRSS	At 7 months: RTX group vs baseline: Reduction in mRSS 14.4 ± 1.5 vs 18.1 ± 1.6 v $p = 0.0002$ no decline in FVC ($p = 0.5$), improvement in DLCO ($p = 0.03$) Control group: decline in FVC ($p = 0.01$)
	Daoussis, 2010 [64]	RCT	8 dcSSc	Y ($n = 6$)	375 mg/m^2 weekly 4 weeks, at 0 and 24 weeks	48 weeks	Efficacy assessment	At 48 weeks RTX group vs baseline: Reduction in mRSS 8.37 ± 6.45 vs 13.5 ± 6.84, $p < 0.001$ Improvement in FVC ($p = 0.0018$) and DLCO ($p = 0.017$)
	Melissaropoulos, 2015 [65]	OL	30 dcSSc	N	At 0, 6, 12 and 18 months*	7 years	Long term efficacy and safety assessment	Treatment vs baseline: Lung function improvement FVC: 86.2 ± 5.5 vs 78.2 ± 3.6, $p = 0.018$; DLCO: 62.4 ± 4.5 vs 57.3 ± 3.2, $p = 0.012$ Reduction in mRSS, ($p < 0.001$) 5 deaths not proven to be treatment-related

Abbreviations: RCT, randomized controlled trial; OL, open label; MCNCC, multicentre nested case-control; Y, yes; N, no; sc, subcutaneous; FVC, forced vital capacity; DLCO, diffusing capacity for carbon monoxide; TCZ, tocilizumab; INF, infliximab; RTX, rituximab; AEs, adverse events; IL-6, interleukin-6 and MPDN, methylprednisolone.
*Dose not specified.

Table 3. Clinical trials investigating the efficacy of biological therapy in SSc.

3. Targeting pathogenic processes in systemic sclerosis

3.1. Targeting cytokines

3.1.1. Interleukin-6

Multiple lines of evidence indicate that IL-6 is a critical interleukin in SSc. Animal models have confirmed this hypothesis. Saito et al. demonstrated that in the bleomycin mouse model, the IL-6 knockout (KO) variety had reduced fibrotic bleomycin-induced lung fibrosis, and a significant decrease in the total inflammatory cell count, namely macrophages and neutrophils, in bronchoalveolar lavage fluid, compared with the wild type (WT) mice ($p < 0.05$). Moreover, lung tissue pathology, on day 21 after bleomycin treatment, showed significant fibrotic changes with increased collagen content in WT mice compared with IL-6 KO mice ($p < 0.05$) [14]. Kitaba et al. obtained similar results with IL-6 KO bleomycin mice having reduced dermal fibrosis comparing with the WT mice [15].

In a recent work by Khan et al., serum IL-6 levels were determined in 39 patients with diffuse cutaneous SSc (dcSSc), 29 patients with limited cutaneous SSc (lcSSc) and 15 healthy controls. Serum IL-6 levels were higher in dcSSc patients, especially in the subgroup with thrombocytosis and elevated C-reactive protein levels, compared with dcSSc with normal platelets count, lcSSc and controls ($p < 0.001$). IL-6 expression was higher in dermal fibroblasts and endothelial cells especially in patients with early dcSSc (<3 years since disease onset) [16].

The relationship between serum IL-6 levels and clinical outcomes was also addressed. Serum IL-6 levels positively correlated with modified Rodnan skin score (mRSS) at the time of disease onset (Spearman's $p = 0.514$, $p = 0.001$). In addition, serum IL-6 levels at presentation also correlated with the mRSS at 36-month follow-up (Spearman's $p = 0.795$, $p < 0.001$), which may reflect a predictive role for IL-6 levels regarding the extent of skin involvement in early diffuse patients. Furthermore, these authors also showed that higher levels of IL-6 (≥10 pg/mL) at disease presentation predicted mortality in dcSSc, with a 15-year survival of 30% in patients with high IL-6 levels vs 93% survival among patients with low IL-6 serum levels ($p = 0.021$). These results reinforce and define a subset of SSc patients in which IL-6 plays a relevant role and support the rationale for specific anti-IL6 therapeutics in SSc [16].

Tocilizumab is a humanized anti-IL6 receptor antibody that binds to both the soluble and the membrane bound IL-6 receptor, and is approved for the treatment of rheumatoid arthritis amongst other immune-mediated diseases [17]. The first report of SSc patients treated with tocilizumab was published in 2010, demonstrating its benefits in two dcSSc patients, one with lung fibrosis and the other with renal crisis. Monthly treatment with tocilizumab for 6 months reduced skin sclerosis in both patients, with skin biopsies showing a reduced number of cells in the dermis and vascular walls, and reduced the immunohistochemical staining for α-smooth muscle actin (SMA) after treatment. Internal organ involvement remained stable, namely lung and renal impairment [18]. Other cases were subsequently reported, reinforcing the role of tocilizumab as a valuable treatment option in dcSSc, improving skin thickness, halting lung fibrosis and reducing the patient's Global Disease Activity scores [19, 20].

In a European League Against Rheumatism (EULAR) Systemic Sclerosis Trials and Research Group (EUSTAR) observational study, 15 SSc patients with refractory polyarthritis and myopathy were treated with tocilizumab for 5 months, with significant improvement in the 28-joint count Disease Activity Score in 10 patients. No significant change was seen in lung or skin involvement [19].

Another mini-series evaluated the effect of tocilizumab in three dcSSc patients with interstitial lung disease. After treatment for 6 months, the skin score improved in all three patients, and the patients' global assessment also improved. In two patients, there was a halt in the progression of lung fibrosis, on lung high-resolution CT scan (HRCT) and lung function tests [20].

The first clinical trial assessing the effects of subcutaneous tocilizumab in dcSSc (faSScinate) was done in 35 hospitals in five different countries (Canada, France, Germany, United Kingdom and United States of America) and was published in 2015. In this phase II study, 87 patients with early dcSSc (disease duration ≤5 years) were enrolled, 43 patients were treated with tocilizumab and 44 with placebo for 48 weeks. The change in the mRSS at 24 weeks was −3.92 in the tocilizumab group and −1.22 in the placebo group (difference of −2.70, 95% CI −5.85 to 0.45, $p = 0.0915$). Also, fewer patients assigned for tocilizumab treatment had an absolute decline of forced vital capacity (FVC) of more than 10%, compared with patients treated with placebo [21]. Given these encouraging results, there is an on-going 2-year randomized double-blinded controlled clinical trial, across 120 global study sites, which will assess the efficacy and safety of subcutaneous tocilizumab in early dcSSc. The primary outcome measure is the change in mRSS at 48 weeks [22].

3.1.2. *Tumour necrosis factor α*

Tumour necrosis factor α (TNF-α) is a pro-inflammatory cytokine that plays an important role in the pathogenesis of many autoimmune diseases. Anti-TNF-α agents are approved for the treatment of rheumatoid arthritis, seronegative spondyloarthropathies and inflammatory bowel diseases [7]. Contrasting with its well-proven role in other inflammatory diseases, the relevance in SSc and in profibrotic conditions is still conflicting.

Some animal models have shown a benefit from TNF-α blockade. In a study using the bleomycin mouse model, treatment with etanercept resulted in a significant reduction in dermal sclerosis compared with bleomycin mice not treated with etanercept (dermal thickness 85.83 ± 12.8 vs 126.4 ± 31.3 μm, respectively, $p < 0.05$). Histopathological analysis of the skin revealed a reduction in the collagen content and in infiltrating myofibroblasts (reduced levels of tissue hydroxyproline and α-SMA, $p < 0.05$) and reduced levels of TGF-β (514.4 ± 62,6 vs 716.9 ± 49.1, treated mice vs non-treated, $p < 0.05$) [23].

The efficacy of anti-TNF-α agents was also assessed in SSc patients. In an open-label study, 16 patients with dcSSc were treated with infliximab 5 mg/kg (five infusions at weeks 0, 2, 6, 14 and 22). There was no significant improvement in the mRSS, but there was a trend towards a decline between the peak score at 6 weeks (OR 29, 95% CI 11–44) and the 22-week time point (OR 17, 95% CI 6–46, $p = 0.10$). A limiting factor was the frequency of adverse events (total of 127, with 21 considered serious events and 19 definitively related to infliximab treatment). Eight patients (50%) discontinued infliximab prematurely [24].

In addition, a EUSTAR consensus meeting on the role of anti-TNF-α therapy in SSc concluded that its use in SSc should be discouraged, although it can be considered for patients with inflammatory arthritis overlap. These conclusions were based on a review of data on anti-TNF-α therapy from 79 EUSTAR centres. From a total of 65 patients treated with TNF-α inhibitors, 48 patients (74%) improved, but their main clinical manifestation was inflammatory arthritis. In seven patients (11%), the disease worsened mostly due to progression of lung fibrosis, and in two patients (15%), there was no change in the outcome [25].

Furthermore, there is evidence in the literature of progression of lung fibrosis in patients with rheumatoid arthritis, mainly related to lung alveolitis after treatment with TNF-α antagonists [26], and in the last few years, some similar cases in SSc have been reported. Recently, Allanore et al. reported a case of a patient with a 5-year diagnosis of lcSSc with established interstitial lung disease with relatively well-preserved lung function (FVC of 72% predicted and diffusing capacity for carbon monoxide (DLCO) of 52%), treated with azathioprine and with progressively disabling inflammatory polyarthritis. Treatment with adalimumab was started with improvement in the articular symptoms, but worsening of the lung disease after 6 months of treatment, requiring long-term oxygen therapy and resulting in death from respiratory failure [27].

Due to these reports, anti-TNF-α therapy is now seldom used in SSc patients, based on recommendations by experts and despite the absence of randomized controlled trials.

3.1.3. Interleukin-1

The role of interleukin-1 (IL-1) in the pathogenesis of SSc has been addressed in a few studies. The IL-1 role in proliferation and collagen production of fibroblasts is well established. After IL-1 stimulation, normal fibroblasts produce various cytokines, including IL-6, IL-8, TNF-α and PDGF. IL-1α is elevated in the serum of SSc patients, and it is constitutively produced by SSc fibroblasts, as demonstrated by Maekawa et al. [28]. In this study, IL-1α levels were significantly higher in SSc patients compared with healthy controls ($p = 0.0017$), although the stratification of SSc patients according to disease subsets (limited vs diffuse) did not show a significant difference in serum IL-1α levels. Furthermore, Kawaguchi et al. demonstrated that inhibition of IL-1α in SSc fibroblasts resulted in decreased fibroblast proliferation, decreased IL-6 production and procollagen synthesis, whilst overexpression of IL-1α in normal fibroblasts resulted in an SSc phenotype fibroblast [29].

Considering these results, a phase I/II double-blinded placebo-controlled trial is on-going in patients with early dcSSc in order to assess the effects of rilonacept (IL-1 Trap), an anti-IL-1 antibody, currently used for autoinflammatory syndromes such as cryopyrin-associated periodic syndromes. In this study, the primary outcome is the 4-gene biomarker expression in the skin, and the secondary outcome is the reduction of skin thickness measured by mRSS. Farina et al. previously described the 4-gene biomarker as highly predictive of mRSS in patients with early dcSSc. It includes two TFG-β-regulated genes: cartilage oligomeric matrix protein (COMP) and thrombospondin-1 (THS1), and two interferon (IFN)-regulated genes: interferon-induced 44 (IFI44) and sialoadhesin (SIG1). The central hypothesis is that if IL-1 is a key cytokine leading to fibrosis in SSc, its inhibition will downregulate the expression of the 4-gene biomarker in the skin [30, 31].

3.1.4. Interleukin-13

Substantial experimental evidence has shown that interleukin-13 (IL-13) has a significant role in SSc as a profibrotic cytokine that interplays with other mediators such as TGF-β [2, 6, 32].

Fichtner-Feigl et al. have recently defined the pathway of IL-13-induced fibrosis via TGF-β in an *in vivo* bleomycin model of fibrosis. Firstly, this process involves the induction of a cell-surface IL-13 receptor (IL-13Rα_2) by IL-13 and TNF-α. In a second phase, IL-13 signalling through this receptor induces activation of the TGFB1 promoter. Prevention of IL-13Rα_2 expression via IL13Rα_2 gene silencing or blockade of the IL-13Rα_2 signalling leads to marked downregulation of TGF-β production and collagen deposition in bleomycin-induced lung fibrosis [32].

Fuschiotti et al. analysed the ability of SSc patients' CD4+ and CD8+ T-cells to produce cytokines following *in vitro* activation. There was a dysregulation in IL-13 production by effector CD8+ T-cells in SSc, not present in the healthy control group or in rheumatoid arthritis patients ($p < 0.001$). This dysregulated IL-13 production also correlated with the extent of skin fibrosis, with dcSSc showing higher levels of IL-13 compared with lcSSc ($p < 0.01$) [33].

Supporting this work, Bleperio et al. also concluded that in the bleomycin-induced mouse model, IL-13 levels were elevated and its neutralisation led to attenuation of bleomycin-induced pulmonary fibrosis and to a decrease in C10 levels (a chemotactic factor for mononuclear phagocytes) [34].

Moreover, in another work from Fuschiotti et al., circulating IL-13 producing CD8+ T-cells in SSc expressed skin-homing receptors and induced a profibrotic phenotype in normal fibroblasts which was inhibited by an anti-IL13 antibody. The histopathological analysis showed a dermal inflammatory infiltration of CD8+ T-cells and the IL-13 accumulation was higher in the early phases of the disease (duration <3 years) [35].

Tralokinumab is an interleukin-13 neutralising humanized monoclonal antibody used in uncontrolled severe asthma. It seems to be particularly effective in the subgroup of patients with higher baseline levels of periostin, an IL-13-induced protein in the airways, which is also elevated in SSc patients [36]. Yang et al. showed that after bleomycin treatment, WT mice had marked cutaneous fibrosis, increased expression of periostin and increased numbers of myofibroblasts, while these changes were not seen in periostin−/− mice (PN−/−). Moreover, fibroblasts of PN−/− mice showed reduced expression of α-SMA and procollagen type-Iα1 induced by TGF-β. Also, SSc patients had elevated expression of periostin in the skin compared with healthy controls [37]. Tralokinumab is currently under evaluation in a phase II dose-ranging study for patients with idiopathic pulmonary fibrosis [38].

Altogether, there is significant research supporting a possible role for tralokinumab in SSc treatment, especially in patients with interstitial lung disease.

3.1.5. Interleukin-17

Interleukin-17 (IL-17) is a cytokine secreted by a distinct T-cell subset called T helper 17 (TH17) cells, which leads to activation of fibroblasts and subsequent secretion of pro-inflammatory cytokines such as IL-6 and IL-8, and to an increased surface expression of Intercellular Adhesion Molecule 1 (ICAM-1). In a work by Kurasawa et al., IL-17 was found to be overexpressed in peripheral blood cells and in lymphocytes from the skin and lungs of SSc patients, compared with samples from patients with systemic lupus erythematosus, autoimmune inflammatory myositis and healthy donors. Furthermore, IL-17 overproduction significantly correlated with an early disease stage and an enhanced proliferation of fibroblasts and IL-1 production in SSc patients [39]. Altered IL-17 expression in SSc has also been reported elsewhere, with studies documenting a decrease in regulatory T-cell (Treg) levels, as well as a functional deficiency, accompanied by an increase in CD4+CD25+FoxP3+ T-cells and IL-17 levels, potentially causing an immune imbalance between Treg and Th17 cells [40, 41].

Recently, studies have started looking at several biological agents that target IL-17 (ixekizumab) and its receptor (brodalumab), especially in psoriatic arthritis, but currently there are no data available on its use in SSc [42].

3.2. Targeting morphogenic regulators

3.2.1. Transforming growth factor-β

Transforming growth factor-β (TGF-β) has been recognised as the central mediator of fibrosis in SSc and the persistence of TBG-β signalling is a key feature in SSc pathogenesis [43]. TGF-β is secreted from monocytes, lymphocytes and fibroblasts in the latent form and sequestered in the extracellular matrix. In its active form, TGF-β promotes collagen gene expression and sustained fibrosis via SMAD (mothers against decapentaplegic) 2/3 signalling and epithelial-mesenchymal transition through a SMAD-independent pathway [44, 45].

Examining the role of TGF-β in fibrosis, Sargent et al. assessed TGF-β responsive gene expression in the skin of SSc patients. This TGF-β responsive signature was found only in patients with the diffuse subset and correlated with higher mRSS and with a higher prevalence of interstitial lung disease. There was no association between disease duration, specific autoantibodies or any other clinical manifestation and TGF-β-expression gene signature [43].

The blockade of TGF-β pathways has been shown to prevent collagen synthesis in SSc fibroblasts. Ihn et al. evaluated the levels of active and latent TGF-β and its receptor from cultured dermal fibroblasts of 10 patients with early dcSSc (<2 years disease duration). They also examined the expression of human α2(I)-collagen messenger RNA (mRNA) and its transcriptional activity both before and after blocking TGF-β signalling with anti-TGF-β antibodies or with a TGF-β anti-sense oligonucleotide. SSc fibroblasts produced an equivalent amount of TGF-β as control fibroblasts (0.381 ± 0.031 vs 0.435 ± 0.082, respectively), although SSc fibroblasts had a significantly increased expression of TGF-β receptors ($p < 0.01$). Furthermore, the blockage of TGF-β signalling resulted in a dose-dependent decrease of α2(I)-collagen mRNA expression [44].

Given the role of TGF-β in SSc pathogenesis and the availability of commercial anti-TGF-β antibodies, some recent trials tested their safety and efficacy in the treatment of SSc.

In a multi-centre randomised placebo-controlled trial, 45 early dcSSc patients were treated with CAT-192 (Metelimumab), a recombinant human antibody that neutralises active human

TGF-β1 (doses of 0.5, 5 or 10 mg/kg, in a total of four administrations, every 6 weeks). The primary endpoint was to evaluate safety and tolerability of CAT-192; secondary outcomes included mRSS, Systemic Sclerosis Health Assessment Questionnaire, organ-based manifestations, levels of collagen propeptides (N propeptide and type I and type III collagen) and skin levels of mRNA for procollagen I and III, TGF-β1 and TGF-β2. No changes in mRSS or in any other clinical variables assessed were documented, including the levels of biomarkers in the serum and the mRNA analysis of skin biopsies, independently of the dose used. Moreover, there were more serious adverse events, including deaths, than in the placebo group (four deaths in the treatment group vs zero in the placebo group) [46].

Contrasting with CAT-192 that has a weak neutralising effect and is monospecific for TGF-β1, fresolimumab is a high-affinity neutralising antibody that targets all three TGF-β isoforms. In an open-label trial, 15 patients with early dcSSc were divided in two groups and treated with fresolimumab (either two infusions of 1 mg/kg 4 weeks apart, or one infusion of 5 mg/kg). The skin expression of TGF-β-regulated genes was assessed, as well as skin thickening using mRSS. At weeks 3 and 7 after treatment, there was a downregulation of all the TGF-β-regulated biomarker genes studied, namely thrombospondin-1 (THBS1), cartilage oligomeric protein (COMP), Serpin Family E Member 1 (SERPINE1) and connective tissue growth factor (CTGF) in both groups. There was also a parallel improvement in mRSS, with a mean change in mRSS in both groups of −6 ($p = 0.0005$) and −9.5 ($p = 0.0024$), at weeks 11 and 17, respectively, compared with baseline. SMA staining on skin biopsies also decreased significantly ($p < 0.01$, comparing week 4 to baseline). Regarding safety, one patient died of congestive heart failure 12 weeks after fresolimumab treatment. The most significant adverse events were bleeding episodes (11 patients, two of them with gastrointestinal bleeding) and anaemia in 10 patients (66.7%) [47]. By considering these results and fresolimumab's effect as an antifibrotic agent, further studies are needed to determine the safety profile of fresolimumab and its effects on organ involvement in SSc.

3.3. Targeting of cellular subpopulations

3.3.1. T-cells

As described previously, activated T-cells play an important role in SSc pathogenesis. Abatacept is a soluble fusion protein consisting of an extracellular domain of the human cytotoxic T-lymphocyte-associated antigen 4 (CTLA4), linked to the modified fragment crystallizable (FC) region of IgG1. It inhibits T-cell activation by binding CD80/CD86 on antigen presenting cells, blocking its interaction with CD28 on T-cells. It is currently approved for the treatment of rheumatoid arthritis [7].

In mouse models of bleomycin-induced dermal fibrosis and chronic graft-vs-host disease (early and inflammatory stages of SSc), abatacept prevented skin fibrosis and it was also effective in treating established fibrosis. Activated T-cells, B-cells and monocytes infiltrating the skin were reduced, along with IL-6 and IL-10 levels. However, abatacept did not have any efficacy reducing dermal fibrosis in Tsk-1 mice (inflammatory-independent mouse model of SSc) reinforcing the concept that inhibition of T-cell response by abatacept can only prevent and reduce inflammation-driven dermal fibrosis. Moreover, abatacept did not protect against bleomycin-induced dermal fibrosis in CB17-SCID mice, further supporting the idea that T-cells have a role in the anti-fibrotic effect of abatacept [48].

Some case reports and observational studies have shown the benefit of abatacept in SSc patients. In a small clinical report of four patients with dcSSc refractory to conventional therapy, abatacept was administered intravenously at weeks 0, 2 and 4, and then every 4 weeks. All four patients had severe progression of skin thickness, and two of them had interstitial lung disease under conventional therapy (cyclophosphamide and low-dose prednisolone). After adding abatacept, a decrease in mRSS was achieved in all patients (average of 1.3 units/month) and lung function improved 6 months after starting abatacept. Furthermore, these effects were sustained even after tapering the other treatments [49]. In an observational EUSTAR study in 20 SSc patients with refractory polyarthritis and myositis, treatment with abatacept for a mean of eleven months showed benefits in polyarthritis with a reduction of the 28-joint count Disease Activity Score but it showed no efficacy in muscle involvement. There was also no difference in mRSS, but only half of these patients had dcSSc and the mean baseline mRSS was only 5 [19].

In addition, Chakravarty et al. carried out a pilot study in 10 early dcSSc patients (seven treated with abatacept at 0, 2, 4 and every 4 weeks, for 24 weeks; three patients treated with placebo). Compared to placebo, patients treated with abatacept showed a greater improvement in absolute mRSS (−8.6 vs −2.3, p = 0.059) and a higher mean percentage of change in mRSS (−33% vs −6.2%, respectively, p = 0.31). No changes in the other variables were documented, namely in lung function tests. There were no serious adverse events [50].

Recently, the same group performed a randomised placebo-controlled clinical trial to evaluate the effect of abatacept and to assess safety outcomes in 10 SSc patients (seven treated with abatacept for 24 weeks and three with placebo). Improvement in mRSS was defined as ≥30% from baseline; skin biopsies were obtained for differential gene expression and intrinsic gene expression subset assignment (inflammatory signature, fibroproliferative signature and normal-like signature). This included biopsies from four healthy controls [51].

There was a trend towards improvement in mRSS in the treatment group at week 24, when compared to the baseline (−8.6 ± 7.5, p = 0.0625), but not to the placebo group (−2.3 ± 15, p = 0.75). When accounting for repeated measures over the eight visits of the study, there was a significant difference between the two groups, with a decrease estimate of −9.8 (95% CI −16.7 ± 3.0, p = 0.0014) in mRSS. Five of the patients in the treatment group and one in the placebo group showed a decrease in mRSS ≥ 30%. Adverse events were similar in both groups, with one serious adverse event in the treatment group (supraventricular tachycardia), considered to be unrelated to the study drug and the patient completed the study. Patients who improved with abatacept mapped to the inflammatory intrinsic subset of skin gene expression at baseline and showed decreased gene expression after treatment, mainly in genes related to CD28 T-cell co-stimulation, whereas non-improvers and the placebo group showed stable or reverse inflammatory gene expression [51].

Given these data, the same group is currently conducting a larger multi-centre placebo-controlled trial for subcutaneous abatacept in early dcSSc. In addition to safety assessment, the primary outcome of this trial is variation in mRSS [52].

3.3.2. B-cells

The findings of pre-clinical and clinical works suggest an important role for B-cells in the physiopathology of SSc. SSc patients have an altered blood B-cell homeostasis, with studies showing expanded naive B-cells, activated but diminished memory B-cells, and chronic hyper-reactivity of memory B-cells [53, 54]. Additionally, DNA microarrays of gene expression patterns in skin biopsies of dcSSc patients have revealed a B-lymphocyte signature when compared to healthy controls, and this was present in both affected and unaffected skin [55].

B-cell infiltration was also found in lung biopsies of SSc patients with interstitial lung disease (ILD). Lafyatis et al. analysed pulmonary tissue of 11 patients with dcSSc (four with non-specific interstitial pneumonia and seven with a usual interstitial pneumonia pattern). Tissue was stained for CD20, CD3 and CD68 and compared with lung biopsies from four healthy controls. Lung tissue from SSc patients showed a variable but intense infiltration of B-cells arranged in lymphoid aggregates as well as in a diffuse pattern. Staining tended to be more intense in patients with the usual interstitial pneumonia (UIP) pattern, but the correlation was not statistically significant, possibly due to the small sample size. These data suggest that B-cells could be important in the pathogenesis of ILD in SSc, and considering the variability of B-cell infiltration, anti-CD20 therapy can be a therapeutic option at least in a subset of patients with SSc [56].

Contributing to probable relevancy of B-cells in SSc, serum levels of B-cell activating factor (BAAF) were also shown to be elevated in SSc patients, correlating with the extent of skin fibrosis. BAAF is a member of the tumour necrosis factor (TNF) superfamily and plays an important role in the survival and maturation of B-cells. It influences all stages of B-cell differentiation, from development, selection and homeostasis of naive primary B-cells to the maintenance of long-lived bone marrow plasma cells. BAAF excess rescues self-reactive B-cells from anergy, contributing to autoimmunity. Matsushita et al. examined BAAF levels in the serum of 21 SSc patients (both diffuse and limited subsets) and related the results to clinical features of the patients. Serum BAAF levels were significantly higher in patients with SSc when compared with healthy controls [median 1.26 ng/mL (0.32 – 1.37) vs 0.78 ng/mL (0.39.1.37), respectively, $p < 0.001$], and patients with dcSSc had higher levels than lcSSc ($p < 0.05$). BAAF levels in SSc correlated positively with mRSS ($r = 0.415$, $p < 0.005$). A longitudinal study of BAAF levels for 6 years classified SSc patients as follows: 7 patients had decreased BAAF levels, 11 had unchanged levels and 3 had increased levels. Decreased BAAF levels were associated with a significant decrease in mRSS from baseline to 2 years (36%, $p < 0.05$), 4 years (45%, $p < 0.05$) and 6 years (54%, $p < 0.05$). In the three patients in whom BAAF levels remained high, there was no change in mRSS, and new onset/worsening of internal organ involvement (renal crisis and deterioration of ILD) was documented. In the group in whom BAAF levels remained unchanged, mRSS tended to decrease, but it was not statistically significant [57].

The levels of BAAF receptor were also higher in SSc compared to controls (mean 81 ± 40 vs 43 ± 7, $p < 0.05$). Moreover, BAAF mRNA expression in affected skin from SSc patients was significantly upregulated in early SSc patients (disease duration <3 years) compared with late SSc patients (>6 years disease duration) and normal controls ($p < 0.005$ and $p < 0.0001$, respectively). The expression of BAAF mRNA in the skin of late SSC and normal controls was not significantly different. To evaluate the role of BAAF in B-cell function of SSc, B-cells were stimulated with BAAF and the amounts of IL-6 and IgG were determined. SSc B-cells produced 38% more IL-6 and 35% more IgG than B-cells from healthy controls [57].

B-cell depletion has been proven to be effective in reversing skin fibrosis both in animal models of SSc and in small case series and clinical trials. Studies in the tsk mouse model showed that B-cell depletion by an anti-CD20 antibody inhibited the development of autoimmunity and skin fibrosis when initiated early in the course of disease. In a study by Hasegawa et al., B-cell depletion using an anti-mouse CD20 monoclonal antibody before (at day 3 after birth) and after disease development (day 56) resulted in reduced skin fibrosis, decreased autoantibody generation and decreased levels of hypergammaglobulinemia in new born mice, but not in adult mice with established disease [58].

Rituximab is a chimeric anti-CD20 monoclonal antibody largely used in rheumatology for the treatment of RA, SLE and more recently for Anti-neutrophil cytoplasmic antibody (ANCA)-positive vasculitis [7]. In an open-label trial, Bosello et al. treated nine dcSSc patients with rituximab, and analysed long-term safety, skin score and serum levels of IL-6. After treatment, at 6 months, there was an improvement in mRSS from 21.1 ± 9.0 to 12.0 ± 6.1 ($p = 0.001$), with a median decrease of 43.3% (range from 21.1 to 64.0%), a parallel fall in IL-6 serum levels (from 3.7 ± 5.3 to 0.6 ± 0.9 pg/mL, $p = 0.02$) and an improvement in the Health Assessment Questionnaire (HAQ) score (from 0.9 ± 0.7 to 0.4 ± 0.5, $p = 0.01$). The FVC and DLCO levels showed no significant difference at follow-up compared with baseline. Nevertheless, none of the patients had a clinically significant reduction in FVC values (>10%). Moreover, none of the patients had new or progressive cardiac involvement, renal crisis or symptoms suggesting progressive gastrointestinal disease [59].

Smith et al. obtained similar results in a 24-week open-label clinical trial in eight dcSSc patients. Rituximab induced effective B-cell depletion in all patients and improved the skin score from 24.8 ± 3.4 to 14.3 ± 3.5 ($p < 0.001$) at 24 weeks. Parameters of internal organ involvement remained stable, namely lung function tests. Histopathological study of the skin revealed a decrease in the mean hyalinised collagen score from 60 ± 6.5 to 7.1 ± 7.2 ($p < 0.0001$) and abolished myofibroblast positivity [4/7 vs 0/8, (χ^2 test $p = 0.013$)] [60].

In another small pilot study, Lafyatis et al. assessed rituximab safety, clinical efficacy and resulting skin B-cell and autoantibody depletion in 15 patients with early dcSSc (less than 18 months prior to trial entry). The mRSS did not change significantly between baseline and 6 months. Similarly, both predicted FVC and DLCO remained unchanged at 6 months after treatment. Nevertheless, none of the patients showed evidence of progression of major organ involvement. Circulating B-cell depletion was achieved in all patients at 3 months, with recovery at 6–12 months. Also, most patients showed complete depletion of skin B-cells, with an average quantification per specimen at baseline of 10.4, compared with 3.4 at 6 months. Autoantibody levels declined modestly but the changes were not consistent during follow-up [61].

In a large observational case-control series of 63 SSc patients (both diffuse and limited) from the EUSTAR cohort, mRSS decreased significantly from 18.1 ± 1.6 to 14.4 ± 1.5 ($p = 0.0002$) and there was also a significant decrease in the mean percentage of change from baseline of −15.0 ± 5.3% ($p = 0.008$) on follow-up at 7 months. Furthermore, in patients with SSc-related

ILD, FVC was stable after treatment, compared with baseline (60 ± 2.4 vs 61.3 ± 4.1%, $p = 0.5$), whereas DLCO significantly improved (41.1 ± 2.8 vs 44.8 ± 2.7%, $p = 0.03$). In contrast, matched controls from the EUSTAR database showed a decline in FVC in both the mean percentage of predicted value ($p = 0.02$) and in absolute change ($p = 0.01$) [62].

Focusing on lung fibrosis, Daoussis et al. studied eight dcSSc patients with ILD treated with rituximab, during a 2-year follow-up [63]. Similarly to previous results from a smaller scale study from the same group [64], there was a significant increase from baseline in both FVC (mean 68.13 ± 19.69 vs 75 ± 19.73, $p = 0.0018$) and DLCO (mean 52.25 ± 20.71 vs 62 ± 23.21, $p = 0.017$), reinforcing the benefits of rituximab treatment in SSc-associated ILD. In a larger population of 30 patients, the same group performed a 7-year follow-up open-label multi-centre study, with results supporting the benefits of continuous rituximab treatment for skin involvement and SSc-related ILD. Patients were treated at baseline, 6, 12 and 18 months. Both FVC and DLCO improved after 2 years (mean FVC: 86.2 ± 5.5 vs 78.2 ± 3.6, $p = 0.018$; mean DLCO: 62.4 ± 4.5 vs 57.3 ± 3.2, $p = 0.012$, treatment vs baseline, respectively). There was a trend towards stabilisation after 2 years of treatment (mean FVC 84.3 ± 6.5 at 5 years, $p = 0.04$). However, in three patients who had an initial improvement or stabilisation of lung function with continuous treatment, there was deterioration in the lung function tests after 3 years of rituximab cessation and they did not respond to retreatment. Corroborating previous results, an early improvement in mRSS was also achieved at all time-points compared with baseline ($p < 0.001$) [65].

Considering the role of B-cells in SSc and positive results associated with its depletion, several clinical trials are on-going with rituximab and belimumab, an anti-B-lymphocyte stimulator monoclonal antibody used in patients with SLE, but no preliminary results are yet available [66].

In the study Rituximab in Systemic Sclerosis (RECOVER) the primary outcome is the treatment of polyarthritis (through analogy with rheumatoid arthritis), and the secondary outcomes are improvements in mRSS, lung function tests and quality of life [67].

Another on-going trial aims to validate an infusion protocol-based treatment for early diffuse SSc with rituximab, using a dose of 1000 mg intravenously, at day 1 and 15 and then at week 26–28, together with a corticosteroid regimen consisting of intravenous methylprednisolone 100 mg, 30 minutes prior to both infusions. Clinical variables will be assessed after 28 weeks, namely survival rate, presence of heart and lung failure and antibody titres [68].

Based on pre-clinical data and anecdotal reports, which suggest that modulation of the immune system may be an effective strategy for treating pulmonary arterial hypertension in SSc, patient recruitment is currently underway for a randomised double-blinded placebo-controlled trial (phase II) to evaluate the effects of rituximab on this severe manifestation of the disease. The primary outcome is the change in pulmonary vascular resistance measured by right heart catheterisation, assessed at week 24. Patients will still receive concurrent stable-dose standard therapy with a prostanoid, endothelin receptor antagonist and/or phosphodiesterase-5 inhibitor. In a sub-study, cardiac magnetic resonance will be used to evaluate changes in right ventricular end diastolic volume index and stroke volume, as measures of right ventricular function [69].

4. Conclusions

The interplay of vasculopathy, fibrosis, inflammation and autoimmunity makes SSc a complex disease. The growing understanding of its pathogenesis has increased the identification of potential targets, and thereby the use of specific therapies such as biological agents. Although most studies and clinical trials are restricted to a subgroup of SSc patients, mainly with the early diffuse cutaneous subset, the results are encouraging for some biologicals, especially B-cell depleting agents and anti-IL6 drugs for skin and lung involvement.

While tocilizumab has shown benefits in reducing skin fibrosis and halting progression of interstitial lung disease, data on rituximab are more consistent in relation to improvement of lung fibrosis, at least in early disease stages, although the benefits in later phases are not clear.

Apart from anti-IL6 antagonists, other biologicals targeting cytokines are not yet valuable options for SSc treatment. All three cytokines, IL-17, IL-13 and IL-1, are relevant in fibrosis mechanisms, but the clinical utility of their antagonists in SSc is still unknown. Anti-TNF-α therapy can be beneficial in a highly selected subgroup of patients with inflammatory arthritis overlap, although its use is not recommended for SSc, due to concerns related to worsening interstitial lung disease.

Other therapeutic approaches such as T-cell target therapy (abatacept) have had good results, although limited to skin fibrosis and arthritis, and without any proven benefits for SSc organ-based complications. Additionally, despite the key role of TGF-β in the pathogenesis of SSc, clinical use of TGF-β antagonists did not show any benefits regarding internal organ involvement, and there were serious treatment-related adverse events.

Although some of the results from clinical trials in SSc are compelling, primary outcomes mostly address only skin fibrosis and lung disease, probably reflecting the lack of validated internal organ assessment outcome measures, especially for gastrointestinal and cardiac complications. Nevertheless, randomised clinical trials are necessary to validate new therapies as the standard of care in clinical practice. Hence, apart from better insights into disease mechanisms, which will help to identify new therapeutic targets, improvement in clinical trial design, with better cohort definition and updating of traditional clinical end-point assessment, will provide more robust results to inform the clinical applicability of biological therapies in SSc.

Based on the complexity of SSc pathogenesis and early indicators from the studies up to date, it seems likely that future treatment approaches may be built around targeting multiple pathways simultaneously. This may means combined therapy using both biologicals and small molecule inhibitors, such as tyrosine kinases, although issues related to adverse events and cost would have to be addressed.

Author details

Joana Caetano[1], Susana Oliveira[1] and José Delgado Alves[1,2*]

*Address all correspondence to: jose.alves@nms.unl.pt

1 Systemic Autoimmune Diseases Unit, Department of Medicine IV, Fernando Fonseca Hospital, Amadora, Portugal

2 CEDOC/NOVA Medical School, Lisbon, Portugal

References

[1] Gabrielli A, Avvedimento EV, Krieg T. Scleroderma. New England Journal of Medicine. 2009;**360**:1989-2003

[2] Stern E, Denton CP. The pathogenesis of systemic sclerosis. Rheumatic Diseases Clinics of North America. 2015;**41**:367-382

[3] Denton CP. Advances in pathogenesis and treatment of systemic sclerosis. Clinical Medicine. 2015;**6**:s58–s63

[4] Allanore Y, Simms R, Distler O. Systemic sclerosis. Nature Reviews. 2015;**1**:1-21

[5] Denton CP, Ong VH. Target therapies for systemic sclerosis. Nature Reviews Rheumatology. 2013;**9**:451-464

[6] Rogers JL, Serafin DS, Timoshchenko RG, et al. Cellular targeting in autoimmunity. Current Allergy and Asthma Reports. 2012;**12**(6):495-510

[7] Rosman Z, Shoenfeld Y, Zandman-Goddard G, et al. Biologic therapy for autoimmune diseases: An update. BMC Medicine. 2013;**11**:88

[8] Conti F, Ceccarelli F, Massaro L, et al. Biological therapies in rheumatic diseases. Clinica Terapeutica. 2013;**164**(5):e413-428

[9] Abraham DJ, T. Krieg T, Distler J. Overview of pathogenesis of systemic sclerosis. Rheumatology. 2009;**48**:iii3–iii7

[10] Gourh P, Arnett FC, Assassi S, et al. Plasma cytokine profiles in systemic sclerosis: Associations with autoantibody subsets and clinical manifestations. Arthritis Research & Therapy. 2009;**11**:R147

[11] Zuber JP, Spertini F. Immunological basis of systemic sclerosis. Rheumatology. 2006;**45**: iii23–iii25

[12] Kanna D, Distler JHW, Sandner P, et al. Emerging strategies for treatment of systemic sclerosis. Journal of Systemic Sclerosis and Related Disorders. 2016;**1**:186-193

[13] Lafatatis R. Transforming growth factor β—at the centre of systemic sclerosis. Nature Reviews Rheumatology. 2014;**10**:706-719

[14] Saito F, Tasaka S, Inoue K, et al. Role of Interleukin-6 in Bleomycin-Induced lung inflammatory changes in mice. American Journal of Respiratory Cell and Molecular Biology. 2008;**38**:566-571

[15] Kitaba S, Murota T, Terao M, et al. Blockade of Interleukin-6 Receptor alleviates disease in mouse model of scleroderma. The American Journal of Pathology. 2012;**180**(1):165-176

[16] Khan K, Xu S, Nihtyanova S, et al. Clinical and pathological significance of interleukin 6 overexpression in systemic sclerosis. Annals of the Rheumatic Diseases. 2012;**71**: 1235-1242

[17] O'Reilly S, Cant R, Ciechomska M, et al. Interleukin-6: A new therapeutic target in systemic sclerosis? Clinical & Translational Immunology. 2013;**2**(4):e4

[18] Shima Y, KuwaharaY, Murot H, et al. The skin of patients with systemic sclerosis softened during the treatment with anti-IL-6 receptor antibody tocilizumab. Rheumatology. 2010;**49**:2408-2412

[19] Elhai M, Meunier M, Matucci-Cerinic M, et al. Outcomes of patients with systemic sclerosis-associated polyarthritis and myopathy treated with tocilizumab or abatacept: A EUSTAR observational study. Annals of the Rheumatic Diseases. 2013;**72**:1217-1220

[20] Fernandes das Neves M, Oliveira S, Amaral M, et al. Treatment of systemic sclerosis with tocilizumab. Rheumatology. 2015;**54**:371-372

[21] Khanna D, Denton CP, Jahreis A, et al. Safety and efficacy of subcutaneous tocilizumab in adults with systemic sclerosis (faSScinate): A phase 2, randomised, controlled trial. Lancet. 2016. **387**(10038):2630-40

[22] US National Library of Medicine. Clinical Trials. Gov [Internet]. Available from: https://clinicaltrials.gov/ct2/show/NCT02453256

[23] Koca SS, Isik A, Ozercan IH, et al. Effectiveness of etanercept in bleomycin-induced experimental scleroderma. Rheumatology. 2008;**47**:172-175

[24] Denton CP, Engelhart M, Tvede N, et al. An open-label pilot study of infliximab therapy in diffuse cutaneous systemic sclerosis. Annals of the Rheumatic Diseases. 2009;**68**: 1433-1439

[25] Distler JHW, Jordan S, Airò P, et al. Is there a role for TNF-α antagonists in the treatment of SSc? EUSTAR expert consensus development using the Delphi technique. Clinical and Experimental Rheumatology. 2011;**29**(Suppl. 65):S40–S45

[26] Ostor AJ, Crisp AJ, Somerville MF, et al. Fatal exacerbation of rheumatoid arthritis associated fibrosing alveolitis in patients given infliximab. British Medical Journal. 2004;**329**:1266

[27] Allanore Y, Devos-Francois G, Caramella C, et al. Fatal exacerbation of fibrosing alveolitis associated with systemic sclerosis in a patient treated with adalimumab. Annals of the Rheumatic Diseases. 2006;**65**:834-835

[28] Maekawa T, et al. Serum levels of interleukin-1α in patients with systemic sclerosis. The Journal of Dermatology. 2013;**40**(2):98-101

[29] Kawaguchi Y, McCarthy SA, Watkins SC, et al. Autocrine activation by interleukin 1alpha induces the fibrogenic phenotype of systemic sclerosis fibroblasts. The Journal of Rheumatology. 2004;**31**(10):1946-1954

[30] US National Library of Medicine. Clinical Trials. Gov [Internet]. Available from: http://www.clinicaltrials.gov/ct2/show/NCT01538719

[31] Farina G, Lafyatis D, Lemaire R, et al. A four-gene biomarker predicts skin disease in patients with diffuse cutaneous systemic sclerosis. Arthritis & Rheumatism. 2010;**62**(2): 580-588

[32] Fichtner-Feigl S, Strober W. Kawakami K, et al. IL-13 signaling through the IL-13α2 receptor is involved in induction of TGF β1 production and fibrosis. Nature Medicine. 2006;**12**:99-106

[33] Fuschiotti P, Medsger TA, Morel PA. Effector CD8-T cells in systemic sclerosis patients produce abnormally high levels of Interleukin-13 associated with increased skin fibrosis. Arthritis & Rheumatism. 2009;**60**:1119-1128

[34] Belperio JA, Dy M, Burdick MD, et al. Interaction of IL-13 and C10 in the pathogenesis of Bleomycin-Induced pulmonary fibrosis. American Journal of Respiratory Cell and Molecular Biology. 2002;**27**:419-427

[35] Fuschiotti P, Larregina AT, Johnan H, et al. IL-13-producing CD8+ T cells mediate dermal fibrosis in patients with systemic sclerosis. Arthritis & Rheumatology. 2013;**65**(1):236-246

[36] Kraft M. Asthma phenotypes and interleukin 13 moving closer to personalized medicine. New England Journal of Medicine. 2011;**365**:1141-1144

[37] Yang L, et al. Periostin facilitates skin sclerosis via PI3K/Akt dependent mechanism in a mouse model of scleroderma. PLoS ONE. 2012;**7**:e41994

[38] US National Library of Medicine Clinical Trials. Gov [Internet]. Available from: http://www.clinicaltrials.gov/ct2/show/NCT01629667

[39] Kurasawa K, Hirose K, Sano H, et al. Increased interleukin-17 production in patients with systemic sclerosis. Arthritis & Rheumatism. 2000;**43**:2455-2463

[40] Radstake TR, van Bon L, Broen J, et al. The pronounced Th17 profile in systemic sclerosis (SSc) together with intracellular expression of TGF-β and IFNγ distinguishes SSc phenotypes. PloS One. 2009;**4**(6):e5903

[41] Yang X, Yang J, Xing X, et al. Increased frequency of Th17 cells in systemic sclerosis is related to disease activity and collagen overproduction. Arthritis Research & Therapy. 2014;**16**:R4

[42] Novelli L, Chimenti MS, Chiricozzi A, et al. The new era for the treatment of psoriasis and psoriatic arthritis: Perspectives and validated strategies. Autoimmunity Reviews. 2014;**13**:64-69

[43] Sargent JL, Milano A, Bhattacharyya S, et al. A TGFb-Responsive gene signature is associated with a subset of diffuse scleroderma with increased disease severity. Journal of Investigative Dermatology. 2010;**130**:694-705

[44] Ihn H, Yamane K, Kubo M, et al. Blockade of endogenous transforming growth factor b signaling prevents Up-Regulated collagen synthesis in scleroderma fibroblasts. Association with increased expression of transforming growth factor b receptors. Arthritis & Rheumatism. 2001;**44**:474-480

[45] Varga J, Pasche B. Transforming growth factor-ß as a therapeutic target in systemic sclerosis. Nature Reviews Rheumatology. 2009;**5**(4):200-206

[46] Denton CP, Merkel PA, Furst DE, et al. Recombinant human Anti-Transforming growth Factor-1 antibody therapy in systemic sclerosis. A multicenter, randomized, Placebo-Controlled Phase I/II Trial of CAT-192. Arthritis & Rheumatism. 2007;**56**:323-333

[47] Rice LM, Padilla CM, McLaughlin SR, et al. Fresolimumab treatment decreases biomarkers and improves clinical symptoms in systemic sclerosis patients. Journal of Clinical Investigation. 2015;**125**(7):2795-2807

[48] Ponsoye M, Frantz C, Ruzehaji N, et al. Treatment with abatacept prevents experimental dermal fibrosis and induces regression of established inflammation-driven fibrosis. Annals of the Rheumatic Diseases. 2015. 2015.DOI:10.1136 and replace for 2016;**75**(12):2142-2149

[49] Paoli FV, Nielsen BD, Rasmussen F, et al. Abatacept induces clinical improvement in patients with severe systemic sclerosis. Scandinavian Journal of Rheumatology. 2014;**43**(4):342-345

[50] Chakravarty EF, Fiorentino D, Bennett D, et al. A pilot study of abatacept for the treatment of patients with diffuse cutaneous systemic sclerosis. Arthritis & Rheumatology. 2011;**63**(Suppl 10):707

[51] Chakravarty EF, Martyanov V, Fiorentino D, et al. Gene expression changes reflect clinical response in a placebo-controlled randomized trial of abatacept in patients with diffuse cutaneous systemic sclerosis. Arthritis Research & Therapy. 2015;**17**:159

[52] US National Library of Medicine. Clinical Trials. Gov [Internet]. Available from: https://clinicaltrials.gov/ct2/show/NCT02161406

[53] Sato S, Fujimoto M, Hasegawa M, et al. Altered blood B lymphocyte homeostasis in systemic sclerosis expanded naive B cells and diminished but activated memory B cells. Arthritis & Rheumatism. 2004;**50**:1918-1927

[54] Sato S, Fujimoto M, Takehara K, et al. Altered B lymphocyte function induces systemic autoimmunity in systemic sclerosis. Molecular Immunology. 2004;**41**(12):1123-1133

[55] Whitfield ML, Finlay DR, Murray J, et al. Systemic and cell type-specific gene expression patterns in scleroderma skin. Proceedings National Academy of Sciences. 2003; **100**(21):12319-12324

[56] Lafyatis R, O'Hara C, Feghali-Bostwick CA, et al. B cell infiltration in systemic sclerosis-associated interstitial lung disease. Arthritis & Rheumatism. 2007;**56**:3167-3171

[57] Matsushita T, Hasegawa M, Yanaba K, et al. Elevated serum BAFF levels in patients with systemic sclerosis enhanced BAFF signaling in systemic sclerosis B lymphocytes. Arthritis & Rheumatism. 2006;**54**:192-201

[58] Hasegawa M, Hamaguchi Y, Yanaba K, et al. B-Lymphocyte depletion reduces skin fibrosis and autoimmunity in the Tight-Skin mouse model for systemic sclerosis. The American Journal of Pathology. 2006;**169**(3):954-966

[59] Bosello S, Santis M, Lama G, et al. B cell depletion in diffuse progressive systemic sclerosis: Safety, skin score modification and IL-6 modulation in an up to thirty-six months follow-up open-label trial. Arthritis Research & Therapy. 2010;**12**:R54

[60] Smith V, Van Praet JT, Vandooren B, et al. Rituximab in diffuse cutaneous systemic sclerosis: An open-label clinical and histopathological study. Annals of the Rheumatic Diseases. 2010;**69**(01):193-197

[61] Lafyatis R, Kissin E, York M, et al. B cell depletion with rituximab in patients with diffuse cutaneous systemic sclerosis. Arthritis & Rheumatism. 2009;**60**:578-583

[62] Jordan S, Distler JW, Maurer B, et al. Effects and safety of rituximab in systemic sclerosis: An analysis from the European Scleroderma Trial and Research (EUSTAR) Group. Annals of the Rheumatic Diseases. 2015;**74**:1188-1194

[63] Daoussis D, Liossis SC, Tsamandas AC, et al. Effect of long-term treatment with rituximab on pulmonary function and skin fibrosis in patients with diffuse systemic sclerosis. Clinical and Experimental Rheumatology. 2012;**30**(Suppl. 71):S17–S22

[64] Daoussis D, Liossis SNc, Tsamandas AC, et al. Experience with rituximab in scleroderma: Results from a 1-year, proof-of-principle study. Rheumatology. 2010;**49**:271-280

[65] Melissaropoulos K, Daoussis D, Antonopoulos I, et al. Rituximab in systemic sclerosis. Results of an up to seven years, open label, Multicenter Study with a Follow-up of 89 Patient-Years. Annals of the Rheumatic Diseases. 2015;**74**:823

[66] US National Library of Medicine. Clinical Trials. Gov [Internet]. Available from: https://clinicaltrials.gov/ct2/show/NCT01670565

[67] US National Library of Medicine. Clinical Trials. Gov [Internet]. Available from: https://clinicaltrials.gov/ct2/show/NCT01748084

[68] US National Library of Medicine. Clinical Trials. Gov [Internet]. Available from: https://clinicaltrials.gov/ct2/show/NCT00379431

[69] US National Library of Medicine. Clinical Trials. Gov [Internet]. Available from: https://clinicaltrials.gov/ct2/show/NCT01086540

Chapter 8

Animal Models of Systemic Sclerosis

Hana Storkanova and Michal Tomcik

Additional information is available at the end of the chapter

http://dx.doi.org/10.5772/intechopen.68551

Abstract

Systemic sclerosis (SSc) is a rare, chronic connective tissue disease affecting the skin, vessels, musculoskeletal system, and internal organs. Despite advances in pharmacotherapy of organ manifestations and new knowledge about the pathogenesis of SSc, there is still no effective universal treatment of this serious disease. The aim of this chapter is to introduce traditional, most commonly used experimental animal models of SSc, clarify their basic pathological mechanism, describe their advantages and limitations, and outline their use in preclinical tests of potential therapeutic agents with subsequent clinical trials in patients with SSc. The existing models have already contributed significantly to preclinical testing of several available biological agents and small molecules, some of which achieved promising results in early clinical studies, and could provide better prospects for patients with this incurable disease.

Keywords: systemic sclerosis, experimental models, biological therapy, small molecules

1. Introduction

Systemic sclerosis (SSc) or scleroderma is a rare, chronic connective tissue disease affecting the skin, vessels, musculoskeletal system, and internal organs. The name of this disease is derived from the Greek words "scleros" and "derma" meaning tough skin and was first used by Gintrac in 1847. The first mention of a stiff skin comes from Hippocrates around 400 BC. SSc affects women more often, usually begins in their 40s, and overall survival is shorter (10-year survival of around 70%). Despite advances in pharmacotherapy of organ manifestations and new knowledge about the pathogenesis of SSc, there is still no effective treatment of this serious disease [1]. The etiology of SSc is still unclear, although there are long known associations between some external factors (mainly silicon compounds and organic solvents) and the development of SSc.

The possibility of biopsy sampling of affected tissues in patients with SSc, in particular as a skin biopsy, helped to a large degree to elucidate the pathogenesis of this disease. Histological analysis of biopsy samples of tissues in different stages of the disease has identified three basic pathological processes and their relative time sequence: vasculopathy, inflammation, and fibrosis. The first pathological changes can be detected at the level of microcirculation, in which damage to the endothelium leads to progressive development of inflammation caused by the activation of cells of both the innate and, subsequently, acquired immunity. Activated cells produce pro-fibrotic cytokines, especially transforming growth factor beta (TGF-β), connective tissue growth factor (CTGF), and platelet-derived growth factor (PDGF). These cytokines activate resident fibroblasts, which increase production of extracellular matrix (ECM) components that lead to remodeling of a functional tissue to a fibrotic one. The fibrotic phase of the pathogenesis of SSc and its severity and extent determine the morbidity and mortality of this disease [2]. The material from skin biopsies has also enabled the analysis of gene and protein expression, epigenetic modifications, and signaling pathways of different target molecules. The potential importance of these candidate molecules must always be first tested and subsequently confirmed, pending their therapeutic use in SSc. For these purposes, we may use in vitro experiments on tissue or cell cultures isolated from tissues explanted from SSc patients and healthy individuals or in vivo experiments using experimental animal models of SSc [3].

Today, there are numerous animal models of SSc. However, none of the available models mimics the full range of pathologies and clinical manifestations of SSc. Experimental animal models help clarify certain pathological mechanisms and only mimic some aspects of SSc. Each model has its advantages and disadvantages. Selection of an appropriate animal model for the analysis of target genes or candidate molecules for therapy must be carefully considered beforehand [4]. Since the skin fibrosis is a dominant and common feature in most patients with SSc, this pathological process is not only a starting point but also the key aspect for the majority of experimental models. With the progress in scientific knowledge and technologies, new models were developed with other dominant features such as activation of immunity and inflammation, vasculopathy, and specific pathological processes in the involved organs, especially the lungs. However, most of available models provide an overlap of the abovementioned pathological mechanisms and a concurrent involvement of several organs characteristic of SSc.

The aim of this chapter is to introduce traditional, most commonly used experimental animal models of SSc, clarify their basic pathological mechanism, describe the advantages and limitations, and outline their use in preclinical tests of potential therapeutic agents with subsequent clinical trials in patients with SSc.

2. Experimental murine models of fibrosis

2.1. Tight skin 1 (Tsk1) mice

Tsk1 mice possess an autosomal dominant mutation, tandem duplication in the gene for fibrillin 1, which is an important regulator of the TGF-β signaling and fibrogenesis. In heterozygous

http://dx.doi.org/10.5772/intechopen.68551

mice (labeled Tsk1), this mutation leads to hyperplasia and thickening of the subcutaneous tissue and fascial layers of the skin without striking thickening of the dermis itself (**Figure 1**). Similarly, hyperplasia of subcutaneous fascia and lipoatrophy can also be detected in the skin of patients with SSc. Tsk1 mice also produce autoantibodies (anti-topoisomerase I, anti-RNA polymerase I, anti-dsDNA) [5–9]. Fibrosis in these mice develops from excessive production of ECM by activated fibroblasts during the activation of TGF-β pathway. The exact mechanism has not yet been elucidated. The progression of fibrosis in Tsk1 mice is mediated by an increased expression of CD19, chronic B-cell activation leading to increased secretion of IL-6, and mast cells. These mechanisms are also applied in the progression of SSc in humans. Tsk1 mice are commonly used as a model mimicking later stages of SSc that are independent of inflammatory infiltrates [10].

The advantage of this model is a detailed documentation and endogenous activation of fibroblasts similar to SSc in humans. The limitations to this model include insufficiently elucidated molecular mechanisms, the absence of vascular phenotype, dominant histological changes in the hypodermis, and some other changes, such as emphysema and kyphosis, which are not part of SSc in humans [4].

2.2. Tight skin 2 (Tsk2) mice

In 1986, a tight skin 2 (Tsk2) mouse model was first described, which is induced by a chemical compound ethylnitrosourea. This compound induces an autosomal dominant mutation localized on the chromosome 1. Only heterozygous individuals (Tsk2/+) survive [11]. The development of phenotypic features of this model occurs mainly between the third and fourth weeks after birth. The gene responsible for the mutation has not yet been precisely identified [12]. However, using in vivo and in vitro genetic tests, previous studies have demonstrated a significant role of missense mutations in the gene for type III collagen alpha 1 (Col3a1) [13]. The Tsk2/+ mice showed elevated levels of type III collagen and changes in the ECM in the

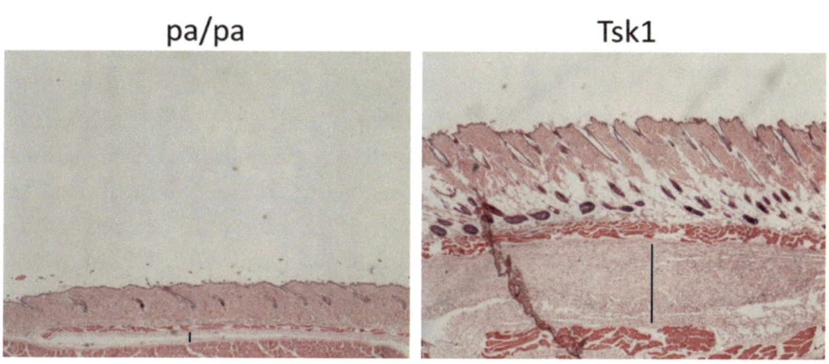

Figure 1. Hyperplasia and thickening of the subcutaneous tissue and fascial layers of the skin without striking thickening of the dermis in Tsk1 mice compared to the wild-type littermates (pa/pa). The sections are stained with hematoxylin-eosin (magnification 20-fold; the black vertical bar represents the thickness of the hypodermis).

dermis, especially during 10 days after birth, which were still prevalent in seventh to eighth month compared with the wild-type littermates. Furthermore, the Tsk2/+ mice demonstrated the presence of mononuclear inflammatory infiltrates [11]. Cultured fibroblasts isolated from Tsk2 mice showed elevated mRNA expression of Col1a1 and Col3a1 gene and overproduction of collagen fibers [14]. Compared with Tsk1 model, the Tsk2 mice are characterized by abundant mononuclear cells infiltrating the dermis and adipose tissue. These mice have excessive thickening of adventitia of the vessels in the heart and lungs along with changes in the alveolar compartment [14, 15].

These findings indicate a significant use of these models for research of fibrotic processes, such as SSc in humans, as this disease is also characterized by an increased expression and accumulation of collagen in dermal fibroblasts [16, 17]. The Tsk2 mouse model has a large number of very similar clinical manifestations to those seen in SSc patients, including skin thickening, increased production of collagen and ECM, and autoimmune responses [11, 18].

2.3. Deletion of the kinase domain of the type II TGF-β receptor in murine fibroblasts (TβRIIΔk-fib)

An experimental mouse model for deactivating the TGF-β signaling has been developed, in which the fibroblasts express a non-signaling mutant type II TGF-β receptor that lacks the intracellular kinase domain (TβRIIΔk) [19]. In in vitro experiments, TβRIIΔk was demonstrated to have inhibitory properties on TGF-β signaling and was characterized as a competitive antagonist of TGF-β1 [20]. TGF-β signaling is mediated through type I and type II TGF-β receptors (TβRI and TβRII), which have a serine/threonine kinase activity and trigger subsequent Smad-dependent or Smad-nondependent signaling. Binding of TGF-β1 to TβRII leads to subsequent phosphorylation of TβRI, which then mediates the activation of downstream signaling pathways [21]. Authors of this model hypothesized that only fibroblasts expressing TβRIIΔk would have distorted TGF-β signaling leading to suppression of genes regulated by this pathway and thus achieve reduced pro-fibrotic effects of TGF-β signaling in these fibroblasts. In in vivo experiments, even though fibroblasts cultured from mouse models expressing TβRIIΔk exhibited resistance to exogenous TGF-β, the TβRIIΔk mice paradoxically and surprisingly developed progressive cutaneous, intestinal, and pulmonary fibrosis [19, 22]. The TβRIIΔk model showed phenotypic properties resembling the properties of the activated TGF-β pathway. Fibrosis was demonstrated in both sexes. From the sixth week after birth, TβRIIΔk mice experienced weight loss and developed pathological changes in the lung, in terms of reduced lung capacity and increased presence of connective tissue and ECM components, compared to wild-type littermates [19]. In 10% of these animals, the acquired damage led to death of an adult mouse around the 16th week of age. At week 12, abnormal thickening of the dermis with the loss of subcutaneous adipose tissue can be demonstrated, which can be especially evident in the lower back of these mice. Furthermore, the TβRIIΔk mice are also characterized by elevated levels of collagen.

This model is used not only for understanding the regulatory effects of non-signaling TGF-β receptors and constitutive activation of TGF-β signaling in vivo but also as a model for genetically determined fibrosis [19].

2.4. Spontaneous age-related organ fibrosis in sirtuin 3-deficient mice

Sirtuin 3 (SIRT3) belongs to the large family of class III histone deacetylases, which alone requires nicotinamide adenine dinucleotide (NAD^+) as a cofactor for its proper enzymatic activity [23]. In mammals, there are seven isoforms/classes of sirtuins (SIRT1-7), which differ in specific binding substrates, different biological functions, and various locations in the cell [24]. SIRT3 is found primarily in the mitochondria, and elevated levels were detected during reduced food intake, so-called caloric restriction, and endurance sports [25]. Proper function of SIRT3 in murine models prevents the development of a number of diseases such as cancer, metabolic syndrome, etc. [26, 27]. Experimental mice deficient for SIRT3 (Sirt3-KO) develop cardiac hypertrophy and contractile dysfunction in adulthood [28]. An association between SIRT3 deficiency and aging was analyzed initially on the development of cardiac fibrosis in three age categories of Sirt3-KO mice. Results showed aggravation of fibrotic cardiac impairment depending on higher age of Sirt3-KO mice. Furthermore, formation of tissue fibrosis in a number of other organs again depending on the age was demonstrated in the Sirt3-KO mice. The older the Sirt3-KO mouse, the more affected organs were observed, including the lung, kidney, and liver, in contrast to the corresponding age-matched control group [29]. Mice that lack or have reduced expression of SIRT3 also develop pulmonary arterial hypertension. Nevertheless, malfunction of SIRT3 is not accompanied by the presence of inflammatory infiltrates, even though mitochondrial damage and the presence of oxidative stress have been detected [30]. Studies on SIRT3 also showed that increased expression of SIRT3 prevents the development of experimentally induced organ fibrosis and promotes the essential role of SIRT3 in maintaining cellular homeostasis of tissues during aging [29, 31].

The model of SIRT3-deficient mice allows for deeper examination of cellular mechanisms involved in the development of organ fibrosis and pulmonary arterial hypertension (PAH) in the absence of inflammatory infiltrates, depending on the age of the mouse.

2.5. Vinyl chloride

Vinyl chloride is a colorless, toxic gas of sweet fragrance, which is an important component in the production of the polymer polyvinyl chloride (PVC). Some individuals, who are exposed to repeated doses of vinyl chloride, develop cutaneous and pulmonary fibrosis. The development of fibrosis is often preceded by the Raynaud's phenomenon [32]. Animal models, particularly mice and rats that are exposed to vinyl chloride, develop the same disease as humans. Injections of vinyl chloride to BALB/cJ retired breeder mice lead to the development of cutaneous fibrosis and dermal inflammation with a substantial presence of mononuclear infiltrates similar to SSc in humans [33].

2.6. TBRI^{CA}; Cre-ER mice

In order to study a variety of genes in in vivo environment with activated TGF-β signaling, which is a central pro-fibrotic cytokine in the pathogenesis of SSc, the TBRI^{CA} mouse model was developed with the mutated form of the TGF-β type I receptor (TBRI^{CA}) in fibroblasts, which leads to its sustained activation independent of the ligand TGF-β. Specific expression in fibroblasts was achieved using a transcription enhancer of proα2(I) collagen gene, which directs the expression exclusively in fibroblasts [34–36]. The attempt to create transgenic mice despite the specific expression of this mutation only in the fibroblasts was not successful, and the mice died during the gestation. Thus, a postnatally induced sustained activation of TBRI using tamoxifen inducible Cre/loxP system was introduced, which leads to progressive generalized dermal fibrosis with overproduction of type I and type III collagen and adnexal atrophy [35]. This model is also characterized by thickening of the walls of the small arteries of the lungs, kidneys, and adrenal glands, as well as the pulmonary artery. Technical and economic demands of this model led to the introduction of alternative solution, in which local skin fibrosis is achieved by subcutaneous injection with a weakened adenovirus with sustained activation of TBRI, which is no longer limited to fibroblasts [35].

The advantages include a well-described pathological mechanism and a possibility of a detailed in vivo analysis of TGF-β signaling in fibroblasts. The limitations comprise only a minimal representation of inflammation and autoimmunity [4].

3. Experimental murine models mimicking immunologic aspects of SSc

3.1. Bleomycin-induced skin fibrosis

This model is a widely used model mimicking the in vivo inflammatory changes present in the early stage of SSc. Bleomycin was originally isolated from *Streptomyces verticillus* and is used in the treatment of various types of tumors [37]. High doses of bleomycin used in cancer therapy have well-known side effects. They cause lung disease, fibrosis, and even SSc-like skin alterations. Therefore, bleomycin is used in murine models of both lung and skin fibroses. Repeated subcutaneous injections in the defined area for 4 weeks lead to dermal fibrosis, which persists even 6 weeks after their administration (**Figure 2**) [38]. Apart from the development of inflammatory infiltrates and fibrosis in the affected skin, there is also a mild lung involvement with fibrosis. Furthermore, this model is characterized by the presence of antinuclear antibodies (ANA), anti-topoisomerase-I, anti-U1 RNP, and anti-histone antibodies, suggesting

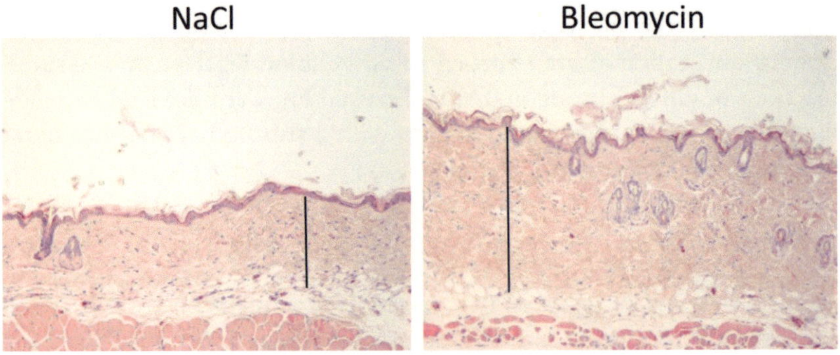

Figure 2. Fibrosis and inflammatory infiltrates in the dermis of mice locally injected with bleomycin compared to control mice injected with saline (NaCl). The sections are stained with hematoxylin-eosin (magnification 100-fold; the black vertical bar represents the thickness of the dermis).

for systemic involvement [39]. Bleomycin injections in the skin induce production of reactive oxygen species, resulting in impairment of endothelial cells and other cell types, and expression of adhesion molecules. This results in increased infiltration of the affected skin with polymorphonuclear cells, T and B lymphocytes, macrophages, eosinophils, and mast cells. Inflammatory infiltrates release increased amounts of pro-fibrotic and pro-inflammatory cytokines (TGF-β, PDGF, MCP-1, IL-4, IL-6, and IL-13), which activate the resident fibroblasts to produce excessive amounts of ECM components leading to cutaneous fibrosis [40].

The model of bleomycin-induced dermal fibrosis is very well documented and described, can be applied to numerous strains of mice, and is easy to use. A limitation of this model is that it is artificially induced, it is not associated with significant systemic involvement, and it tends to overestimate anti-fibrotic effect of anti-inflammatory agents [4].

3.2. Model of chronic sclerodermatous graft-versus-host diseases (SclGvHD)

Chronic graft-versus-host disease (GvHD) occurs in 40–60% of long-term survival patients following hematopoietic cell transplantation. Sclerodermatous (SclGvHD) and cytotoxic GvHD types are the two main subtypes of chronic GvHD [41]. SclGvHD is the fibrosing type, and its clinical manifestations are similar to the symptoms of the early inflammatory phase of diffuse cutaneous SSc. Induction of SclGvHD in mice is carried out in (a) a standard manner, when hematopoietic cells are transplanted into sublethally irradiated BALB/c mice or (b) a modified method, when hematopoietic cells are transplanted into immunodeficient recombinase-activating gene-2 (RAG-2) mice [42]. In both cases, SclGvHD is induced by a transplantation of hematopoietic cells of a donor to a recipient with identical major histocompatibility complex (MHC) but with different minor histocompatibility antigens. After reconstitution of hematopoiesis, SclGvHD is induced in the recipient with inflammation and fibrosis of the skin, lung, liver, kidney, gastrointestinal tract, and parotid gland. Besides inflammation and fibrosis, this model is also characterized by production of autoantibodies against nuclear antigens. In the pathogenesis of chronic SclGvHD, alloreactive CD4 T lymphocytes play a key role [43–47].

The advantage of this model is again a good documentation and systemic manifestations. The disadvantage is the need for sophisticated techniques and experience in dealing with problematic immunocompromised mice [4].

3.3. MRL/lpr murine model with deficient interferon gamma (IFN-γ) receptor (MRL/lpγR−/−)

For understanding and examining immunological aspects of SSc, a mouse model was developed, based on the murine model of MRL/lpr, which primarily mimics the manifestations of systemic lupus erythematosus (SLE) and other pathological mechanisms of other systemic autoimmune diseases. The MRL/lpr mice are characterized by development of inflammatory involvement of tissues, such as immune complex-mediated vasculitis, arthritis, skin disease, and glomerulonephritis, which are accompanied by the production of autoantibodies [48]. On a molecular level, this model is based on a mutation in the gene encoding the Fas receptor belonging to a tumor necrosis factor (TNF) receptor family [49]. However, to induce symptoms of SSc in this model, a subsequent deletion of the interferon gamma (IFN-γ) receptor was introduced. MRL/lpr mice lacking IFN-γ receptor (MRL/lpγR–/–) are protected from the development of glomerulonephritis, which is often the cause of death of MRL/lpr mice. In fact, previous studies demonstrated the essential role of functional IFN-γ receptor for the development of glomerulonephritis in MRL/lpr mice [50]. In MRL/lpγR–/– mice, there is a number of pathological processes and clinical manifestations characteristic of SSc in humans. This mouse model (MRL/lpγR–/–) promotes the development of proliferative vasculopathy, particularly in the lung, and fibrosis in many organs including the skin, lungs, and kidneys [51]. Furthermore, this model is characterized by the presence of autoantibodies and mononuclear infiltrates in the skin, lungs, liver, and heart, accompanied by increased accumulation of collagen. Increased activation of fibroblasts was also observed in MRL/lpγR–/– mice [51].

This mouse model thus mimics the most typical symptoms for SSc, such as vasculopathy, inflammation, and the presence of autoimmunity.

3.4. Fra-2 transgenic mice

Fra-2 is a member of a family of transcription factors called activator protein 1 (AP-1). AP-1 is a heterodimer composed of protein subunits belonging to the family of Fos (c-Fos, Fra-1, Fra-2, FosB) and Jun family (c-Jun, JunB, JunD), which regulate cell proliferation, inflammation, and wound healing via binding of AP-1 to the promoters of target genes [52]. Recent studies have reported a significant role of two members of the AP-1 family, Fra-2, and c-Jun on production of TGF-β and on its autocrine signaling in SSc fibroblasts [53, 54]. Overexpression of Fra-2 was also reported in patients with SSc, specifically in myofibroblasts, endothelial cells, and smooth muscle cells, suggesting a potential importance of Fra-2 in the pathogenesis of SSc [54, 55]. Increased expression of Fra-2 in mice leads to the development of systemic inflammation and fibrosis, especially in the skin and lungs. Fra-2 transgenic mice are also characterized by a vascular phenotype with increased apoptosis of endothelial cells of the capillaries, which appear in the ninth week after birth and lead to serious dysfunction of the small arteries of the skin and lungs. Subsequently, at 12 weeks of age, there is a significant development of dermal fibrosis, which correlates with progressive capillary loss [55]. Fra-2 is also highly expressed in the skin tissue of animal models of SSc. High expression of Fra-2 was detected in myofibroblasts in SSc skin lesions, suggesting a specific role of Fra-2 in fibroblast activation and subsequent transdifferentiation into myofibroblasts. Furthermore, it was demonstrated that silencing of Fra-2 gene leads to reduced production of type I collagen and inhibition of apoptosis but also to the development of angiogenesis in human microvascular endothelial cells [54, 55]. Histological changes of proliferative vasculopathy in the lungs of mice resemble pulmonary arterial hypertension in SSc in humans. Lung fibrosis and pulmonary arterial hypertension then lead to pulmonary insufficiency and increased mortality of mice [54, 55]. Pathological processes that are shared between pulmonary vascular involvement in Fra-2 transgenic mice and SSc in humans are further documented by constitutively activated PDGF signaling in murine pulmonary arteries. The key role of this pathway has been demonstrated by the administration of nilotinib, a tyrosine kinase inhibitor of the PDGF receptor, which prevents the development of proliferative vasculopathy and pulmonary fibrosis in Fra-2 transgenic mice [55].

The advantage of this model is the integration of characteristic vascular and fibrotic manifestations and a similar course of the disease as of SSc in humans. The disadvantages of Fra-2 transgenic mice comprise inadequate characterization of the model and the absence of autoimmunity [4].

3.5. uPAR−/− mice

Urokinase receptor belongs to glycoproteins anchored in the cell membrane via glycosylphosphatidylinositol (GPI) anchor, which is expressed on the surface of fibroblasts, endothelial cells, and lymphohematopoietic cells. The main task of the urokinase-type plasminogen activator receptor (uPAR) is binding the ligand urokinase-type plasminogen activator (uPA) at the interface of cells and matrix. uPA is an important part in the conversion of plasminogen to plasmin and activation of growth factors and matrix metalloproteinases. uPA/uPAR system plays a significant role in fibrinolysis, maintaining cellular homeostasis and angiogenesis. It also participates in many biological processes including differentiation, proliferation, and migration of cells through its interaction with membrane proteins and components of the ECM [56]. Relationship between SSc and uPAR was studied in dermal fibroblasts and endothelial cells obtained from SSc skin lesions, where a decrease in uPAR was detected compared to healthy control cells [57]. Recent studies have demonstrated the effect of inactivation of uPA/uPAR on transdifferentiation of fibroblasts into myofibroblasts and structural and functional changes in vasculature in SSc [58, 59]. uPAR−/− mice mimic fibrotic and vascular manifestations of SSc, which supports a significant role of the uPA/uPAR in the pathogenesis of SSc. In the 12th week, mice with inactivated uPA/uPAR system (uPAR−/−) develop progressive thickening of the skin with increased amount of collagen fibers and the number of activated fibroblasts, as well as the increased presence of perivascular inflammatory infiltrate compared to wild-type littermates. At the same time, fibrosis and perivascular fibrosis in the subcutaneous tissue develop [57]. In the skin of uPAR−/− mice, elevated levels of pro-fibrotic mediators, such as TGF-β and CTGF, were detected. Similar to Fra-2 murine models, uPAR−/− mice have an increased number of apoptotic endothelial cells, reduced number of functional blood vessels, and subsequent development of fibrosis, but do not develop fibroproliferative changes in arteries. During the 24th week, the skin changes stabilize and do not deteriorate [57]. The lung tissue is characterized by interstitial damage, infiltration of inflammatory cells, and excessive deposition of collagen, which is similar to the involvement in SSc patients with interstitial lung disease. Pulmonary involvement is already evident at 12 weeks, with progressive tendencies until the 24th week. This model is also characterized by cardiac involvement, which is also typical for SSc-related cardiomyopathy. This involvement is characterized by damage to cardiomyocytes, differentiation of myofibroblasts, apoptosis of endothelial cells, collagen accumulation, and myocardial fibrosis. However, cardiac involvement occurs later compared to the aforementioned manifestations [57].

Murine models with inactivated uPAR may be used as another preclinical model that mimics vascular changes, fibrosis of tissues similar to those in SSc but again lacks immunological processes typical of this disease [57].

4. Experimental murine models of lung fibrosis

In pulmonary fibrosis, the original functional lung tissue is being replaced by connective tissue which deteriorates the exchange of respiratory gases. The pathogenesis is characterized by damage to epithelial cells and alveolar hyperplasia, accumulation of inflammatory infiltrates, fibroblast hyperplasia, deposition of ECM components, and scarring [60]. Interstitial lung disease in SSc is most commonly characterized by nonspecific interstitial pneumonia (NSIP) or usual interstitial pneumonia (UIP) or organizing pneumonia with later development into NSIP [2]. The most frequently used experimental models of pulmonary fibrosis, which mimic some aspects of the human disease, include induction by bleomycin, silica, fluorescein isothiocyanate, and radiation.

4.1. Bleomycin-induced lung fibrosis

To induce pulmonary fibrosis, bleomycin can be administered intratracheally or intranasally directly into the airways but also by subcutaneous, intraperitoneal, or intravenous injection. The principle of action of bleomycin is described in bleomycin-induced skin fibrosis [61]. The main advantage of the use of bleomycin is its availability, ease of administration, and yet the most accurate induction of symptoms of pulmonary fibrosis within 14–28 days (**Figure 3**). A limitation of this model is the fact that lung fibrosis wanes 28 days after intratracheal administration of bleomycin [61]. Many studies have confirmed that bleomycin-induced experimental pulmonary fibrosis is reversible, unlike pulmonary fibrosis in humans, and after 6 weeks, the animal presents with almost normal lung findings [62].

4.2. Lung fibrosis induced by silica

The instillation of silica into the lungs of mice causes the formation of fibrotic nodes and fibrosis, similar to lesions in humans exposed to long-term inhalation of silica dust and aerosol particles. Silica may be administered via an aerosol or intratracheally via oropharyngeal aspiration [60]. Induction of lung fibrosis is based on the activation of macrophages that phagocytose silica particles and begin to produce the pro-fibrotic cytokines PDGF and

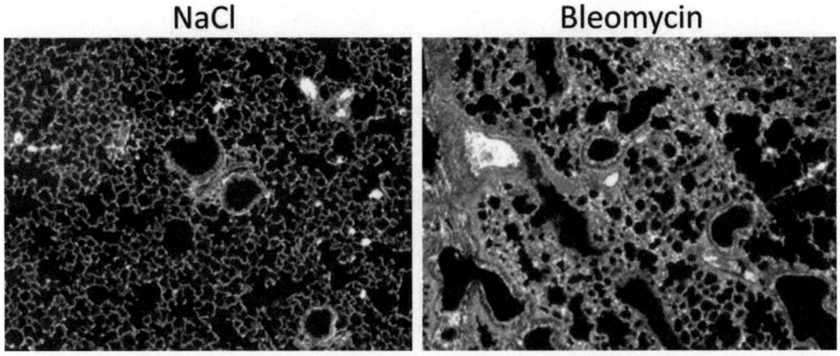

Figure 3. Fibrotic lung tissue (grey colour) of mice after intratracheal administration of bleomycin compared to control mice after intratracheal instillation of saline (NaCl). The sections are stained with sirius red (magnification 100-fold).

TGF-β [61]. The fibrotic response is dependent on the particular strain of mice [63]. The main benefit of this model is that the silica particles are not easily removed from the lungs and cause permanent fibrotic stimuli. The disadvantage of this model is that it lacks the characteristic signs of UIP. The experiment is also expensive and time-consuming due to the need for highly specialized equipment for administration of silica via aerosol and due to the development of the disease only during the 12th to 16th week after exposure [61].

4.3. Lung fibrosis induced by fluorescein isothiocyanate (FITC)

Other chemicals used to induce pulmonary fibrosis include fluorescein isothiocyanate (FITC). FITC is administered directly into the respiratory tract, where it acts as a hapten that binds to the protein present in the lungs, resulting in a new persistent antigen and the subsequent formation of antibodies [61]. This association is used in immunofluorescence for localization of pulmonary fibrosis, which correlates closely with the areas of occurrence of the bound FITC. Administration of FITC increases infiltration of mononuclear cells and neutrophils, in particular in the area of the respiratory tract. In terms of pathogenesis, FITC is linked with the occurrence of acute lung injury, the development of edema, inflammation, and the subsequent development of fibrosis [63]. Induction of lung fibrosis by FITC is based on activation of chemokine receptor type 2 (CCR2) signaling [64]. Release of chemokines CCL12, and to a lesser extent CCL2, causes an increase in the number of fibrocytes expressing CCR2 in the affected lung, which leads to pulmonary fibrosis [65, 66]. FITC further induces increased production of pro-fibrotic cytokine IL-13 [67]. The advantage of this model is the visualization of fibrosis using the characteristic green fluorescence. Pulmonary involvement occurs within 14–28 days and persists for at least 6 months. Unfortunately, this model of pulmonary fibrosis has no characteristic findings of UIP [60].

4.4. Radiation-induced lung fibrosis

Irradiation of mice also leads to the formation of pulmonary fibrosis, without the use of chemicals. Radiation induces direct cell death of type I and type II pneumocytes and the subsequent accumulation of macrophages at the site of damage. Macrophage activation triggers the production of pro-inflammatory and pro-fibrotic cytokines tumor necrosis factor alpha (TNF-α) and TGF-β, which participate in the formation of fibrosis [61]. Radiation-induced fibrosis has findings consistent with UIP and can only be performed in the C57B1/6 mouse model. The disadvantages of this method are the financial and time demands, since the interval from exposure to the development of the first symptoms is 30 weeks [60].

5. Experimental murine models of pulmonary arterial hypertension

Pulmonary arterial hypertension (PAH) is a disease of pulmonary arteries caused by contraction and proliferation of smooth muscle cells of the vascular wall, which may occur alone (primary PAH) or accompany interstitial lung disease (secondary PAH) in SSc [2]. The most frequently used experimental models of PAH include a model induced by semaxanib with chronic hypoxia and monocrotaline and a model of athymic rats.

5.1. PAH induced by chronic hypoxia

Chronic hypoxia, normally induced by the half fraction of inspired oxygen (i.e., FiO_2 10%) for 21 days, leads, unfortunately, only to slight PAH, which is also reversible, unlike PAH in humans, and less pronounced in mice than rats. Furthermore, in mice hypoxia induces perivascular inflammatory infiltrates with the secretion of various pro-inflammatory cytokines and chemokines. Induction of more pronounced and irreversible PAH is achieved by the simultaneous administration of semaxanib (SU5416), a tyrosine kinase inhibitor of the type 1 receptor (Flt) and type 2 receptor (KDR) of vascular endothelial growth factor (VEGF), which was initially developed for cancer treatment [68]. SU5416 is an inhibitor of proliferation and triggers apoptosis of endothelial cells [69]. Paradoxically, however, blocking of VEGFR leads to an expansion of endothelial cells instead of inhibition of their proliferation. This is explained by a compensatory mechanism, when the inhibition of VEGFR is followed by upregulation of other growth factors such as fibroblast growth factor (FGF), and platelet-derived growth factor (PDGF) securing the proliferation of endothelial cells [69]. This model is frequently used for a sufficient understanding of the mechanism of hyperproliferation of endothelial cells, which is a characteristic of plexiform lesions of PAH in humans [70].

5.2. PAH induced by monocrotaline

Monocrotaline (MCTP) is a toxic alkaloid found in the plant *Crotalaria spectabilis*. Monocrotaline must be activated in vivo by liver oxidases to a reactive bifunctional MCTP component that contributes to the development of vascular disease. The response to MCTP depends on the species of animal, since it differs in hepatic metabolism of cytochrome P-450. The preferred animal models include rats, to which MCTP is injected either subcutaneously or intraperitoneally [71]. Subcutaneous injection of MCTP induces changes in the endothelium and smooth muscle cell proliferation in the blood vessels, which are involved in the development of PAH during 3 weeks [72]. The exact mechanism of pathogenesis of PAH induced by MCTP is still not fully understood. A possible cause could include the damage to the endothelium, which triggers rampant progression of severe pulmonary hypertension. Increased pulmonary artery pressure and vascular remodeling causing accumulation of mononuclear inflammatory cells in the tunica adventitia may represent another stimulus to the formation of PAH. This model is used mainly for modeling acute involvement which is easily treatable, that is, unfortunately, completely different from PAH in humans [71].

5.3. PAH in athymic rats

Another commonly used model of PAH is SU5416 treatment of athymic rats. The initial assumption was that the models without T lymphocytes (athymic naked rnu/rnu rats) will exhibit less inflammation with less pronounced PAH. There was, however, paradoxically exactly the opposite, and these models have developed a far higher degree of involvement. Inflammation of the pulmonary artery is induced by activation of macrophages and B cells and the presence of anti-endothelial antibodies. The cause of the development of severe forms of pulmonary hypertension is the absence of anti-inflammatory regulatory T cells, which explains a predisposition for PAH in athymic rats [69].

6. Experimental chicken models of SSc (UCD-200 and UCD-206 chickens)

Chickens of the line UCD-200 were originally isolated from the University of California Leghorn chickens, which had atrophic abnormalities of the comb. This line has systemic manifestations similar to the symptoms of SSc: skin involvement of the comb, neck, and back manifested as edema, Raynaud's phenomenon-like changes, loss of skin adnexa, and skin thickening leading to necrosis [73]. This involvement develops between the first and second weeks after birth and culminates around the second to fourth week of life. Ischemic finger lesions occur in 20% of chickens, and digital ulcerations develop in later stages. There is also an internal organ involvement, particularly of the esophagus, heart, lung, and kidneys and an increased mortality. At around sixth week of age, the chickens develop glomerulonephritis and pericarditis [73, 74]. Histopathological changes are similar to those in SSc and include massive perivascular mononuclear infiltrates, particularly of T and B lymphocytes and deposition of ECM components by activated fibroblasts, signs of obliterative vasculopathy, and apoptosis of endothelial cells with loss of functional capillaries [73]. Subcutaneous adipose tissue is often replaced by collagen. UCD-200 chickens also produce autoantibodies, especially antinuclear, anti-centromere, and anti-phospholipid antibodies, rheumatoid factor, and antibodies to endothelial cells [74, 75]. UCD-206 chickens are similar to the chickens of the line UCD-200. However, they can develop more serious organ involvement [76].

The advantage of this model is the significant systemic involvement covering almost the complete spectrum of pathological processes and the disease course, which is similar to SSc in humans. While this model of SSc affects both sexes equally, in patients with SSc, women are affected more often. Another difference is the composition of mononuclear infiltrates,which consist, in particular, of monocytes/macrophages and T lymphocytes in humans [77]. The limitations of this model include the avian genetic background, which restricts the molecular studies, and, in particular, a very difficult and costly breeding [4].

7. Testing of biological agents and small molecules in preclinical models and clinical setting

One of the first available biological drugs with proven effects in other systemic rheumatic diseases, which were tested in preclinical models of SSc, was the anti-TNF agents. In in vitro experiments, a direct anti-fibrotic effect of TNF-α itself prevailed, while in in vivo experiments, on the contrary, using the TNF inhibitors prevented the development of bleomycin-induced fibrosis, which may be partly explained by the dominant inflammatory component in the model [78, 79]. Results of clinical trials of anti-TNF agents in SSc rather support the anti-fibrotic role of TNF-α itself, judging from progression of fibrosis in anti-TNF-treated SSc patients [80, 81]. Also other clinical trials failed to show significant improvement in skin scores and lung function using etanercept and infliximab, and, thus, the EUSTAR workgroup (EULAR Scleroderma Trials and Research) did not recommend the use of anti-TNF therapy in patients with SSc outside clinical trials [82–84].

The role of B lymphocytes and their depletion has also been studied in experimental models of SSc. Administration of rituximab to 3-day-old Tsk1 mice resulted in a reduction of skin fibrosis, whereas the same application to older, 56-day-old Tsk1 mice did not cause any change [85]. Similar reduction of the skin and pulmonary fibrosis induced by bleomycin was achieved in mice with genetic inactivation of CD19 [86]. Both studies document the effect of depletion of B cells on reduction of fibrosis rather in the early inflammatory phase of experimental SSc. The phase 2 clinical trial and observational study by EUSTAR documented the beneficial effects of rituximab on reduction of skin scores and lung function, but the results will need to be confirmed in a placebo-controlled randomized trial [87–92].

Another, in rheumatology, widely used type of therapy that has been tested in mouse models of SSc was the inhibition of interleukin (IL)-6. Numerous in vitro data demonstrated an increased production of IL-6 by SSc fibroblasts, and its important role as an inducer of activation of fibroblasts and collagen production, and ultimately point to the effective reduction of collagen synthesis through its inhibition [93–95]. In vivo inhibition of IL-6 with antibody against IL-6 receptor reduced the cutaneous fibrosis in a model of bleomycin-induced fibrosis and chronic GvHD, whereas in Tsk1 mice, no improvement was observed, which indicates rather anti-fibrotic effect in the early, inflammatory stage of experimental models of SSc [96–98]. The results of the phase 2/3 double-blind randomized placebo-controlled study faSScinate evaluating efficacy of tocilizumab in 87 patients with an active form of diffuse cutaneous SSc after 48 weeks of treatment showed a trend of reduction in skin scores ($p = 0.06$) and an encouraging stabilization of FVC (forced lung capacity) compared to placebo ($p = 0.09$) [99].

Tyrosine kinases such as the PDGF receptor (platelet-derived growth factor) constitute another interesting target of therapy in SSc. Numerous experimental studies demonstrate the anti-fibrotic effects of imatinib mesylate, a multikinase inhibitor (inhibitor of the kinases PDGFR, c-Abl, and c-Kit). In vitro, imatinib reduced the expression of pro-inflammatory and pro-fibrotic genes and collagen production by SSc fibroblasts [100, 101]. In vivo imatinib therapy prevented the development of cutaneous fibrosis induced by bleomycin and in Tsk1 mice and prevented the development of pulmonary, renal, and hepatic fibrosis, as well as reduced established dermal fibrosis [100, 102]. Similar results were obtained in vivo with other PDGFR inhibitors, such as nilotinib and dasatinib [103]. The first promising results from an open clinical trial with imatinib in SSc demonstrated significant improvement in skin scores and FVC after 12 months, however, with numerous side effects, particularly edema. Unfortunately, these findings were not confirmed in two other randomized placebo-controlled clinical trials, one of which was closed for numerous early side effects, and the other failed to show significant improvement in skin scores, and was accompanied by numerous side effects as well [104–106].

Another interesting target of anti-fibrotic therapies investigated in in vitro and in vivo experiments in SSc is a vasoactive small molecule riociguat, a stimulator of soluble guanylate cyclase (sGC). Treatment with riociguat led to a significant improvement in the primary outcome (6-min walking test) after 16 weeks of treatment of pulmonary arterial hypertension in the phase 3 PATENT-1 trial and also met a number of secondary outcomes [107]. In vitro experiments with riociguat resulted in a reduction of collagen synthesis by SSc fibroblasts in a dose-dependent manner. In in vivo experiments, riociguat prevented the development of cutaneous fibrosis induced by bleomycin, in Tsk1 mice, in a TβRI mouse model, and in SclGvHD in which it even reduced the gastrointestinal fibrosis. In the bleomycin-induced skin fibrosis model, riociguat was also shown to reduce the established fibrosis [108–110]. Effectiveness of riociguat in skin and pulmonary involvement is currently being evaluated in an ongoing phase 2 placebo-controlled randomized clinical trial RISE in patients with early diffuse cutaneous SSc.

8. Conclusion

Currently, there are several well-characterized experimental models through which we can study various pathological processes of SSc. The knowledge gained through animal models of SSc may bring new information and clarify previously unexplained pathogenic mechanisms of SSc. Animal models also serve as a promising tool for developing and testing new candidate molecules for the treatment of SSc. It must be stressed that none of the currently available experimental models includes all aspects of SSc in humans. Most of established models represent several pathologic mechanisms at once. Almost all models, except for a few focused only on vasculopathy, are characterized by severe tissue fibrosis. Conversely, only a few models are acceptable for studying damage to small arteries. It is therefore very important to carefully consider the selection of a suitable model or a combination of several models before commencing specific in vivo experiments. When the aim is to completely analyze the pathogenesis of the disease, it is suitable to prioritize models that mimic a wide spectrum of pathologies of SSc, such as Fra-2 transgenic mice or chicken lines UCD-200/206. For testing a new anti-fibrotic agent, it is preferable to start with a well-characterized model, such as bleomycin-induced fibrosis for inflammation and Tsk1 mice for fibrosis independent of inflammation. Ideally, both abovementioned models should be used for testing, and, subsequently, the efficiency should be checked on a more complex model, such as Fra-2 transgenic mice [4].

Systemic sclerosis represents a great unmet medical need due to its substantial morbidity and mortality and, to date, still missing efficient disease-modifying therapies. Finding novel effective therapeutic approaches requires better and more complex understanding of the pathogenesis of this heterogeneous multisystem disorder. The currently existing animal models of SSc, with their abovementioned limitations, still continue to serve as the basis for the vital preclinical studies of presently available and novel candidate targeted therapies before they can be used in clinical trials in humans. Furthermore, they will be essential for further in-depth analysis of the hallmark pathogenic mechanisms in SSc and for progress in hypothesis-driven and discovery research. In addition, with recent advances in genetic approaches, mapping of the human and murine genome, and novel data from the high-throughput sequencing of the biopsy samples from different subsets of SSc patients and healthy volunteers, there is a new window of opportunity for currently existing animal models to be further explored and used in more suitable and elaborate way and thus lead to vital progress in understanding the pathogenesis of SSc and providing new candidate therapies. Furthermore, the recent use of conditional genetic strategies in murine SSc models, through which particular genes of interest can be turned on/off in determined cell lineages at defined points of time, enables also for assessment of genes, which would have had lethal consequences if manipulated on germ-line level. These approaches also provide novel possibilities to examine modifications to specific cell lineages only and to assess their effect in experimental settings other than prevention (of induction of particular pathology), such as reversal or treatment (of established pathology). Progress in research strategies and new developments in existing animal models will inevitably lead to discovery of novel and more sophisticated animal models of SSc. In the future, a combination of genetic and induction strategies can lead to creation of experimental models which accurately, and to a greater extent, mimic SSc in humans and could lead to substantial clarification of pathological mechanisms and the discovery of a universal causal treatment of SSc. Nevertheless, the existing models have already contributed significantly to preclinical testing of several available biological agents and small molecules, some of which achieved promising results in early clinical studies and could provide better prospects for patients with this incurable disease.

Acknowledgements

This chapter was supported by grant projects AZV 16-33542A, AZV 16-33574A, SVV 260263, PRVOUK and the Ministry of Health of the Czech Republic [Research Project No. 00023728].

Author details

Hana Storkanova and Michal Tomcik*

*Address all correspondence to: michaltomcik@yahoo.com

Department of Rheumatology, First Faculty of Medicine, Institute of Rheumatology, Prague, Czech Republic

References

[1] Gabrielli A, Avvedimento EV, Krieg T. Mechanisms of disease: Scleroderma. The New England Journal of Medicine. 2009;**360**(19):1989-2003

[2] Varga J, Abraham D. Systemic sclerosis: A prototypic multisystem fibrotic disorder. The Journal of Clinical Investigation. 2007;**117**(3):557-567. 2007/03/03

[3] Denton CP, Black CM. Scleroderma—Clinical and pathological advances. Best Practice & Research. Clinical Rheumatology. 2004;**18**(3):271-290. 2004/05/26

[4] Beyer C, Schett G, Distler O, Distler JH. Animal models of systemic sclerosis: Prospects and limitations. Arthritis and Rheumatism. 2010;**62**(10):2831-2844. 2010/07/10

[5] Siracusa LD, McGrath R, Ma Q, Moskow JJ, Manne J, Christner PJ, et al. A tandem duplication within the fibrillin 1 gene is associated with the mouse tight skin mutation. Genome Research. 1996;**6**(4):300-313. 1996/04/01

[6] Green MC, Sweet HO, Bunker LE. Tight-skin, a new mutation of the mouse causing excessive growth of connective tissue and skeleton. The American Journal of Pathology. 1976;**82**(3):493-512. 1976/03/01

[7] Menton DN, Hess RA, Lichtenstein JR, Eisen A. The structure and tensile properties of the skin of tight-skin (Tsk) mutant mice. Journal of Investigative Dermatology. 1978;**70**(1):4-10. 1978/01/01

[8] Menton DN, Hess RA. The ultrastructure of collagen in the dermis of tight-skin (Tsk) mutant mice. Journal of Investigative Dermatology. 1980;**74**(3):139-147. 1980/03/01

[9] Baxter RM, Crowell TP, McCrann ME, Frew EM, Gardner H. Analysis of the tight skin (Tsk1/+) mouse as a model for testing antifibrotic agents. Laboratory Investigation. 2005;**85**(10):1199-1209. 2005/08/30

[10] Saito E, Fujimoto M, Hasegawa M, Komura K, Hamaguchi Y, Kaburagi Y, et al. CD19-dependent B lymphocyte signaling thresholds influence skin fibrosis and autoimmunity in the tight-skin mouse. The Journal of Clinical Investigation. 2002;**109**(11):1453-1462. 2002/06/05

[11] Christner PJ, Peters J, Hawkins D, Siracusa LD, Jimenez SA. The tight skin 2 mouse. An animal model of scleroderma displaying cutaneous fibrosis and mononuclear cell infiltration. Arthritis and Rheumatism. 1995;**38**(12):1791-1798

[12] Phelps RG, Daian C, Shibata S, Fleischmajer R, Bona CA. Induction of skin fibrosis and autoantibodies by infusion of immunocompetent cells from tight skin mice into C57BL/6 Pa/Pa mice. Journal of Autoimmunity. 1993;**6**(6):701-718

[13] Long KB, Li Z, Burgwin CM, Choe SG, Martyanov V, Sassi-Gaha S, et al. The Tsk2/+ mouse fibrotic phenotype is due to a gain-of-function mutation in the PIIINP segment of the Col3a1 gene. The Journal of Investigative Dermatology. 2015;**135**(3):718-727

[14] Christner PJ, Hitraya EG, Peters J, McGrath R, Jimenez SA. Transcriptional activation of the alpha1(I) procollagen gene and up-regulation of alpha1(I) and alpha1(III) procollagen messenger RNA in dermal fibroblasts from tight skin 2 mice. Arthritis and Rheumatism. 1998;**41**(12):2132-2142

[15] Jimenez SA, Christner PJ. Murine animal models of systemic sclerosis. Current Opinion in Rheumatology. 2002;**14**(6):671-680

[16] Jimenez SA, Feldman G, Bashey RI, Bienkowski R, Rosenbloom J. Co-ordinate increase in the expression of type I and type III collagen genes in progressive systemic sclerosis fibroblasts. The Biochemical Journal. 1986;**237**(3):837-843

[17] Kahari VM, Vuorio T, Nanto-Salonen K, Vuorio E. Increased type I collagen mRNA levels in cultured scleroderma fibroblasts. Biochimica et Biophysica Acta. 1984;**781**(1-2):183-186

[18] Gentiletti J, McCloskey LJ, Artlett CM, Peters J, Jimenez SA, Christner PJ. Demonstration of autoimmunity in the tight skin-2 mouse: A model for scleroderma. Journal of Immunology. 2005;**175**(4):2418-2426

[19] Denton CP, Zheng B, Evans LA, Shi-wen X, Ong VH, Fisher I, et al. Fibroblast-specific expression of a kinase-deficient type II transforming growth factor beta (TGFbeta) receptor leads to paradoxical activation of TGFbeta signaling pathways with fibrosis in transgenic mice. The Journal of Biological Chemistry. 2003;**278**(27):25109-25119

[20] Brand T, MacLellan WR, Schneider MD. A dominant-negative receptor for type beta transforming growth factors created by deletion of the kinase domain. The Journal of Biological Chemistry. 1993;**268**(16):11500-11503

[21] Schmierer B, Hill CS. TGFbeta-SMAD signal transduction: Molecular specificity and functional flexibility. Nature Reviews Molecular Cell Biology. 2007;**8**(12):970-982

[22] Thoua NM, Derrett-Smith EC, Khan K, Dooley A, Shi-Wen X, Denton CP. Gut fibrosis with altered colonic contractility in a mouse model of scleroderma. Rheumatology. 2012;**51**(11):1989-1998

[23] Imai S, Armstrong CM, Kaeberlein M, Guarente L. Transcriptional silencing and longevity protein Sir2 is an NAD-dependent histone deacetylase. Nature. 2000;**403**(6771): 795-800

[24] Nakagawa T, Guarente L. Sirtuins at a glance. Journal of Cell Science. 2011;**124**(Pt 6): 833-838

[25] Hebert AS, Dittenhafer-Reed KE, Yu W, Bailey DJ, Selen ES, Boersma MD, et al. Calorie restriction and SIRT3 trigger global reprogramming of the mitochondrial protein acetylome. Molecular Cell. 2013;**49**(1):186-199

[26] Finley LW, Carracedo A, Lee J, Souza A, Egia A, Zhang J, et al. SIRT3 opposes reprogramming of cancer cell metabolism through HIF1alpha destabilization. Cancer Cell. 2011;**19**(3):416-428

[27] Hirschey MD, Shimazu T, Jing E, Grueter CA, Collins AM, Aouizerat B, et al. SIRT3 deficiency and mitochondrial protein hyperacetylation accelerate the development of the metabolic syndrome. Molecular Cell. 2011;**44**(2):177-190

[28] Sundaresan NR, Gupta M, Kim G, Rajamohan SB, Isbatan A, Gupta MP. Sirt3 blocks the cardiac hypertrophic response by augmenting Foxo3a-dependent antioxidant defense mechanisms in mice. The Journal of Clinical Investigation. 2009;**119**(9):2758-2771

[29] Sundaresan NR, Bindu S, Pillai VB, Samant S, Pan Y, Huang JY, et al. SIRT3 blocks aging-associated tissue fibrosis in mice by deacetylating and activating glycogen synthase kinase 3beta. Molecular and Cellular Biology. 2016;**36**(5):678-692

[30] Paulin R, Dromparis P, Sutendra G, Gurtu V, Zervopoulos S, Bowers L, et al. Sirtuin 3 deficiency is associated with inhibited mitochondrial function and pulmonary arterial hypertension in rodents and humans. Cell Metabolism. 2014;**20**(5):827-839

[31] Lam AP, Gottardi CJ. beta-catenin signaling: A novel mediator of fibrosis and potential therapeutic target. Current Opinion in Rheumatology. 2011;**23**(6):562-567

[32] Yamakage A, Ishikawa H. Generalized morphea-like scleroderma occurring in people exposed to organic solvents. Dermatologica. 1982;**165**(3):186-193

[33] Christner PJ, Artlett CM, Conway RF, Jimenez SA. Increased numbers of microchimeric cells of fetal origin are associated with dermal fibrosis in mice following injection of vinyl chloride. Arthritis and Rheumatism. 2000;**43**(11):2598-2605

[34] Bou-Gharios G, Garrett LA, Rossert J, Niederreither K, Eberspaecher H, Smith C, et al. A potent far-upstream enhancer in the mouse pro alpha 2(I) collagen gene regulates expression of reporter genes in transgenic mice. Journal of Cell Biology. 1996;**134**(5):1333-1344. 1996/09/01

[35] Sonnylal S, Denton CP, Zheng B, Keene DR, He R, Adams HP, et al. Postnatal induction of transforming growth factor beta signaling in fibroblasts of mice recapitulates clinical, histologic, and biochemical features of scleroderma. Arthritis and Rheumatism. 2007;**56**(1):334-344

[36] Denton CP, Zheng B, Shiwen X, Zhang Z, Bou-Gharios G, Eberspaecher H, et al. Activation of a fibroblast-specific enhancer of the proalpha2(I) collagen gene in tight-skin mice. Arthritis and Rheumatism. 2001;**44**(3):712-722. 2001/03/27

[37] Umezawa H, Ishizuka M, Maeda K, Takeuchi T. Studies on bleomycin. Cancer. 1967;**20**(5):891-895. 1967/05/01

[38] Yamamoto T, Takagawa S, Katayama I, Yamazaki K, Hamazaki Y, Shinkai H, et al. Animal model of sclerotic skin. I: Local injections of bleomycin induce sclerotic skin mimicking scleroderma. The Journal of Investigative Dermatology. 1999;**112**(4):456-462. Epub 1999/04/14

[39] Yoshizaki A, Iwata Y, Komura K, Ogawa F, Hara T, Muroi E, et al. CD19 regulates skin and lung fibrosis via Toll-like receptor signaling in a model of bleomycin-induced scleroderma. The American Journal of Pathology. 2008;**172**(6):1650-1663. 2008/05/10

[40] Yamamoto T, Nishioka K. Cellular and molecular mechanisms of bleomycin-induced murine scleroderma: Current update and future perspective. Experimental Dermatology. 2005;**14**(2):81-95. 2005/02/01

[41] Vogelsang GB, Lee L, Bensen-Kennedy DM. Pathogenesis and treatment of graft-versus-host disease after bone marrow transplant. Annual Review of Medicine. 2003;**54**:29-52. 2002/10/03

[42] Ruzek MC, Jha S, Ledbetter S, Richards SM, Garman RD. A modified model of graft-versus-host-induced systemic sclerosis (scleroderma) exhibits all major aspects of the human disease. Arthritis and Rheumatism. 2004;**50**(4):1319-1331. 2004/04/13

[43] Jaffee BD, Claman HN. Chronic graft-versus-host disease (GVHD) as a model for scleroderma. I. Description of model systems. Cellular Immunology. 1983;**77**(1):1-12

[44] Claman HN, Jaffee BD, Huff JC, Clark RA. Chronic graft-versus-host disease as a model for scleroderma. II. Mast cell depletion with deposition of immunoglobulins in the skin and fibrosis. Celluar Immunology. 1985;**94**(1):73-84. 1985/08/01

[45] Howell CD, Yoder T, Claman HN, Vierling JM. Hepatic homing of mononuclear inflammatory cells isolated during murine chronic graft-vs-host disease. Journal of Immunology. 1989;**143**(2):476-483. 1989/07/15

[46] Levy S, Nagler A, Okon S, Marmary Y. Parotid salivary gland dysfunction in chronic graft-versus-host disease (cGVHD): A longitudinal study in a mouse model. Bone Marrow Transplantation. 2000;**25**(10):1073-1078. 2000/06/01

[47] Li J, Helm K, Howell CD. Contributions of donor CD4 and CD8 cells to liver injury during murine graft-versus-host disease. Transplantation. 1996;**62**(11):1621-1628. 1996/12/15

[48] Andrews BS, Eisenberg RA, Theofilopoulos AN, Izui S, Wilson CB, McConahey PJ, et al. Spontaneous murine lupus-like syndromes. Clinical and immunopathological manifestations in several strains. The Journal of Experimental Medicine. 1978;**148**(5):1198-1215

[49] Kono DH, Theofilopoulos AN. Genetics of systemic autoimmunity in mouse models of lupus. International Reviews of Immunology. 2000;**19**(4-5):367-387

[50] Haas C, Ryffel B, Le Hir M. IFN-gamma is essential for the development of autoimmune glomerulonephritis in MRL/Ipr mice. Journal of Immunology. 1997;**158**(11):5484-5491

[51] Le Hir M, Martin M, Haas C. A syndrome resembling human systemic sclerosis (scleroderma) in MRL/lpr mice lacking interferon-gamma (IFN-gamma) receptor (MRL/lpr-gammaR−/−). Clinical and Experimental Immunology. 1999;**115**(2):281-287

[52] Wagner EF, Eferl R. Fos/AP-1 proteins in bone and the immune system. Immunology Reviews. 2005;**208**:126-140. 2005/11/30

[53] Fichtner-Feigl S, Strober W, Kawakami K, Puri RK, Kitani A. IL-13 signaling through the IL-13alpha2 receptor is involved in induction of TGF-beta1 production and fibrosis. Nature Medicine. 2006;**12**(1):99-106

[54] Reich N, Maurer B, Akhmetshina A, Venalis P, Dees C, Zerr P, et al. The transcription factor Fra-2 regulates the production of extracellular matrix in systemic sclerosis. Arthritis and Rheumatism. 2010;**62**(1):280-290

[55] Maurer B, Busch N, Jungel A, Pileckyte M, Gay RE, Michel BA, et al. Transcription factor fos-related antigen-2 induces progressive peripheral vasculopathy in mice closely resembling human systemic sclerosis. Circulation. 2009;**120**(23):2367-2376

[56] Blasi F, Carmeliet P. uPAR: A versatile signalling orchestrator. Nature Reviews Molecular Cell Biology. 2002;**3**(12):932-943

[57] Manetti M, Rosa I, Milia AF, Guiducci S, Carmeliet P, Ibba-Manneschi L, et al. Inactivation of urokinase-type plasminogen activator receptor (uPAR) gene induces dermal and

pulmonary fibrosis and peripheral microvasculopathy in mice: A new model of experimental scleroderma? Annals of the Rheumatic Diseases. 2014;**73**(9):1700-1709

[58] Bernstein AM, Twining SS, Warejcka DJ, Tall E, Masur SK. Urokinase receptor cleavage: A crucial step in fibroblast-to-myofibroblast differentiation. Molecular Biology of the Cell. 2007;**18**(7):2716-2727

[59] Kanno Y, Kaneiwa A, Minamida M, Kanno M, Tomogane K, Takeuchi K, et al. The absence of uPAR is associated with the progression of dermal fibrosis. The Journal of Investigative Dermatology. 2008;**128**(12):2792-2797

[60] Moore BB, Hogaboam CM. Murine models of pulmonary fibrosis. American Journal of Physiology. Lung Cellular and Molecular Physiology. 2008;**294**(2):L152-L160

[61] Degryse AL, Lawson WE. Progress toward improving animal models for idiopathic pulmonary fibrosis. The American Journal of the Medical Sciences. 2011;**341**(6):444-449

[62] Chung MP, Monick MM, Hamzeh NY, Butler NS, Powers LS, Hunninghake GW. Role of repeated lung injury and genetic background in bleomycin-induced fibrosis. American Journal of Respiratory Cell and Molecular Biology. 2003;**29**(3 Pt 1):375-380

[63] Moore B, Lawson WE, Oury TD, Sisson TH, Raghavendran K, Hogaboam CM. Animal models of fibrotic lung disease. American Journal of Respiratory Cell and Molecular Biology. 2013;**49**(2):167-179

[64] Moore BB, Paine R, 3rd, Christensen PJ, Moore TA, Sitterding S, Ngan R, et al. Protection from pulmonary fibrosis in the absence of CCR2 signaling. Journal of Immunology. 2001;**167**(8):4368-4377

[65] Moore BB, Kolodsick JE, Thannickal VJ, Cooke K, Moore TA, Hogaboam C, et al. CCR2-mediated recruitment of fibrocytes to the alveolar space after fibrotic injury. The American Journal of Pathology. 2005;**166**(3):675-684

[66] Moore BB, Murray L, Das A, Wilke CA, Herrygers AB, Toews GB. The role of CCL12 in the recruitment of fibrocytes and lung fibrosis. American Journal of Respiratory Cell and Molecular Biology. 2006;**35**(2):175-181

[67] Korfhagen TR, Swantz RJ, Wert SE, McCarty JM, Kerlakian CB, Glasser SW, et al. Respiratory epithelial cell expression of human transforming growth factor-alpha induces lung fibrosis in transgenic mice. The Journal of Clinical Investigation. 1994;**93**(4):1691-1699

[68] Gomez-Arroyo J, Saleem SJ, Mizuno S, Syed AA, Bogaard HJ, Abbate A, et al. A brief overview of mouse models of pulmonary arterial hypertension: Problems and prospects. American Journal of Physiology. Lung Cellular and Molecular Physiology. 2012;**302**(10):L977-L991

[69] Nicolls MR, Mizuno S, Taraseviciene-Stewart L, Farkas L, Drake JI, Al Husseini A, et al. New models of pulmonary hypertension based on VEGF receptor blockade-induced endothelial cell apoptosis. Pulmonary Circulation. 2012;**2**(4):434-442

[70] Sakao S, Tatsumi K. The effects of antiangiogenic compound SU5416 in a rat model of pulmonary arterial hypertension. Respiration; International Review of Thoracic Diseases. 2011;**81**(3):253-261

[71] Stenmark KR, Meyrick B, Galie N, Mooi WJ, McMurtry IF. Animal models of pulmonary arterial hypertension: The hope for etiological discovery and pharmacological cure. American Journal of Physiology. Lung Cellular and Molecular Physiology. 2009;**297**(6):L1013-L1032

[72] Firth AL, Choi IW, Park WS. Animal models of pulmonary hypertension: Rho kinase inhibition. Progress in Biophysics and Molecular Biology. 2012;**109**(3):67-75

[73] Gershwin ME, Abplanalp H, Castles JJ, Ikeda RM, van der Water J, Eklund J, et al. Characterization of a spontaneous disease of white leghorn chickens resembling progressive systemic sclerosis (scleroderma). Journal of Experimental Medicine. 1981;**153**(6):1640-1659. Epub 1981/06/01

[74] Wick G, Andersson L, Hala K, Gershwin ME, Selmi C, Erf GF, et al. Avian models with spontaneous autoimmune diseases. Advances in Immunology 2006;**92**:71-117. Epub 2006/12/06

[75] Sgonc R, Gruschwitz MS, Dietrich H, Recheis H, Gershwin ME, Wick G. Endothelial cell apoptosis is a primary pathogenetic event underlying skin lesions in avian and human scleroderma. Journal of Clinical Investigation. 1996;**98**(3):785-792. Epub 1996/08/01

[76] Sgonc R, Wick G. Pro- and anti-fibrotic effects of TGF-beta in scleroderma. Rheumatology (Oxford). 2008;**47**(Suppl 5):v5-v7. Epub 2008/09/17

[77] Zhang Y, Gilliam AC. Animal models for scleroderma: An update. Current Rheumatology Reports. 2002;**4**(2):150-162

[78] Koca SS, Isik A, Ozercan IH, Ustundag B, Evren B, Metin K. Effectiveness of etanercept in bleomycin-induced experimental scleroderma. Rheumatology. 2008;**47**(2):172-175

[79] Mauviel A, Daireaux M, Redini F, Galera P, Loyau G, Pujol JP. Tumor necrosis factor inhibits collagen and fibronectin synthesis in human dermal fibroblasts. FEBS Letters. 1988;**236**(1):47-52

[80] Allanore Y, Devos-Francois G, Caramella C, Boumier P, Jounieaux V, Kahan A. Fatal exacerbation of fibrosing alveolitis associated with systemic sclerosis in a patient treated with adalimumab. Annals of the Rheumatic Diseases. 2006;**65**(6):834-835

[81] Ramos-Casals M, Perez-Alvarez R, Perez-de-Lis M, Xaubet A, Bosch X, Group BS. Pulmonary disorders induced by monoclonal antibodies in patients with rheumatologic autoimmune diseases. The American Journal of Medicine. 2011;**124**(5):386-394

[82] Denton CP, Engelhart M, Tvede N, Wilson H, Khan K, Shiwen X, et al. An open-label pilot study of infliximab therapy in diffuse cutaneous systemic sclerosis. Annals of the Rheumatic Diseases. 2009;**68**(9):1433-1439

[83] Distler JH, Jordan S, Airo P, Alegre-Sancho JJ, Allanore Y, Balbir Gurman A, et al. Is there a role for TNFalpha antagonists in the treatment of SSc? EUSTAR expert consensus

development using the Delphi technique. Clinical and Experimental Rheumatology. 2011;**29**(2 Suppl 65):S40-S45

[84] Lam GK, Hummers LK, Woods A, Wigley FM. Efficacy and safety of etanercept in the treatment of scleroderma-associated joint disease. The Journal of Rheumatology. 2007;**34**(7):1636-1637

[85] Hasegawa M, Hamaguchi Y, Yanaba K, Bouaziz JD, Uchida J, Fujimoto M, et al. B-lymphocyte depletion reduces skin fibrosis and autoimmunity in the tight-skin mouse model for systemic sclerosis. The American Journal of Pathology. 2006;**169**(3):954-966

[86] Komura K, Yanaba K, Horikawa M, Ogawa F, Fujimoto M, Tedder TF, et al. CD19 regulates the development of bleomycin-induced pulmonary fibrosis in a mouse model. Arthritis and Rheumatism. 2008;**58**(11):3574-3584

[87] Bosello S, De Santis M, Lama G, Spano C, Angelucci C, Tolusso B, et al. B cell depletion in diffuse progressive systemic sclerosis: Safety, skin score modification and IL-6 modulation in an up to thirty-six months follow-up open-label trial. Arthritis Research & Therapy. 2010;**12**(2):R54

[88] Daoussis D, Liossis SN, Tsamandas AC, Kalogeropoulou C, Kazantzi A, Sirinian C, et al. Experience with rituximab in scleroderma: Results from a 1-year, proof-of-principle study. Rheumatology. 2010;**49**(2):271-280

[89] Daoussis D, Liossis SN, Tsamandas AC, Kalogeropoulou C, Paliogianni F, Sirinian C, et al. Effect of long-term treatment with rituximab on pulmonary function and skin fibrosis in patients with diffuse systemic sclerosis. Clinical and Experimental Rheumatology. 2012;**30**(2 Suppl 71):S17-S22

[90] Lafyatis R, Kissin E, York M, Farina G, Viger K, Fritzler MJ, et al. B cell depletion with rituximab in patients with diffuse cutaneous systemic sclerosis. Arthritis and Rheumatism. 2009;**60**(2):578-583

[91] Smith V, Piette Y, van Praet JT, Decuman S, Deschepper E, Elewaut D, et al. Two-year results of an open pilot study of a 2-treatment course with rituximab in patients with early systemic sclerosis with diffuse skin involvement. The Journal of Rheumatology. 2013;**40**(1):52-57

[92] Smith V, Van Praet JT, Vandooren B, Van der Cruyssen B, Naeyaert JM, Decuman S, et al. Rituximab in diffuse cutaneous systemic sclerosis: An open-label clinical and histopathological study. Annals of the Rheumatic Diseases. 2010;**69**(1):193-197

[93] Allanore Y, Saad M, Dieude P, Avouac J, Distler JH, Amouyel P, et al. Genome-wide scan identifies TNIP1, PSORS1C1, and RHOB as novel risk loci for systemic sclerosis. PLoS Genetics. 2011;**7**(7):e1002091

[94] Kadono T, Kikuchi K, Ihn H, Takehara K, Tamaki K. Increased production of interleukin 6 and interleukin 8 in scleroderma fibroblasts. The Journal of Rheumatology. 1998;**25**(2):296-301

[95] Kawaguchi Y, Hara M, Wright TM. Endogenous IL-1alpha from systemic sclerosis fibroblasts induces IL-6 and PDGF-A. The Journal of Clinical Investigation. 1999;**103**(9):1253-1260

[96] Desallais L, Avouac J, Frechet M, Elhai M, Ratsimandresy R, Montes M, et al. Targeting IL-6 by both passive or active immunization strategies prevents bleomycin-induced skin fibrosis. Arthritis Research & Therapy. 2014;**16**(4):R157

[97] Kitaba S, Murota H, Terao M, Azukizawa H, Terabe F, Shima Y, et al. Blockade of interleukin-6 receptor alleviates disease in mouse model of scleroderma. The American Journal of Pathology. 2012;**180**(1):165-176

[98] Le Huu D, Matsushita T, Jin G, Hamaguchi Y, Hasegawa M, Takehara K, et al. IL-6 blockade attenuates the development of murine sclerodermatous chronic graft-versus-host disease. The Journal of Investigative Dermatology. 2012;**132**(12):2752-2761

[99] Khanna D, Denton CP, Jahreis A, van Laar JM, Frech TM, Anderson ME, et al. Safety and efficacy of subcutaneous tocilizumab in adults with systemic sclerosis (faSScinate): A phase 2, randomised, controlled trial. Lancet. 2016;**387**(10038):2630-2640

[100] Distler JH, Distler O. Imatinib as a novel therapeutic approach for fibrotic disorders. Rheumatology. 2009;**48**(1):2-4

[101] Distler JH, Jungel A, Huber LC, Schulze-Horsel U, Zwerina J, Gay RE, et al. Imatinib mesylate reduces production of extracellular matrix and prevents development of experimental dermal fibrosis. Arthritis and Rheumatism. 2007;**56**(1):311-322. 2006/12/30

[102] Akhmetshina A, Venalis P, Dees C, Busch N, Zwerina J, Schett G, et al. Treatment with imatinib prevents fibrosis in different preclinical models of systemic sclerosis and induces regression of established fibrosis. Arthritis and Rheumatism. 2009;**60**(1):219-224

[103] Akhmetshina A, Dees C, Pileckyte M, Maurer B, Axmann R, Jungel A, et al. Dual inhibition of c-abl and PDGF receptor signaling by dasatinib and nilotinib for the treatment of dermal fibrosis. FASEB Journal. 2008;**22**(7):2214-2222. 2008/03/11

[104] Pope J, McBain D, Petrlich L, Watson S, Vanderhoek L, de Leon F, et al. Imatinib in active diffuse cutaneous systemic sclerosis: Results of a six-month, randomized, double-blind, placebo-controlled, proof-of-concept pilot study at a single center. Arthritis and Rheumatism. 2011;**63**(11):3547-3551

[105] Prey S, Ezzedine K, Doussau A, Grandoulier AS, Barcat D, Chatelus E, et al. Imatinib mesylate in scleroderma-associated diffuse skin fibrosis: A phase II multicentre randomized double-blinded controlled trial. The British Journal of Dermatology. 2012;**167**(5):1138-1144

[106] Spiera RF, Gordon JK, Mersten JN, Magro CM, Mehta M, Wildman HF, et al. Imatinib mesylate (Gleevec) in the treatment of diffuse cutaneous systemic sclerosis: Results of a 1-year, phase IIa, single-arm, open-label clinical trial. Annals of the Rheumatic Diseases. 2011;**70**(6):1003-1009

[107] Shanmugam E, Jena A, George M. Riociguat: Something new in pulmonary hypertension therapeutics? Journal of Pharmacology & Pharmacotherapeutics. 2015;**6**(1):3-6

[108] Beyer C, Reich N, Schindler SC, Akhmetshina A, Dees C, Tomcik M, et al. Stimulation of soluble guanylate cyclase reduces experimental dermal fibrosis. Annals of the Rheumatic Diseases. 2012;**71**(6):1019-1026

[109] Beyer C, Zenzmaier C, Palumbo-Zerr K, Mancuso R, Distler A, Dees C et al. Stimulation of the soluble guanylate cyclase (sGC) inhibits fibrosis by blocking non-canonical TGFβ signalling. Ann Rheum Dis. 2015 Jul;**74**(7):1408-16.

[110] Dees C, Beyer C, Distler A, Soare A, Zhang Y, Palumbo-Zerr K et al. Stimulators of soluble guanylate cyclase (sGC) inhibit experimental skin fibrosis of different aetiologies. Ann Rheum Dis. 2015 Aug;**74**(8):1621-5.